GUIDE TO ORTHOPAEDICS
1 TRAUMA

GUIDE TO ORTHOPAEDICS
1. TRAUMA

K.L.G. MILLS

MA MB BChir(Camb) BSc(Lond) FRCS(Eng) FRCS(Edin)
FRCS(Canada) LRCP(Lond)
Consultant Orthopaedic Surgeon, Grampian Health Board,
Scotland
Clinical Senior Lecturer, University of Aberdeen
Formerly Senior Lecturer in Orthopaedics, University of
Dundee

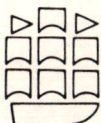

CHURCHILL LIVINGSTONE
EDINBURGH LONDON MELBOURNE AND NEW YORK 1981

CHURCHILL LIVINGSTONE
Medical Division of Longman Group Limited

Distributed in the United States of America by
Churchill Livingstone Inc., 19 West 44th Street,
New York, N.Y. 10036, and by associated companies,
branches and representatives throughout the world.

First published 1981

ISBN 0 443 02018 3

British Library Cataloguing in Publication Data
Guide to orthopaedics.
  1: Trauma
  1. Orthopedia
  I. Mills, Kenneth L G
  617'.3   RD731   79-41480

Printed in Singapore by Singapore Offset Printing Pte Ltd

Preface

This book aims to be a wide-ranging presentation of the whole field of trauma in a compact form designed for the young man training as a specialist orthopaedic surgeon and with a specialty examination in mind. It is hoped that it will also prove useful to the practising orthopaedic surgeon who wishes to survey a particular field or to identify some authoritative reference quickly.

It is a 'bouquet of other men's flowers' and its only originality lies in the collection of facts and references in a compact form. It does not aim to replace standard textbooks of trauma, orthopaedics or operative surgery.

The references have been incorporated at the end of sections for ease of access. They have been selected from journals and volumes which are likely to be stocked by libraries of the Western world and are as up to date as possible. From them the searcher after knowledge should be able to obtain other references to other and older authoritative texts.

The treatments under each heading are those commonly practised and are listed in an order reflecting common practice in Scotland in the 1970s. However, it is not the primary purpose of this book to detail methods of management and the reader will find more information about aspects of treatment from the references. To have been more encyclopaedic would have increased the size of the book to unmanageable proportions.

The author's enthusiasms, preferences, weaknesses and areas of ignorance will be evident to those who are better informed. Criticisms and advice from readers will be welcomed.

1981   K.L.G.M

Acknowledgements

My thanks are due to the following:

My colleagues in the various surgical disciplines in the Royal Infirmary, Aberdeen, who have helped in the revision of those parts of the typescript pertaining to their specialty.

My orthopaedic colleagues who have helped to revise the musculo-skeletal sections.

The typists who have faithfully deciphered my writing—Mrs Alice Macgregor and Mrs Hilda Grieve.

Mr Nigel Lukins, Medical Artist, Royal Infirmary, Aberdeen who has prepared the diagrams.

Dr Lawrence and his staff in the Medical Library, Royal Infirmary, Aberdeen, who have helped to obtain all the necessary references.

The diagrams have come from various sources. I thank the following for their permission to use their original material:

Dr F. W. Braisdell and *Surgery, Gynaecology and Obstetrics* for Figure 1

Mr W. F. Walker, Consultant General Surgeon, Ninewells Hospital, Dundee for Figures 4 to 9

Mr Graham Page, Royal Infirmary, Aberdeen for Figure 2

Drs R. B. Salter and W. R. Harris and *Journal of Bone and Joint Surgery* for Figure 10

Dr J. B. Lynch and Messrs Little, Brown and Company for Figure 12

Mr D. J. Brain, Consultant Otolaryngologist, Birmingham for Tables 1 and 2

Mr C. Blaiklock, Consultant Neurosurgeon, Royal Infirmary, Aberdeen, for Figure 15

Annals of the Royal College of Surgeons of England for Figure 24

Mr I. F. K. Muir, Mr T. L. Barclay, Consultant Plastic Surgeons and Messrs Lloyd Luke Medical Books for Figures 13 and 14

Mr J. Hughes, Strathclyde University for material on Prosthetics and Faulty Gait

Mr H. N. Burwell and *Journal of Bone and Joint Surgery* for Figures 26 to 33

Contributors

Bennett, Fiona M, MB, ChB, FRCS (Edin), DO
Consultant Ophthalmologist,
Grampian Health Board
Clinical Senior Lecturer in Ophthalmology,
University of Aberdeen

Blaiklock, Christopher T, MBBS, FRCS (Eng),
MRCP D Obst, RCOG
Consultant Neurosurgeon,
Grampian Health Board
Clinical Senior Lecturer in Surgery,
University of Aberdeen

Clarke, Peter B, OBE, TD, BSc, MB, ChB,
FDSRCS (Eng, Edin and Glasg)
Consultant Oral Surgeon,
Grampian Health Board
Honorary Civil Dental Consultant Royal Navy
Clinical Senior Lecturer in Surgery,
University of Aberdeen.

Davidson, Alan I, MB, ChB, ChM,
FRCS (Edin), D Obst, RCOG
Consultant Surgeon,
Grampian Health Board
Clinical Senior Lecturer in Surgery,
University of Aberdeen

Engeset, J, MB, ChB, ChM, FRCS (Edin)
Senior Lecturer in Surgery,
University of Aberdeen
Honorary Consultant Surgeon,
Grampian Health Board

Foote, Andrew V, MB, ChB, ChM,
FRCS (Edin)
Consultant Thoracic Surgeon,
Grampian Health Board
Clinical Senior Lecturer in Surgery,
University of Aberdeen

Garvie, W H H, MB, ChB, FRCS (Edin),
FRCS (Eng)
Consultant Urological Surgeon,
Grampian Health Board
Clinical Senior Lecturer in Surgery,
University of Aberdeen

Muir, Ian F K, MBE, VRD, MS, MBBS,
FRCS (Edin), FRCS (Eng), LRCP
Consultant Plastic Surgeon,
Grampian Health Board
Clinical Senior Lecturer in Surgery,
University of Aberdeen

Page, Graham, MB, ChB, MCh, FRCS (Edin)
Senior Surgical Registrar,
Grampian Health Board

Troup, Ian M, MB, ChB, D Med Rehab Eng
Consultant
Dundee Limb Fitting Centre,
Tayside Health Board

Wills, Leslie, C, MB, ChB, FRCS (Edin)
Consultant E.N.T. Surgeon,
Grampian Health Board
Clinical Senior Lecturer in Surgery,
University of Aberdeen

Contents

Contents

SHOCK AND HEMORRHAGE

With the assistance of G. Page

Pathogenesis of shock

Definition
Inadequate perfusion of tissues which is often fatal if untreated.

Mechanisms

Failure of pumping action of heart
Coronary thrombosis
Cardiac tamponade
Hyperkalemia
Tension pneumothorax

Block in circulation
Pulmonary embolism
Major vein thrombosis
Whitman-Waters syndrome

Loss of circulating blood volume
Hemorrhage
Burns
Diarrhoea and vomiting
Sepsis
Anaphylaxis

Loss of vascular tone
Fainting
Adrenal apoplexy
Spinal anesthesia
Hypotensive drugs

Effects of diminished circulating blood volume

Fall in BP
Baro-receptors stimulated
Sympathetic venous constriction
  Skin and spleen etc. empty
  This alone will compensate for 10% B.V. reduction

Rise in pulse rate
Withdrawal of intercellular fluid into capillaries

Diminished cardiac output
Provoked by fall in central venous pressure
Lessened stroke volume
Chemoreceptors in aortic and carotid bodies stimulated by stagnant hypoxia
These cause temporary rises in blood pressure (Mayer Waves)
Circulation to brain, heart and kidneys is maintained (in that order)
Pulmonary artery pressure may fall by 50%
Upper alveoli not perfused
Diminished coronary blood flow impairs cardiac efficiency

Desaturation of venous blood
Provoked by tissues extracting more oxygen
Metabolic acidosis produced (rise in pyruvate and lactate)
Anemic hypoxia stimulates chemoreceptors
Oxygen dissociation curve shifts to right

Effects of hemorrhage

Chronic
Plasma or red cell replacement keeps pace with loss so long as iron stores last. Then hypochromic anemia and increased cardiac output.

Acute
Withdrawal of intercellular fluid into capillaries
Peripheral vasoconstriction
Rise in output of
  Catecholamines, Angiotensin, Corticosteroids, Aldosterone
Rise in fibrinogen, platelets, white cells; coagualability of blood
Metabolic acidosis

Clinical effects of shock

Fainting	Pallor
Breathlessness	Weak rapid pulse
Weakness	Thirst
Coldness	Oliguria

Treatment of shock
Diagnose cause

Restore blood volume (care with cardiac infarcts)
Treat cause
Pressor agents doubtful value
Vasodilator agents unproven

Hormonal response to shock

Emergency response

Adrenalin output from adrenal medulla
Effects: Vasoconstriction in skin and renal
        vessels
        Vasodilation in muscle, heart and brain
        Speeds up heart
        Promotes gluconeogenesis
        Increased hypothalamic output of ACTH

Nor-adrenalin output from adrenal medulla
Effects: Vasoconstriction in splanchnic and renal
        vessels
        Vasodilation in coronary vessels

Subsequent responses

A.D.H. release from posterior pituitary by a fall in extra-cellular fluid volume
Effect: Re-absorption of water from kidney
      tubules

A.C.T.H. release from anterior pituitary by hypothalamic impulses and increased circulatory adrenalin
Effect: Increased output of corticosteroids

Growth hormone release from anterior pituitary. Mechanism uncertain
Effect: Not yet defined

Peripheral effects

Glucocorticoid output from adrenal cortex
Effects: Gluconeogenesis from muscle protein
Leucopenia
Increased capillary resistance
Suppression of inflammatory response
Increased insulin resistance of muscle cells

Aldosterone output from adrenal cortex
Effect: Retention of sodium in renal tubules

Angiotensin output from juxta glomerular apparatus in response to renal hypotension
Effect: Peripheral vasoconstriction and rise in
      blood pressure

Erythropoetin output from kidney in response to decreased renal oxygenation
Effect: Raised output of red cells from bone
      marrow

Glucagon output from pancreas in response to early hypoglycemia
Effect: Raised blood glucose levels

Insulin output from pancreas in response to hyperglycemia
Effect: Diminution of blood glucose levels

Development of shock process

Likely in   Old or ill patients
               Hypothermia
               Crushed limbs
Speeded by Alcohol
               Anesthesia
               Too rapid re-warming
               Delayed restoration of blood volume

'Sick cell' syndrome
Histamine and Kinins released from damaged or
    under-perfused tissues
Rise in blood levels of
    (a) fibrinolysins
    (b) urea
    (c) potassium
    (d) pyruvate and lactate
Hypoxia disturbs cellular enzyme systems:
    (1) Oxidase mechanisms in mitochondria
    (2) ADP → ATP change inhibited
    (3) Potassium leaves cells, sodium enters
    (4) Cell breakdown increases nitrogen loss
    (5) Pyruvate and lactate levels rise within cells

Further deterioration
Fall in body temperature

Adrenals
Failure of stress response due to hypotension and
    cortical necrosis

Kidneys
Hypotension, acidosis ± hemolysis may lead to renal tubular necrosis

Intestines
Failure of mucin production
Mucosal ulceration
Bacterial invasion
Further fluid loss

References
Flear C T, Singh C M 1973 Hyponatremia and sick cells. British Journal of Anaesthesia 45: 976-994
Giddings A E B 1974 Control of plasma glucose in the surgical patient. British Journal of Surgery 61: 787-792
Imamura M et al 1975 Liver metabolism and glucogenesis in trauma and sepsis. Surgery 77: 868-880
Meguid M M et al 1974 Hormone substrate interrelationships following trauma. Archives of Surgery 109: 776-783
Moyer C A, Butcher H R 1967 Burns, shock and plasma volume regulations. Chapters 1-3 C. V. Mosley Co. St. Louis
Stoner H B 1969 Response to trauma. Annals of Royal College of Surgeons of England 44: 308-323
Walker W F, Johnston I D A 1971 The metabolic basis of surgical care, Chapter 4. Heineman Medical Books, Chichester
Wright P D, Johnston I D A 1975 The effects of surgical operation on growth hormone levels in plasma. Surgery 77: 479-486

Shock lung

General features
Clearly recognised only in recent decades
Worse with soft tissue injuries elsewhere

Clinical features
Massive loss of blood volume from
  Trauma
  Thoracic surgery
  Post-partum
Hyperventilation. Restlessness
Cough
Raised pCO_2
Near normal pO_2, then falling

Radiological features
Patchy opacification of lungs
Tendency to confluence

Pathological features
Fall in cardiac output
Reduction in pulmonary blood flow
Excessive desaturation of venous blood
Damage to capillary walls
Platelet microembolism as part of disseminated intravascular coagulation

SCHEME OF DEVELOPMENT OF SHOCK LUNG

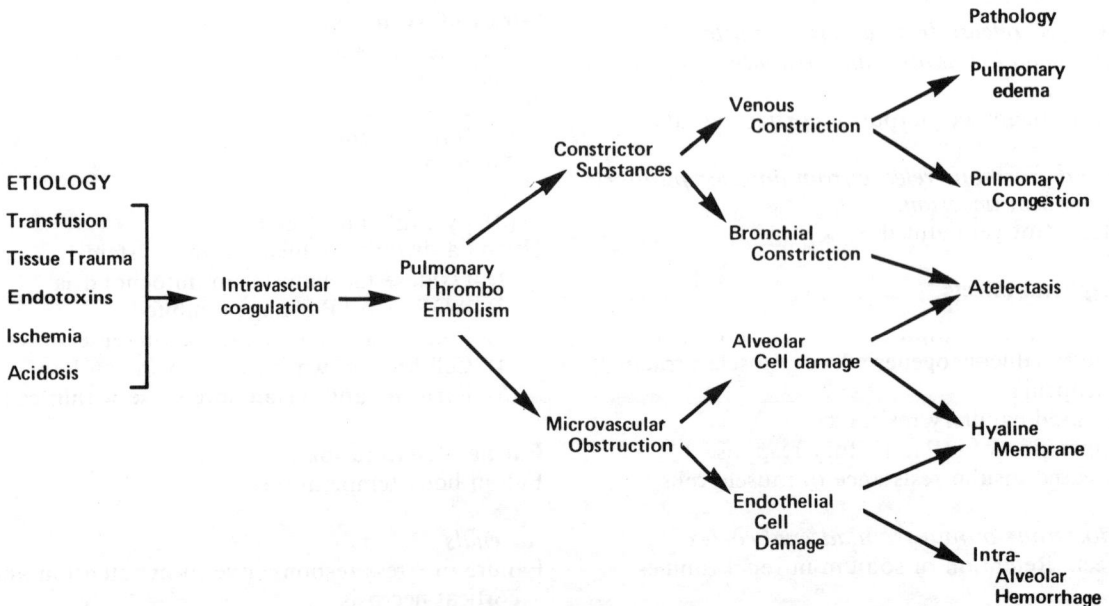

Fig. 1 Scheme of development of shock lung.

Release locally of
  Serotonin
  Histamine
  A.T.P. and A.D.P.
Causing local vasoconstriction

Respiration
Poor CO_2 output causing hyperventilation
Little change in O_2 uptake
Decreased surfactant activity
Lung phospholipid synthesis is depressed

Treatment
Restoration of blood volume
Artificial ventilation – even hyperventilation
Respiratory physiotherapy
Antibiotics, steroids, heparin

Experimental
Methysergide, aspirin
See Figure 1

References
Blaisdell F W, Lim R C, Stallone R J 1970 The mechanism
  of pulmonary damage following traumatic shock. Surgery,
  Gynaecology and Obstetrics 130: 15-22
Prys-Roberts C 1974 Respiratory problems of the seriously
  injured patient. Injury 5: 67-78

Shock kidney

Spectrum of damage
From: Transient depression of the glomerular
  filtration rate
To: Total renal failure
Kidneys respond to hypotension with oliguria and
  tolerate total ischemia for 15 minutes at 37°C
Solute load is inversely proportional to the
  adequacy of resuscitation
Cortico-medullary shunting of blood is now
  thought to be more apparent than real.
Failing kidneys shown by:
  rising blood urea
  falling sodium clearance
  blood urea/urine urea ratio rising

Renal tubular damage exacerbated by:
Hemolysis
Myoglobinemia
Sulfonamide crystalluria
Pyelonephritis
Renal tubular acidosis etc.

High output renal failure
May occur without preceding oliguria
  (but usually follows long continued oliguria)

Evidence
Specific gravity of urine is low
blood urea is rising
average urine volumes continue.

Treatment
Restore blood volume
Restore normal blood pressure
Restore electrolyte balance
Promote diuresis

Reference
Shires T G, Carrico C J, Canizaro P C 1973 Shock,
  Chapter 3. W. B. Saunders Co. Philadelphia, London,
  Toronto

Septic shock

Synonyms
Bacteremic shock, endotoxic shock
  gram-negative septicemia, gram-positive
  septicemia, septicemic shock

General features
Uncommon, but more frequently recognised
Other diseases often present
High death rate (-50% +)
Gram-negative septicemia commoner in old
  people

Clinical features
(1) Normovolemic circulation: (Hyperdynamic)
      Normotensive. Warm extremities.
      Tachycardia. No sweating.
(2) Hypovolemic circulation: (Hypodynamic)
      Hypotension. Cold, pale extremities.
      Sweating. Cyanosis.

Common features
Moderate pyrexia
Hyperventilation
Clear mind

Predisposing conditions
Abdominal sepsis
Pelvic sepsis (abortion sepsis, etc.)
Urinary tract surgery
Respiratory sepsis
Large burns

Pathological features
Bacteremia present
Exact mechanisms still unknown
Possible causes:
    Exotoxins – gram-positive bacteria
    Endotoxins – gram-negative bacteria
High cardiac output
Shift of hemoglobin/oxygen dissociation curve to
    left
Tissues unable to utilise oxygenated hemoglobin
Metabolic acidosis follows

Respiratory changes
Moderate hypoxia
Pulmonary function diminished
Patchy infiltrates
Secondary infection

Treatment
Resources of I.C.U. required

Primary
Remove or drain foci of sepsis
Culture blood

Adjuvants
Antibiotics –
    Large doses intravenously
    Maintenance of circulatory volume
    Steroids
    Hypovolemia – vasopressors helpful
    Normovolemia – vasodilators helpful

References
Hershey S G, Del Guerico L R M, McConn R, Editors
    1971 Septic Shock in Man. Little, Brown and Company,
    Boston
Shires T G, Carrico C J, Canizaro P C 1973 "Shock",
    Chapter 7. W. B. Saunders Co., Philadelphia, London,
    Toronto

Unexpected hemorrhage

Causes

Local
Division of arteries
Division of veins
Slipping of ligatures
Sepsis
Movement of surgical devices (metal or plastic)
Vessel invasion by tumour

Hemostatic failure
Undiagnosed congenital bleeding disorder
Thrombocytopenia
Anticoagulant drugs
Massive transfusion
Liver disease
Disseminated intravascular coagulation
Inhibitors of coagulation,
    a. Factor VII inhibitor,
    b. D.L.E. inhibitor
Dysproteinemia

Consider
History of trauma, surgery, dentistry
Family history
Drug history
Examination
    Purpura – (platelet vascular disorder)
    Bruising/hemarthrosis (coagulation disorder)
    Nature of blood flow from wound

Investigations
10 ml citrated blood   }
 4 ml sequestrene blood }   adequate for
 1) Prothrombin test
 2) Kaolin cephalin clotting time
 3) Thrombin time
 4) Platelet count and blood film

Later
Fibrinogen titre
Urinary Fibrin degradation products

Intra-vascular coagulation

Synonyms
Consumption coagulopathy
Disseminated intravascular coagulation (D.I.C.)
Intravascular coagulation-fibrinolysis syndrome
    (I.C.F.)

General Features
Recognised in recent years
A spectrum of severity from subclinical effects to
    death
Hemorrhage is both a cause and effect

Disorders in which defibrination syndrome has been described:

Infections
Gram negative sepsis
Gram positive sepsis more rarely
Rickettsial (Rocky Mountain spotted fever)
Malaria

Obstetrics
Septic abortion
Saline induced abortion
Abruptio placentae
Prolonged retention of dead fetus
Amniotic fluid embolus

Malignancies
Carcinomas (Prostate, pancreas, lung, colon,
  ovary)
Acute leukemias under treatment

Massive tissue injury
Trauma
Thoracic surgery with cardiac bypass
Fat embolism

Vascular and circulatory disorders
Local: Aortic aneurysm resection
General: Shock, cardiac arrest

Immunologic
Hemolytic transufsion reaction
Anaphylaxis

Miscellaneous
Snake bite
Purpura fulminans
Heat stroke

Clinical features
Persistent uncontrollable hemorrhage after
  surgery or injury
Respiratory insufficiency
Diminishing renal function
High mortality
Survival often followed by sepsis

Pathological features
Abnormally rapid consumption of fibrinogen
  with intravascular embolisation and clotting

Haematological
All clotting factors reduced
Thrombocytopenia
Fragmentation hemolysis
Fibrin monomers in circulation
Reduced plasminogen levels
Increased urinary fibrinogen degradation
  products

Macroscopy
Lungs: Heavy, congested
          hemorrhagic, atelectatic
Kidneys: Pale and swollen

Microscopy
Platelet and fibrin plugs in lungs, kidneys, liver
Acute tubular necrosis of kidneys
Centrilobular necrosis of liver

Treatment
Difficult to balance coagulants/anticoagulants
Vigorous treatment of underlying condition
if hemorrhage is dominant:
  Fresh blood transfusion
  Concentrated clothing factors
if thrombosis dominates:
  Heparin
  Epsilon amino caproic acid

References

Hassman G C, Keim H A, 1974 Disseminated intravascular
  coagulation (D.I.C.) in orthopaedic surgery. Clinical
  Orthopaedics 103: 118-132
Lerner R G 1976 The defibrination syndrome. Medical
  Clinics of North America 60: 871-880

Fluid replacement in shock

Blood
  For: Full volume retained in cardiovascular
             system
           Oxygen carrying capacity better than
             any other fluid
  Against: Cross matching time
           Infection
           Transfusion reactions
           Storage difficulties

Auto-transfusion
  For: No transfusion reactions
           No blood bank required
           No cross matching required
           Cheap
  Against: Only possible in
             major surgery
             chest or abdominal trauma
           or pre-operative donations required
           Filtering required
           Infection

Plasma
> For: Rapid availability
> No cross matching
> Provides protein
> Against: Infective hepatitis risk in pooled plasma
> Requires mixing in sterile water

Dextran
> For: Sterile. No cross matching
> No special storage requirements
> Retained intravascularly
> Diminishes phlebothrombosis
> Against: Allergy
> Thrombocytopenia
> Minor interference with hemostasis and
> cross matching

Saline/Dextrose
> For: Cheap. Sterile
> No special storage
> Against: Rapidly lost from intravascular
> compartment
> No oxygen carrying capacity
> May overload heart and lungs
> Dextrose does not meet full energy
> requirements

References
Allen J G 1971 Commercial blood in our national blood program. Archives of Surgery 102: 122-126
Cowell H R, Swickard J W 1974 Auto-transfusion in children's orthopaedics. Journal of Bone and Joint Surgery 56A: 908-912

Dextran

Glucose polymers of varying molecular sizes formed by leuconostoc mesenteroides

Common commercial forms
Dextran 70: Average molecular weight of 70,000
Used chiefly for blood volume as an adjunct to blood and plasma expansion
Dextran 40: Average molecular weight of 40,000
Used for improvement of micro-circulation

Effects
All dextrans exert colloidal osmotic pressure
Large molecules: ($>$100,000 M.W.)
Increase viscosity of blood
Cause erythrocyte aggregation
Interfere with cross-matching

Ingested by reticulo-endothelial system
Slowly metabolised
Small molecules: ($<$40,000 M.W.)
Leak out into urine and extracellular fluid
Decrease viscosity of blood by
1. Haemodilution
2. Decreasing aggregation and rigidity of erythrocytes
3. Decreasing platelet adhesiveness
Diminish thrombosis by
1. Coating platelets and vessel walls
2. Reducing plasma fibrinogen level

Side effects

1. Increased bleeding tendency
To be avoided –
at end of large transfusions
in hemorrhagic diseases
in anti-coagulant therapy

2. Overloading of circulation
Careful monitoring required

3. Allergy and anaphylaxis
To be avoided in those with such a previous history

4. Nephrotoxicity
To be avoided in early renal failure

Indications
Circulatory replacement. Before compatible blood is available. (maximum dose 1500 ml)
To improve micro-circulation:
Vascular surgery
Phlebothrombosis
Hypothermic procedures

References
Atik M 1969 The uses of dextron in surgery. A current evaluation. Surgery 65: 548-562
Data J L, Nies A S 1974 Dextran 40. Annals of Internal Medicine 81: 500-504

Intravenous therapy

General considerations
Upper limbs are less likely to give thrombo embolic problems

Venepuncture can nearly always be achieved with care,
   i.e. Tourniquet inflated to near systolic pressure
      Arm dependent
      Good lateral lighting

Situations of failure
Obese patients
Hypovolemic hypotension
Infants

Immediate remedy
Subclavian puncture ⎫
External jugular puncture ⎬ in adults
Scalp vein puncture   in infants
Dissection of peripheral veins
   Antecubital fossa
   Lower end of radius
   Medial malleolus
   Groin
   Delto-pectoral groove
Poor flow after successful venepuncture
   may be due to
      Venespasm
      Limb flexion
      Constricting bandages etc
Overcoming venespasm
Application of external pressure to bag fluid
Raising head of pressure of fluid
Venous tubing pump
Warming fluid
Warming limb or whole patient
Injection of 1% procaine into vein
Poor flow after initial good flow for 1+ hours
Thrombophlebitis
Extravasation of fluid around vein
Development of proximal hematoma
Corrected by changing site of venepuncture

Central vein cannulation

Purposes
Monitoring central venous pressure
Massive rapid fluid replacement
Long term fluid therapy
Intravenous alimentation

Sites
Antebrachial vein
Subclavian vein
External jugular vein
Femoral vein   ⎫ Least desirable
Long saphenous vein ⎬ site in groin.

Problems
Sepsis
Central vein thrombosis

Precautions
Extreme care in setting up infusion with
Sterile precautions
Well fixed dressings
No disturbance of dressings
Rewithdrawal of cannula on first sign of sepsis
   or thrombosis and replacement with new
   materials at a new site

Other general problems of venepuncture

Accidental arterial puncture
Air embolism, particularly in central veins
Plastic cannula embolisation
Administration
   of mis matched blood
   of incorrect doses of drugs
   of incorrect drugs
   of incompatible drugs

References

Bernard R W, Stahl W M 1971 Subclavian vein catheterisation. A prospective study. Annals of Surgery 173: 184-200

Drabinsky M 1976 Retreival of embolised central venous catheters by a Dormia ureteral stone dislodger with a straight filiform tip. Chest 69: 435-437

Hegarty M M 1977 Hazards of subclavian vein cannulation. Practical considerations and an unusual case report. South African Medical Journal 52: 240-243

Mogil R A, Delaurentis D A, Rosemund G P 1967 The infraclavicular venepuncture. Archives of Surgery 95: 320-324

2

METABOLIC CHANGES OF TRAUMA

With the assistance of G. Page

Water balance

Volumes of body compartments (Average 70 Kg man)
Total body 50 litres
   Intra cellular 35 litres
   Extra cellular 15 litres
     Interstitial water 11.5 litres
     Plasma water 3.5 litres

Measurement
Total water: D_2O distribution
Extracellular water: Inulin or Thiosulphate
   distribution
Plasma volume: Evans Blue dye or I^{131}
Percentage of body water compared to total
   weight falls as the percentage of body fat rises

Balance

Input
Fluid drink: Variable
Water in food: 300-400 ml
Water formed from oxidation
   of food: 12 ml/100 calories

Output
Urine: Variable
Feces
Sweat   } Insensible loss   1000 ml daily
Breath   }   in temperate climate

Classification of dehydration

Water depletion
Primary dehydration
Intracellular fluid most affected
Mainly potassium and water lost
Effects: Thirst
        Oliguria

Salt depletion
Secondary dehydration
Extracellular fluid most affected
Mainly sodium and water lost
Effects: Circulatory disturbances

Excessive water loss

Lungs
Metabolic acidosis   produces hyper-
Heavy exercise at high altitude   ventilation

Gastro-intestinal tract
Vomiting
Diarrhoea
Nasogastric suction
Fistulae
Intestinal obstruction: fluid sequestrates in lumen
   of bowel

Renal disease
  (1) Nephrogenic Diabetes Insipidus. (Renal
      tubules do not respond to A.D.H)
      Fanconi's syndrome
      Any chronic renal disease
  (2) Diuretic phase of acute renal failure
  (3) Potassium depletion

Endocrine changes
Pituitary injury: Deficient production of A.D.H.
Adrenal failure: Loss of Na^+ Cl^- HCO_3^-
Hyperparathyroidism: And any condition giving
   hypercalcuria
Diabetes Mellitus. Osmotic diuresis with glucose

Skin
Excessive sweating. High environmental
   temperature.
Pyrexia

Alcohol
Inhibits ADH production
Causes pyrexia

Deficient water intake

Causes
No available water
Nausea
Esophageal obstruction
Deficient thirst mechanism –
   Coma
   Weakness
   Lethargy

Effects of loss of body water
0-5%: Thirst and discomfort
       Impaired efficiency
5-10%: Headache, apathy, extreme thirst
>10%: Hypotension, collapse, medical aid
   required
20%: Survival unlikely

Laboratory studies
D_2O dilution will give total body water
Weight loss
Raised levels of urea and electrolytes in serum

Raised hemoglobin and packed cell volume (P.C.V.)
Raised urinary specific gravity

Treatment
Water to drink if possible
Intravenous water as 5% Dextrose
  or N/$_3$ Saline in 4% Dextrose

Deficient water output

Causes
Failure of sweating
  Heat stroke
  Drugs
  Skin paint
Renal failure

Water intoxication

Causes
Renal failure acute or chronic
Pituitary damage: diabetes insipidus
Hysterical overdrinking
Excess intravenous fluid

Effects
Nausea and vomiting
Light headedness
Confusion, convulsions
Pulmonary edema, cardiac failure

Laboratory studies
Weight rise
Fall in serum urea and electrolytes
  Hemoglobin and packed cell volume
  Plasma protein concentration

Treatment
Oral hypertonic saline
Intravenous 100 ml. 5% saline hourly until serum sodium rises to 120 mmol/l

Acid-base balance

pH of body tissues maintained within close limits.
  i.e. 7.33-7.45 Limits of life 6.4-8.1

Control of body pH
(1) Buffer systems in blood
  (a) Bicarbonate $H_2CO_3 \rightleftharpoons H^+ + HCO_3^-$
        $NaHCO_3$ $Na^+ + HCO_3^-$
  (b) Phosphate NaH_2PO_4 $H^+ + NaHPO_4^-$
        $Na_2HPO_4 \rightleftharpoons 2Na^+ + HPO_4^-$
  (c) Haemoglobin H Hb $H^+ + Hb^-$
  (b) Protein H (Protein) $H^+ + Protein^-$
(2) (a) Respiratory control: Lungs regulate carbon dioxide level
  (b) Renal control: Renal tubules regulate bicarbonate and phosphate levels

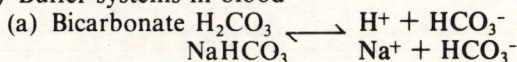

Ionic Concentrations in Body Fluids

Extracellular ions

			mmol/litre
Na	143	Cl	103
K	5	HCO$_3$	27
Ca	2.5	HPO$_4$	1
Mg	1.0	SO$_4$	1
Others	3.5	Protein	16
		Organic acids	6
	155		155

Intracellular ions

K	150	HPO$_4$	95
Mg	45	SO$_4$	15
		HCO$_3$	15
		Protein	70
	195		195

Tissue fluids ions

Na	143	Cl	110
K	5	HCO$_3$	30
Ca	2.5	HPO$_4$	3
Mg	1.0	SO$_4$	1
Others	3.5	Organic acids	6
	155		155

Average range in extracellular fluid

		mmol/litre
Na$^+$	135 -	145
K$^+$	3.5-	5.5
Ca^{++}	2.3-	2.7
HCO$_3$	20 -	30
Cl	95 -	105
Urea	2.3-	7.3

Normal levels
  CO$_2$: 10.6 —13.3 KPa
  pCO$_2$: 4.5 — 6.0 KPa
  pH : 7.33— 7.45
Standard bicarbonate : 21-25 mmol/litre
Actual bicarbonate   : 21-25 mmol/litre

Base excess or deficit : ± 3 mmol/litre
Buffer Base   : 38-48 mmol/litre

Astrup's formula
0.3 × Base Deficit × Body Weight in kg
    = ml 8.4% NaHCO₃required for correction
    of metabolic acidosis

Respiratory acidosis

Causes
(1) Depressed respiratory centre
        Asphyxia
        Cardiac arrest
        Electrocution
        Cerebral concussion
            or hemorrhage
        Barbiturate poisoning etc
(2) Defects in efferent nerve pathway
        C.N.S. damage
        Polyneuropathies
        Myasthenia gravis
        Anesthetic relaxants
(3) Defects in effector mechanisms
        Obstructed airway
        Myopathies
        Fractured ribs
        Pulmonary pathology

Effects
Drowsiness/coma
Sweating
Hypertension
Peripheral vasodilation

Respiratory alkalosis

Causes
Hyperventilation
    High altitude
    Voluntary
    Hysterical
    Mechanical
    Encephalitis

Effects
Pallor
Hypotension
Tetany

Metabolic acidosis

Causes
Ingestion of excess acids
Increased production of ketoacids (Diabetes)
Aspirin poisoning

Retention of H⁺ ions (Chronic renal failure
    oliguria)
Loss of OH⁻ ions Vomiting
                    Diarrhoea
                    Fistulae
Exercise

Effects
Drowsiness/Coma
Increased depth and frequency of respiration
Increased urinary ammonium

Metabolic alkalosis

Causes
Ingestion of excess alkali (milk-alkali syndrome)
Loss of gastric acid.
    Vomiting (especially pyloric stenosis)
    Fistulae (especially high small bowel)
Hyperaldosteronism (Conn's syndrome)
Hypercorticism (Cushing's syndrome)

Effects
Phasic respiration
Tetany

Reference
Walker W F, Johnston I D A 1971 The metabolic basis of
    surgical care, Chapter 6. William Heinneman Medical
    Books, Ltd., Chichester.

Nitrogen balance

In health: Nitrogen input = Nitrogen output

Daily nitrogen input

$$\frac{\text{g of dietary protein}}{6.25} = \text{g of Nitrogen}$$

Daily nitrogen output
Skin + Feces = 1.5g
Urine: Creatinine
       Peptides
       Ammonia ⎱ 2.0g
       Amino Acids ⎰
       Uric Acid
       Urea: Variable

24 hour nitrogen output in g
   = Urinary Urea Nitrogen in g + 3.5
Further correction of ± 2g N for change of 0.8
  mmol./litre of blood urea nitrogen must be
  made

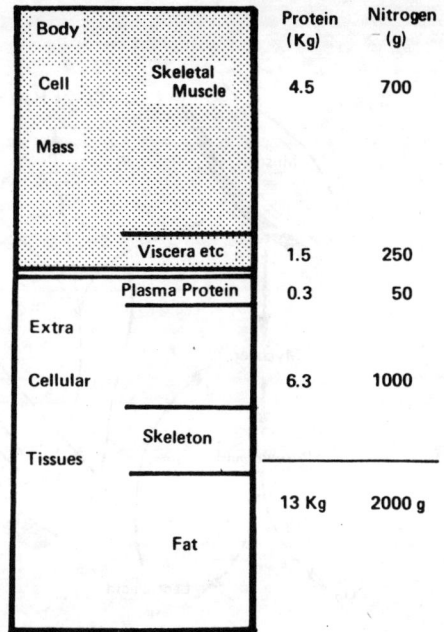

Fig. 2 Distribution of body constituents.

Adult energy and nitrogen requirements

	Kcals/24 hr	MJ	Nitrogen, g/24 hr
At rest	1500-2000	6.25-8.33	7.5-10.0
Post operative	2000-3500	8.33-14.6	10-15
Hypercatabolic states	3500-5000	14.6-20.8	15-25
Major burns	>5000	>20.8	>25
Fever	Add 2000/C°	+ 8.33	+ 10

See Figures 2, 3-9

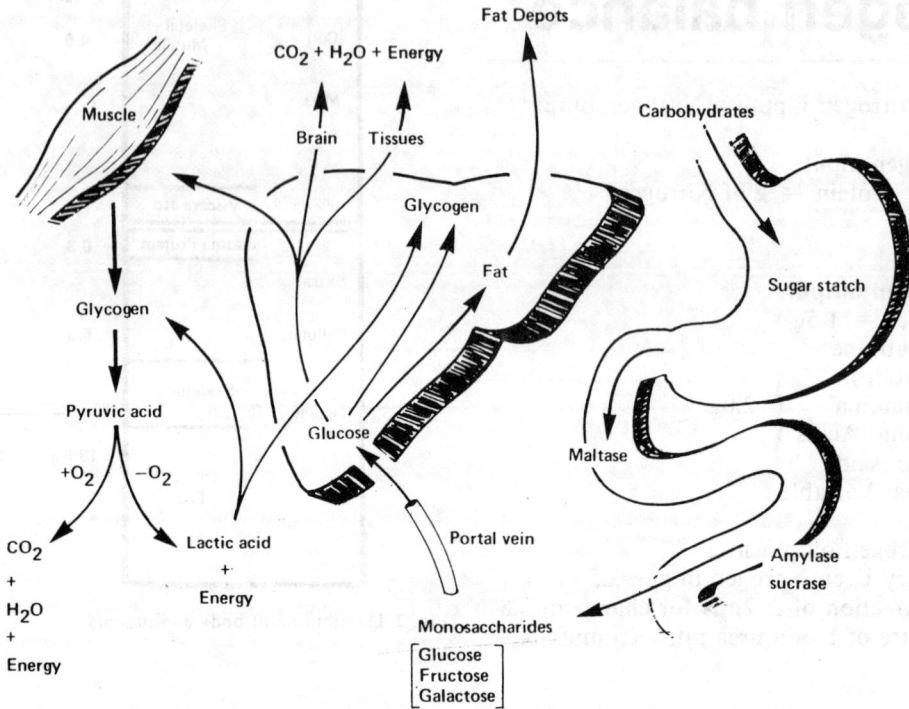

Fig. 3 Normal carbohydrate metabolism.

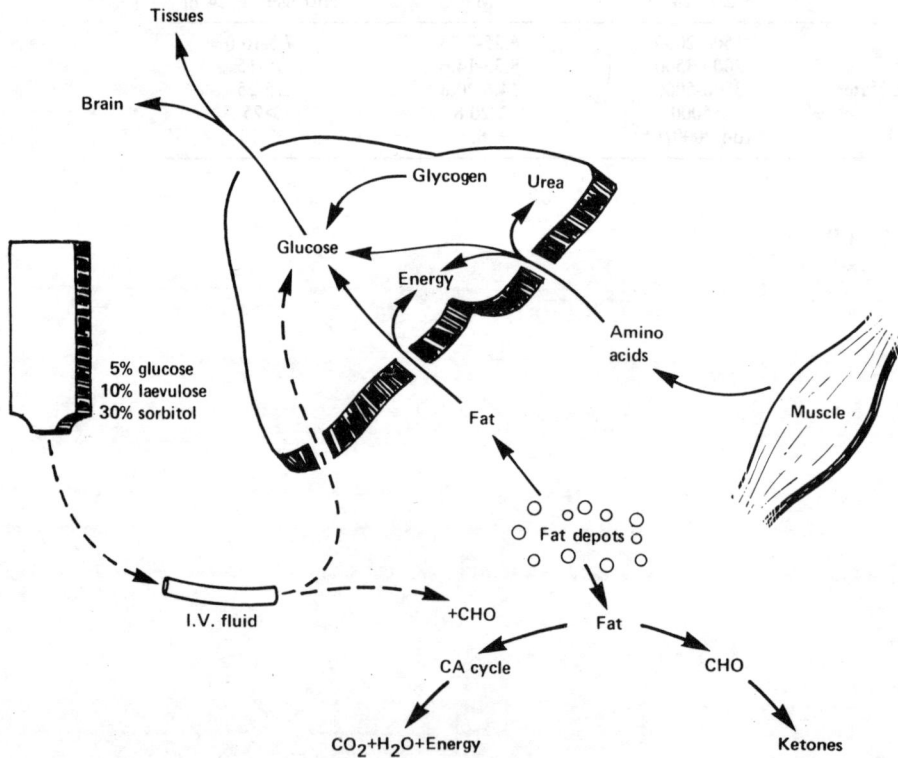

Fig. 4 Carbohydrate metabolism after trauma.

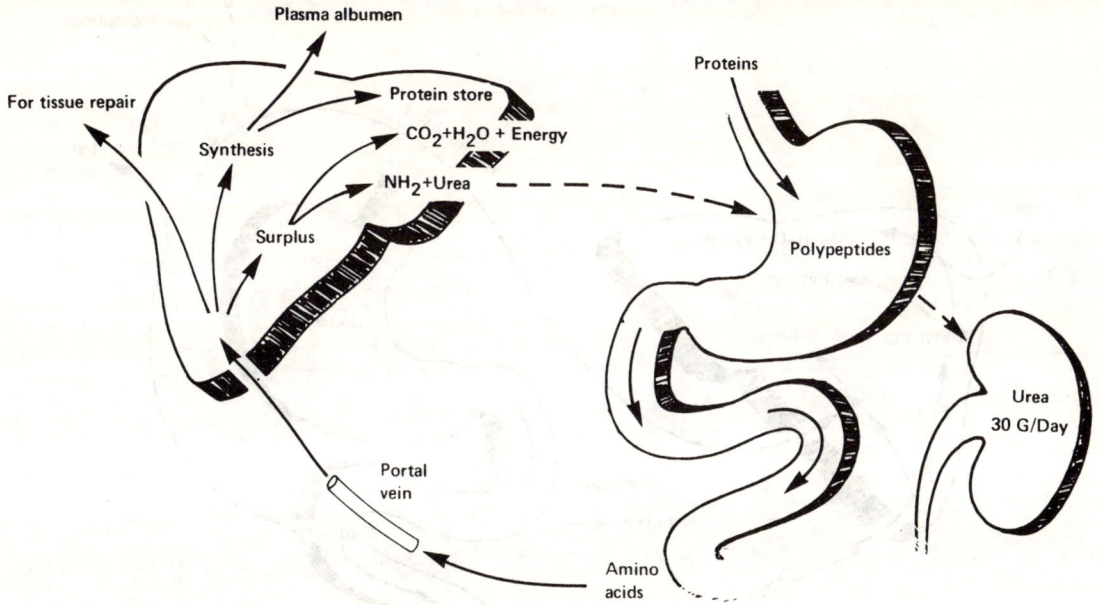

Fig. 5 Normal protein metabolism.

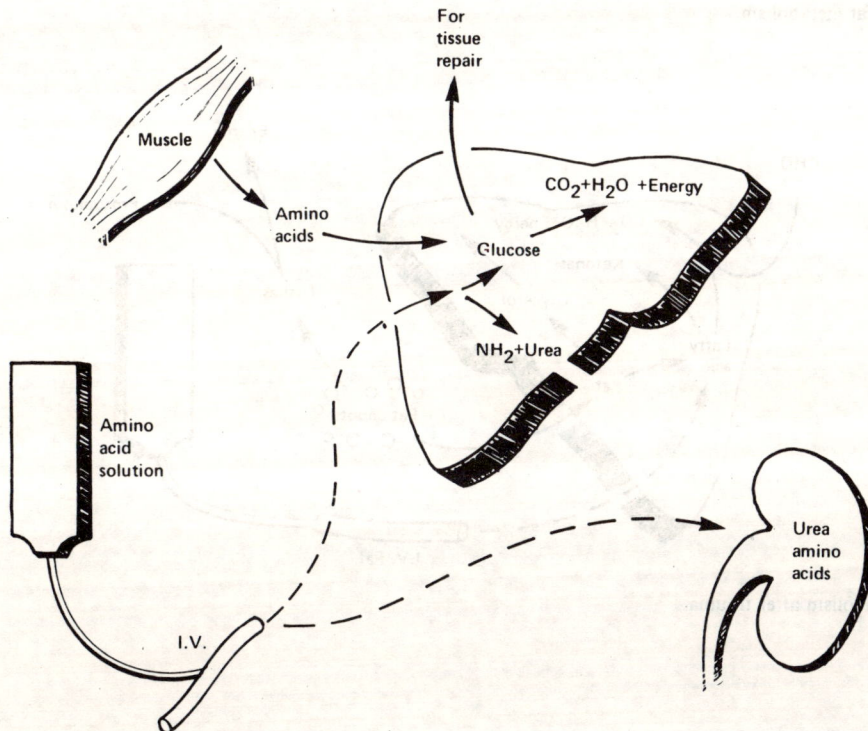

Fig. 6 Protein metabolism after trauma.

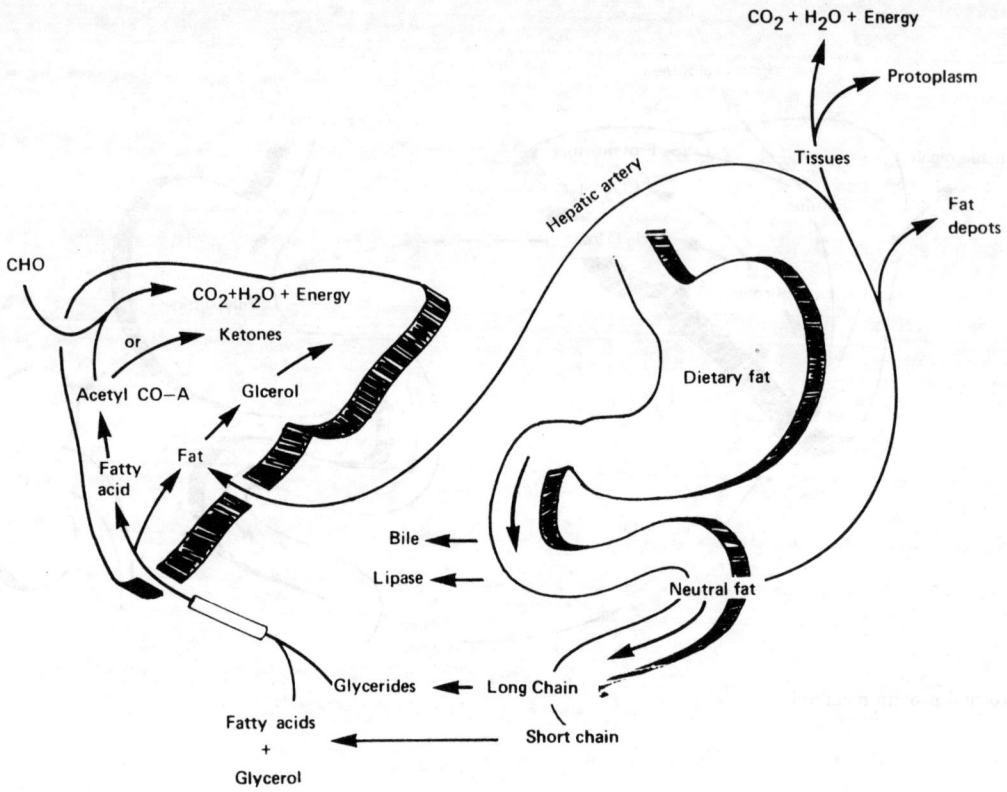

Fig. 7 Normal fat metabolism.

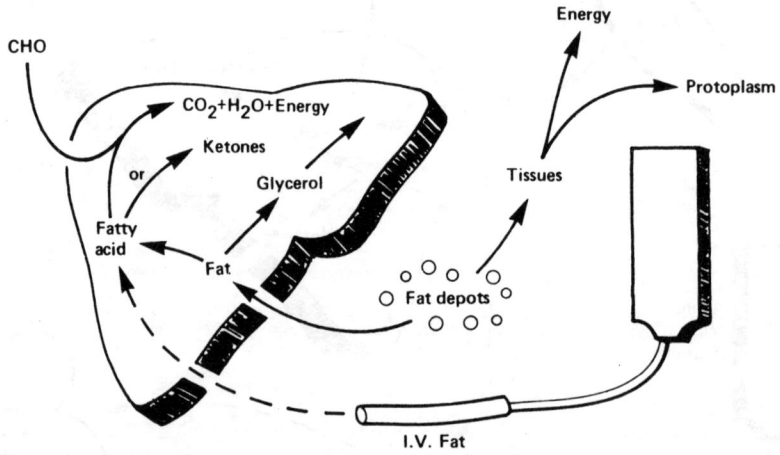

Fig. 8 Fat metabolism after trauma.

Indications for intravenous nutrition

Additional to oral and tube feeding
  Multiple injuries +/- sepsis
  Severe burns
Malabsorption syndromes
  Dysphagia
  Carcinoma of esophagus or stomach
  Esophageal stricture
Pre-operative preparation
  Pyloric stenosis
  Crohn's disease
  Ulcerative colitis
Post-operative conditions
  Peritonitis and sepsis
  Fistulae
  Prolonged ileus
Contra-indications
  Hepatocellular disease
  Renal failure (40g protein daily can be safely
  used)

Laboratory control

Daily
Body weight
Fluid balance chart
Serum: Na$^+$, K$^+$, Cl$'$, HCO$'_3$, urea, creatinine
  glucose
Blood: Hemoglobin, white cell count,
      culture unexplained-pyrexia
Urine: Na$^+$, K$^+$, urea, protein, glucose
Nitrogen balance

Twice weekly
Serum: Osmolarity
      Ca$^+$, Mg$^+$, PO$_4'$, lactate
      Iron, Folate, B12
      Liver function tests

Complications

Sepsis
Biochemical irregularities glucose, phosphate,
  potassium, acid base, etc.
Allergies
Incompatibilities of additives
Displacement of catheter

Reference

Lee H A, 1974 Intravenous nutrition. British Journal of
  Hospital Medicine 11, 719-728

Average electrolyte composition of gastro intestinal secretions

	Vol/24 hr	Na	K	Cl	HCO$_3$
Gastric	2500	60	9	98	
Bile	500	149	5	101	40
Pancreatic	700	141	5	77	120
Ileostomy (recent)	300	129	11	116	
Ileostomy (adapted)		46	3	21	
Diarrhoea	Variable	75	3	21	
Sweat		50	7	40	

M.Mols per Litre for columns Na, K, Cl, HCO$_3$

Constituents of common intravenous solution

Volume	Designation	g NacL	g KCl	Na	Cl	K	HCO$_3$	Calories
1000 ml.	Normal saline	9	-	150	150	-	-	-
	N/3 saline in 4% dextrose	3	-	50	50	-	-	160
	n/5 saline in 4% dextrose	1.8	-	30	30	-	-	160
	5% dextrose	-	-	-	-	-	-	200
	Hartman's Solution	7.0	0.4	131	110	5	29*	-
	M/6 sodium lactate	9.0	-	167	-	-	167*	-
400 ml.	Plasma	4.0	0.5	70	35	5	30	-
5 ml.	KCl ampoule	-	1	-	-	13	-	-

M. Mol per Litre for columns Na, Cl, K, HCO$_3$

* Lactate

Types of renal failure

1. Pre-renal

Hypovolemia
Burns
Diarrhoea and vomiting
Diabetic coma
Trauma

Prolonged hypotension
Cardiogenic
Bacteremic
Adrenal failure

2. Renal

Acute
Glomerulonephritis
Pyelonephritis
Hemolysis:
    Crush syndrome
    Mismatched transfusion
    Malaria
    Drugs and poisons
Eclampsia
Thrombocytopenic microangiopathy

Chronic
Polycystic disease
Diabetes
Tuberculosis
Amyloidosis/myelomatosis
Prolonged hypercalcemia

3. Post-renal

Congenital
Ureteral achalasia
Urethral valves
Urethral phimosis or stricture

Acquired
Prostatic hypertrophy
Vesical calculi
Carcinoma of bladder

Ureteral blockage
Bilateral calculi
Peri-ureteric fibrosis
Acccidental ligation
Blood clot
Crystals (Sulphonamide)

Reference
Linseth R E, et al. 1975 Acute renal failure following trauma. Journal of Bone and Joint Surgery 57A, 831-835

Treatment of renal failure

Establishment of diagnosis
Fall in renal output
SG or urine fixed at 1008-1012
Red cells, granular and epithelial casts present
Urine concentration of sodium above 40 mmol/litre
Urine/Plasma urea ratio <5
No increase in urine output on
    Raising of blood pressure or,
    20g Mannitol intravenously

Management
Chart fluid and electrolyte balance
Replace no more than the known daily loss
Correct hyperkalemia

Methods
1. 10-30 ml. 10% calcium gluconate intravenously over 15 minutes
2. 200 ml 50% glucose + 16 units insulin intravenously
3. 20-30 g resin by mouth or nasogastric tube, or intra-rectally
4. Hemodialysis
Correct acidosis: 8.4% sodium bicarbonate intravenously. Volume calculated by Astrup's formula.
Give 200g carbohydrate daily to reduce protein metabolism
Anticipate infection
Watch for gastric ulceration, thrombocytopenia, hypoprothrombinemia
Conserve arteries and veins

Fructose

A Hexose occurring naturally in fruit
Levo-rotatory isomer of glucose Synonym:
 Laevulose
Forms insulin when polymerised
Found in man in seminal vesicles
Metabolised independently of insulin
1 litre of 5% solution provides 200 calories

Effects in man
70% converted to glucose (Insulin required for
 further metabolism)
10% converted to muscle or liver glycogen
20% lost in urine
Inhibits gluconeogenesis in liver
Raises serum lactate and urate levels to cause a
 **metabolic acidosis ($>$600 g/24 hours
 dangerous)**

Therapeutic uses
1. Provision of calories in intravenous nutrition
 without provoking hyperglycemia (partly
 effective)
2. Detoxication of acute alcoholism (unproven)

Contra-indications
Children
Metabolic acidosis
History of gout

References
Leutenegger A F, Goschke H, Stutz K, et al 1977
 Comparison between glucose and a combination of glucose,
 fructose and xylitol as carbohydrates for total parenteral
 nutrition of surgical intensive care patients. American
 Journal of Surgery 133: 199-205
Levy R, Elo T, Hanenson I B 1977 Intravenous fructose
 treatment of acute alcohol intoxication. Archives of
 Internal Medicine 137: 1175-1177

Mannitol solution

Hydrogenated mannose
10% or 25% solution used for osmotic diuresis
Not metabolised

Indications
Prophylaxis of oliguria
Hepato-renal failure
Drug overdosage

Reduction of intracranial or intraocular
 pressure
Reduction of refractory edema

Contra-indications
Impaired renal function
Severe congestive cardiac failure
Metabolic edema with an associated capillary
 fragility

Dosage
50-200 g/24 hours

Test dose
0.2g/kg given intravenously in 3-5 minutes
 should produce a renal output $>$40 ml/hr.

References
Miller J D, Leech P 1975 Effects of mannitol and steroid
 therapy on intra-cranial volume – pressure relationships in
 patients. Journal of Neurosurgery, 42: 274-281
Powell W J, et al 1976 The protective effect of
 'Hyperosmotic' mannitol in myocardial ischaemia and
 necrosis. Circulation 54: 603-615
Powers S R, et al 1977 Hypertonic mannitol in the therapy of
 the acute respiratory distress syndrome. Annals of Surgery,
 185: 619-624

Sorbitol

Produced by hydrolysis of glucose
Breakdown produces fructose and glucose
Used as an artifical sweetener in commercial
 foods

Indications
Source of calories:
 8% higher than glucose or fructose
 Used in 10% or 20% solutions. (0.5g/min)
Osmotic diuretic

Side effects
Venous irritant (from a high pH)
Hyperglycemia (in large doses)
Bolus injection causes severe discomfort

References
Lee H A, et al 1972 Sorbitol: Some aspects of its metabolism
 and role as an intravenous nutrient. In: Wilkinson A W,
 Parenteral nutrition, pp 121-137. Edinburgh, Churchill-
 Livingstone

Alterations in oxygen transport

Code: P_{50} = Pressure of Oxygen at which Hemoglobin is 50% saturated
D.P.G. = 2:3 diphosphoglycerate
A.T.P. = Adenosine triphosphate
Factors that alter hemoglobin – Oxygen Affinity

Increase in P_{50}
(Shift to right in dissociation curve)

A. Direct effect
Increased (H^+)
Increased pCO_2
Increased D.P.G. or A.T.P. of red cells
Increased hemoglobin concentration
Increased ionic strength
Abnormal hemoglobin
Aldosterone

B. By increased D.P.G.
Decreased (H^+)
Thyroid hormone
Pyruvate kinase deficiency
Increased inorganic phosphate
Cortisol
Young red cells

Decrease in P_{50}
(Shift to left in dissociation curve)

A. Direct effect
Decreased (H^+)
Decreased temperature
Decreased pCO_2
Decreased D.P.G. or A.T.P. of red cells
Decreased Hemoglobin concentration
Decreased ionic strength
Abnormal hemoglobin
Carboxyhemoglobin
Methemoglobin

B. By decreasing D.P.G.
Increased (H^+)
Decreased thyroid hormone
Hexokinase deficiency
Decreased inorganic phosphate
Old red cells
See Figure 3

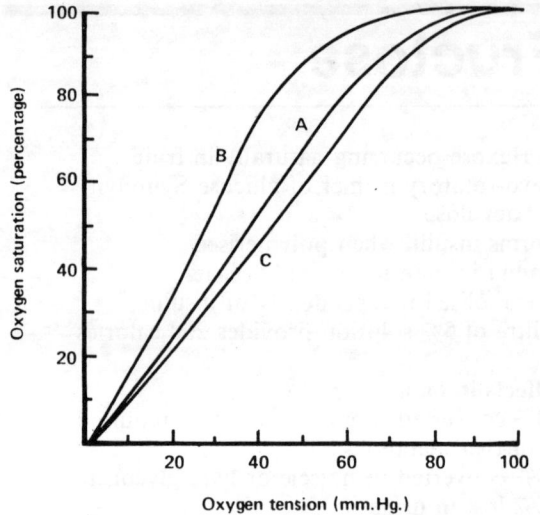

A	=	Normal curve
B	=	Left shifted curve : Increased hemoglobin affinity for oxygen
C	=	Right shifted curve : Decreased hemoglobin affinity for oxygen

Fig. 9 Oxygen—Hemoglobin dissociation curve.

Reference

Shappell S D, Lenfant C J M 1972 Adaptive genetic and iatrogenic alterations of the oxyhaemoglobin dissociation curve. Anaesthesiology 37. 127-139
Walker W F, Johnston I D A 1971 The metabolic basis of surgical care. William Heineman Medical Books Ltd. Chichester

3

GENERAL TOPICS

Organisation for major disasters

Excluding warfare, major civil disasters are
increasing in frequency from:
    Higher speeds of road travel
    Larger numbers of air travellers
    Increasing transport of volatile materials
    Increasing complexity and height of large
        buildings
All regions should design and rehearse a disaster
    plan

Services involved
Best at rescue and first aid:
    Fire
    Police
    Ambulance
Health Services: Doctors and nurses rarely
    required at scene of accident

Triage
Usually at nearest local hospital
Rarely at scene of accident
Experienced senior doctor required for this,
    perhaps from second-line hospital

Categories
1. Dead on arrival
    Desperately injured patients incapable of
        resuscitation. Palliative treatment.
2. Dangerously injured patients who need rapid
    treatment
3. Less seriously injured patients whose treatment
    can be postponed

Communication problems
From site of accident to major receiving hospital
From relatives and/or staff to hospital
From hospital to its off-duty staff

Some solutions
Senior official at site of accident with radio link
    to major hospital
Ex-directory telephone lines to major hospital
Set up information centre and advertise the
    telephone number by radio and television
Use small well defined call out networks for
    essential staff who operate their own call lists
Co-operate with news media

Problems within major hospital
Space
Receiving areas:
    Use unoccupied departments
    Cancel out patient clinics
Ward areas: Disperse moveable patients to home
    or other hospitals
Decide early if hospital resources will be
    overwhelmed

Triage
Dead and dying moved to mortuaries or
    unessential rooms
Dangerously injured resuscitated and order of
    treatment decided
Less seriously injured dispersed to other hospital
    departments
Emotionally injured – require a weeping room
Uninjured relatives and friends require space and
    information

References
Naggan L, 1975 Medical planning for disaster in Israel.
    Injury, 7, 279-et seq
Richardson J W, 1975 Disaster planning. John Wright &
    Sons, Bristol ·
Rutherford W H, 1975 Disaster procedures. British Medical
    Journal 1: 443-445
Rutherford W H, 1972 Experience in the Accident and
    Emergency Department of Royal Victoria Hospital with
    patients from civil disturbances in Belfast 1969-1972 with a
    review of disasters in United Kingdom 1951-1971. Injury 4:
    189-199.
Library: International Civil Defence Organisation.
10-12 Chemin de Surville
12, 13 Petit Lancy, Geneva

Elements of first aid

Move patient out of danger,
    i.e., Fire
            Falling masonry
Protect patient from traffic, crowds, etc.

Breathing
Clear airway
Give artificial respiration
    Mouth to mouth is most efficient

Blood
Stop hemorrhage
Elevate limb if feasible

Apply firm dressings
If arterial:
    Use suitable pressure points
    Apply tourniquet as last resort

Bones
Splint fractures
    Arm: Bound to chest
    Leg: Legs tied together
    Spine: Lay on rigid support

Bystanders
Employ these
To send for further help
To control traffic
To control sight-seers

Transport
Analgesia:
    Intravenous or intramuscular only safe routes
    Mark patient with drug dose time (Forehead
      best)
Position:
    Unconscious patients three quarters face down
      Dentures removed
    Conscious patients supine

Information
Warn receiving hospital if possible
Send details of type of accident, injuries, and
    patients' state in writing if possible.

Reference
First Aid Manual, 1972 Manual of St. John Ambulance
    Association. 3rd Edition. Hills and Lacey, London

Plaster of paris

First used
1852, A. Mathyson, Dutch Army Surgeon,
    rubbed plaster into cotton bandages

Chemistry
Raw state is gypsum-hydrated calcium sulphate
    plus impurities
Surgical state is anhydrous calcium sulphate
    minus impurities
Essential step is heating gypsum to 120°C
$$2\,(CaSO_4\,2H_2O) \longleftrightarrow (CaSO_4)_2\,H_2O + 3H_2O$$
Adding water allows return to crystalline state of
    full hydration
20% added water incorporated in hydration
    lattice

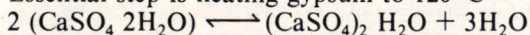

80% of water eventually evaporates
Low temperature and sugar solutions retard
    setting
High temperature and salt or borax solutions
    accelerate setting

Advantages
Safety
Adaptability to size and anatomy of part to be
    splinted
Lack of allergenicity
Speed of application
Price

Disadvantages
Weight
Delay in drying
Porosity
Partial radio-opacity

Mechanical characteristics
Setting time $\times$ 3 at 5°C compared to 55°C
    optimum temperature 25°C
Minimal plaster loss with a soaking time of 3-6
    minutes
Drying may require 7 days if atmosphere is moist
    and cool and if plaster is thick
Movement of cast while setting is occurring
    grossly weakens it
Optimum strength when completely dry – but
    water content at this point is 21%
Failure of a cast is due to different elastic moduli
    in gauze and hydrated calcium sulphate

References
Cameron D M, 1961 Plaster of Paris – A History American
    Journal of Orthopaedics, 3: 8-11
Luck J V, 1944 Plaster of Paris casts. An experimental and
    clinical analysis. Journal of American Medical Association,
    124: 23-29
Schmidt V E, Somerset J H, Porter R E, 1973 Mechanical
    properties of orthopaedic plaster bandages. Journal of
    Biomechanics, 6: 173-185

Cast syndrome

Synonyms
Superior mesenteric artery syndrome
Acute gastric dilatation

General features
Usually follows application of
    Body cast
    Hip spica

Risser jacket
or Scoliosis Surgery
or Spinal Trauma

Clinical features
Persistent vomiting
Distended pain free abdomen
Diminished bowel sounds
No other feature of intestinal obstruction

Radiological features
Gastric and duodenal dilation
Fluid levels in small intestine
Elevated diaphragm

Pathological features
Causation uncertain

Theories
1. Injury to autonomic nerve supply of gut by:
    A. Spinal extension
    B. Retroperitoneal hematoma
2. Compression of third part of duodenum
   between superior mesenteric artery and the
   aorta
Condition is exacerbated by lax abdominal
   musculature

Treatment
Begun on suspicion
Nasogastric tube, intravenous line
Nurse prone or on side
Flex hips if possible
Remove plaster cast or splintage if possible
Surgery:
    Division of ligament of Treitz
    Duodenojejunostomy

References
Evarts C M, Winter R B, Hall J E, 1971 Vascular
  compression of the duodenum associated with the
  treatment of scoliosis. Journal of Bone and Joint Surgery
  53A: 431-444
Schwartz D R, Wirka H W, 1964 The cast syndrome. Journal
  of Bone and Joint Surgery, 46A: 1549-1552
Willet A, 1878 Fatal vomiting following application of the
  plaster of paris bandage in a case of spinal curvature. St.
  Bartholomew's Hospital Reports, 14: 333-335

Crush syndrome

General features
First reported in Second World War
Caused by crushing of major muscle groups
  which are ischemic for long periods

May occur in many accident situations even from
  a forgotten tourniquet

Clinical features
Pain
External wounds
After release – massive swelling of limb
Hypotension
Fall in urinary output
Limb may become gangrenous

Radiological features
Associated fractures

Contrast studies
Angiography may show damage or blockage to
  major vessels but more often no lesion
I.V.P. high dosage infusion with tomography
  required to define kidneys

Pathological features
Mechanism
Crushing of limb and major nerves induces renal
  arteriolar spasm
After release of pressure fluid escapes into
  muscles with associated hypotension
Myoglobins released in large volumes
This precipitates in renal tubules in acid urine to
  block absorption
Acute tubular necrosis

Treatment
Analgesics
Transfusion of fluid and blood
Watch for and treat renal failure
Keep urine alkaline

Limb
Elevate, cool
Wide fascial decompression
Remove dead muscle
Amputation – if patient deteriorates
                if massive muscle necrosis
                is present

References
Bentley G, Jeffreys T E, 1968 The crush syndrome in coal
  miners. Journal of Bone and Joint Surgery, 50B: 588-594
Schreiber S N, Liebowitz M R, Bernstein L M, 1972 Limb
  compression and renal impairment (crush syndrome)
  following narcotic and sedative overdose. Journal of bone
  and Joint Surgery, 54A: 1681-1692

Tourniquets

Types
(1) Cords, bands, etc. dangerous
Less visible
Damage tissues
Huge pressures can be applied

2) Rubber bandages
Pressure uncontrolled
Peripheral nerve damage is frequent – due to
  ischemia or mechanical disruption

3) Pneumatic cuffs
Safer
Pressure controlled
Unlikely to be overlooked

Preliminary exsanguination

Methods
Elevation +/- massage of tissues
Tight bandaging (distal to proximal)
Rubber bandaging
Compression bag
Exsanguination of both legs in an adult
  equivalent to transfusion of 700-800 ml into
  remaining circulation
May lead to congestive cardiac failure in the
  elderly

Duration of application
Safe period undefined in man.
Variable periods of 1-3 hours advocated
If longer periods of ischemia are required:
  a) Consider a 2 stage operation or
  b) Deflate tourniquet for 10-15 minutes
     Exsanguinate and inflate tourniquet again
Tie tourniquet to operating table so that it
  cannot be overlooked

Pressures required to stop blood flow
generally sufficient and safe:
  300 mm. Hg. in arm
  500 mm. Hg. in leg
The larger the limb the higher the pressure
Pressure gradient falls off towards centre of limb
Systolic arterial pressure + 70 mm is effective in
  average limbs

Leakage of blood
Causes:
  Fall of tourniquet pressure
  Movement of tourniquet down a conical limb
    segment
  Medullary venous blood flowing from above
    tourniquet

Reactive hyperemia
Due to tissue metabolites causing vaso-dilation
  Lasts 10-15 minutes
Increases blood loss in wound
Coagulation time increased for up to 1 hour

Overlooked tourniquet
< 8 hours
1. Release tourniquet
   Watch for metabolic acidosis and renal failure
   Perform wide fasciotomies in affected limb
   If no arterial blood flow present explore
     neurovascular bundles at site of tourniquet
2. > 8 hours
   Consider amputation of limb above tourniquet
   Watch for renal failure
   Dialysis may be necessary

References
Bradford E M W, 1969 Haemodynamic changes associated
  with the application of lower limb tourniquets.
  Anaesthesia, 24: 190-197
Burchell G, Stack G, 1973 Exsanguination of the arm and
  hand. The Hand, 5: 124-126
Griffiths J C, Heywood O B, 1973 Biomechanical aspects of
  the tourniquet. The Hand, 5: 113-118
Parke A, 1973 Ischemic effects of external and internal
  pressure on the upper limb. The Hand, 5: 105-112
Sanders R, 1973 The tourniquet: Instrument or weapon? The
  Hand, 5: 119-123

Stress fractures

Synonym
Fatigue fractures

General features
Common
Occur in normal bone in healthy people engaging
  in regular activies without injury
Occur at all ages and in both sexes

Clinical features
Gradual onset of pain in a limb segment
Local tenderness. Slight swelling.
Increased heat. No deformity

Moderate loss of function
Spontaneous recovery with rest over 2-6 weeks

Differential diagnosis

Pain near a joint
Rheumatoid arthritis
Osteoarthritis

Infants
Battered baby
Rickets
Scurvy
Infantile cortical hyperostosis

Youngsters
Osteomyelitis
Osteoid osteoma
Osteogenic sarcoma
Periosteal hematoma

Adults
Tenosynovitis
Gout

Common sites
Metatarsal shaft
Tibial shaft
Pelvis, etc. etc.

Radiological features

Hair line crack in cortex at first
    then Medullary sclerosis
    then Periosteal new bone

Pathological features

All those of a fracture
No abnormal histology
Displacement and angulation very rare
Healing and remodelling in average time for any
    fracture

Treatment

Rest. analgesics
Splintage – plaster cast, etc.

References

Devan W T, Carlton D C 1954 The march fracture persists.
    American Journal of Surgery 87: 227-231
Devas M G, Sweetnam R 1956 Stress fractures of the Fibula.
    Journal of Bone and Joint Surgery 38B: 818-829
Devas M 1975 Stress fractures. Churchill Livingstone,
    London
Maudsley R H 1963 Fatigue fractures of both tibia and
    fibula. Postgraduate Medical Journal 39: 650-652
Provost R A, Morris J M 1969 Fatigue fracture of the
    femoral shaft. Journal of Bone and Joint Surgery 51A:
    487-498
Selakovich W, Love L 1954 Stress fractures of the pubic
    ramus. Journal of Bone and Joint Surgery 36A: 473-576

Re-implantation of severed extremities

General features

Rare to have a patient and the amputated
    extremity available at the same time
Rapid action by a large surgical team is required
Surgery is likely to be prolonged

Clinical features

Other severe injuries may be present
Patient is usually shocked
Only upper limb amputations are worth striving
    for, as lower limb prostheses are so good

Radiological features

Very variable fractures may be present
Pre-operative arteriography not necessary

Pathological features

Warm ischemia time is critical
No chance of success over 6 hours
Distal amputations do better than proximal
    lesions
Crushing of proximal tissues and/or amputated
    part is a contra-indication
Clean-cut distal amputations do best

Treatment

Cool severed part in crushed ice but not enough
    to freeze tissues
Wash through arterial tree with cold heparinised
    Ringers solution
Clean and prepare severed raw surfaces
Stabilise bones by internal fixation
Microvascular techniques to repair first veins,
    then arteries
Repair nerves and tendons
Loosely close skin and elevate limb
Anticoagulate patient for three weeks
Secondary surgery frequently required

References

O'Brien B McC 1976 Reimplantation and reconstructive microvascular surgery. Annals of the Royal College of Surgeons of England 58: 87-103, 171-182

Tamai S et al 1972 Microvascular surgery in orthopaedics and traumatology. Journal of Bone and Joint Surgery 54B: 637-647

Injuries of growth plate

General features

Epiphyseal injuries constitute 15% of all childhood skeletal trauma.

M > F

Summer > Winter

Fractures through the epiphysis and through the epiphyseal plate must be distinguished

Clinical features

Pain and swelling close to a joint

Loss of function

Occasional angulation

Radiological features

Separation (partial or complete) of epiphysis. Crushing injuries may show minimal change

Several injuries of different ages in a young child may indicate abuse

Pathological features

Epiphyses give way through the zone of hypertrophied cells on diaphyseal side of plate

Results:

Rapid thickening of hypertrophied cell layer

Delay in endochondral ossification for four days

Healing in 3 weeks if no ischemia

Classification: (See diagrams)

Type I

Separation of epiphysis

Birth injuries: Femur, humerus

Later life:

Scurvy, osteomyelitis

Slipped upper femoral epiphysis

May become ischemic in upper femur and radius.

Healed in 3 weeks. Except slipped upper femoral epiphysis

Good prognosis if not ischemic

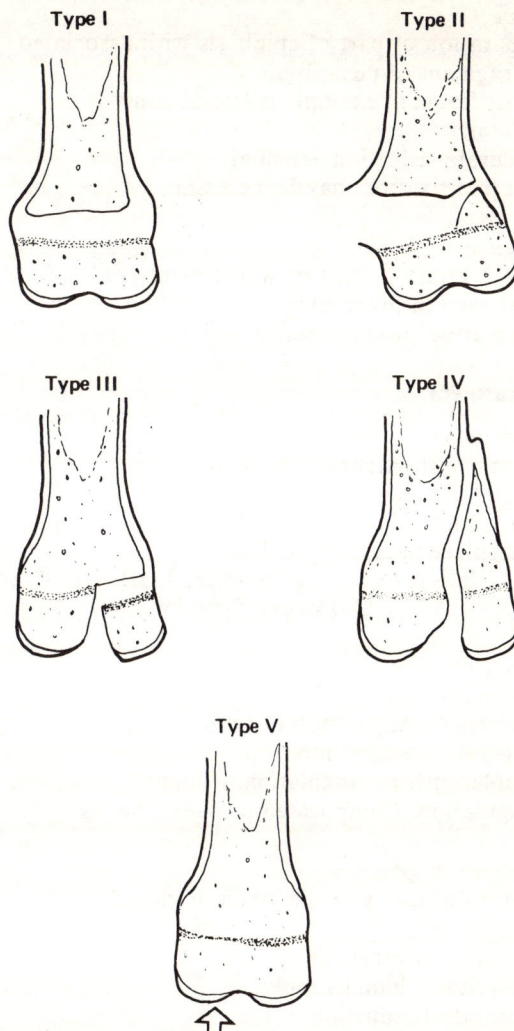

Fig. 10 Classification of growth plate injuries.

Type II

Separation of epiphysis with triangular metaphyseal fragment (Thurston Holland's sign)

Most common of all epiphyseal injuries

Most frequent after 10 years

Easy reduction. Good prognosis

Healed in 3 weeks

Type III

Separation of part of epiphysis

An intra-articular injury

Often lower tibia involved

Accurate reduction essential

Internal fixation may be necessary

Type IV
Separation of part of epiphysis with associated
    fragment of metaphysis
Most frequent example is lateral condyle
    humerus
Accurate reduction essential
Internal fixation may be necessary

Type V
Crush injury of part or whole epiphysis
Best seen in lower tibia
Premature fusion possible

Treatment

Principles
Gentle early accurate reduction
Closed method usually successful
Open method for Types III and IV or complete
    displacement of Type I
Immobilisation 3   weeks Types I, III, III, V
                3-6 weeks Type IV

Complications
Premature fusion:
    Partial – Angulation of limb
    Total – Short limb
Displacement – Angulation of limb
Angulation: Complicated in paired bones

Factors in prognosis
Nature of injury: Type, open or closed
Age of child
Presence of other disease
Integrity of blood supply
Method of reduction

Reference

Salter R B, Harris W R 1963 Injuries involving the
    epiphyseal plate. Journal of Bone and Joint Surgery 45A:
    587–622

Fascial compartment syndromes

Synonyms
Volkmann's Syndrome
Crush syndrome
Exercise ischemia
Phlegmasia cerulea dolens, etc. etc.

General features
Becoming more generally recognised.
Caused by local increase in pressure within
    fascial compartments of limbs
Minor effects:
    Temporary damage
    Intermittent and repetitive
Major effects
    Permanent damage
    May lead to
        death
        loss of limb
        loss of limb function

Causation

*1. Increased volume of contents within
compartment*
Bleeding:
    Injury
    Bleeding disorder
Increased capillary pressure:
    Exercise
    Venous obstruction
Increased capillary permeability:
    Post ischemic swelling
    Injury – Trauma
        Surgery
    Exercise, eclampsia, epilepsy
    Intra-arterial drugs
Muscle hypertrophy
Infiltration by infusion fluids
Nephrotic syndrome

2. Decreased compartment volume
Localised external pressure
Tight dressings
Closure of fascial defects

Diagnostic difficulties
Presence of other painful conditions (i.e.
    fractures)
Variety of initiating mechanisms
Differing rates of development
Differential diagnosis
Presence of plaster casts or dressings

Compartments affected
Commonest:
    Flexor surface of forearm
    Anterior tibial
    Posterior tibial: deep
                      superficial
Less common:
    Peroneal
    Anterior femoral

Posterior femoral
Extensor surface of forearm
Anterior humeral
Posterior humeral

Common clinical features
Continuing pain
Worsened by active or passive movement of
    muscles affected
Venous obstruction distally
Ischemic changes distally
Loss of peripheral pulses
Paresthesia of sensory nerves
Paralysis of affected muscles
Metabolic acidosis:
    locally
    generally on release of
        vascular obstruction

Common pathological features in sequence
Local rise of tissue pressure
Edematous tissues, particularly muscle
Venous obstruction
Arteriolar obstruction
Ischemia of muscle
Death of muscle
Loss of nerve conduction
Loss of axons
Fibrosis and shortening of muscle
Fibrosis of nerve trunks

Systemic manifestations of muscle necrosis
Myoglobinuria   Acidosis
Hypokalemia   Renal failure

Measurement of tissue pressure
Manometer method
Wick method
Measure pressure required to inject saline into
    tissue compartment

References
Matsen F A, Clawson D K 1975 (Editors) Compartmental
    syndromes. Clinical Orthopaedics 113: 3-110
Morimoto K, Harada H 1975 Tissue pressure measurements
    as a determinant for the need of fasciotomy. Clinical
    Orthopaedics 113: 43-57

Injury and pregnancy

General features
Minor injuries to mother common
Major injuries to mother and/or foetus are rare
Injury may lead to rapid termination of
    pregnancy

Foetal injuries
Causes:

1. Before birth from external violence
i.e. Lacerations from stabbing or gun shot
    wounds
Fracture of skull or limbs from fracture of
    maternal pelvis
Exsangination from placental separation or
    division of cord

2. At birth
Vaccum extraction
Forceps application
Cesarian section
Precipitate delivery

Effects
Brachial plexus injuries
Fractures of skull, clavicle, long bones
Facial and cranial hematomata
Exsanguinating cephalo-hematomata in
    hemoglobinopathies

Maternal injuries

Fractures of pelvis from major violence
Results 50% normal delivery
        25% cesarian section
        25% dead baby
Late deformity has minimal effect on later
    pregnancies in the West

Rupture of uterus
Occurs from:
    crushing injuries
    Pelvic fracture
    Seat belts in cars
Fetal death occurs unless the infant is 6 months
    old and rapid cesarian delivery is possible
Later pregnancy: 10% chance of second rupture
    occurring spontaneously if cesarian section not
    performed

Laceration of uterus
Occurs from:
  stabbing
  gun shot wounds
  self induced abortion
Treatment:
  initial observation
  surgery performed only on very clear signs

Rupture of diaphragm
Usually a latent rupture from previous trauma
  months or years earlier
Occurs during later pregnancy or in labour
Treatment: Post delivery surgical repair

Maternal limb fractures
Usually no effect on pregnancy
Internal fixation of leg fractures in late
  pregnancy makes delivery easier

Unconsciousness
Has no effect on fetus provided prolonged
  hypotension and hypoxia are avoided.

References:
Buchsbaum H J 1968- Accidental injury complicating
  pregnancy. American Journal of Obstetrics and
  Gynaecology 102: 752-769
London P S 1974 Injury and pregnancy, Injury 6: 129-140

Fat embolism

Synonym
Respiratory insufficiency syndrome

General features
Present to some degree after every long bone
  fracture
Signs and symptoms most frequent when
  carefully sought, often 12-48 hours after injury
Other causes: Severe soft tissue bruising
              Injury to fatty liver

Clinical features
Respiratory
Tachypnoea
Cyanosis
Blood tinged sputum

Neurological
Anxiety and restlessness
Clouding of consciousness
Coma

Others
Petechial rash
Pyrexia
Tachycardia
(Gurd, 1974)

Differential diagnosis
Head Injury
Pulmonary contusion
Withdrawal syndromes drugs/alcohol
Drug reaction
Pulmonary venous embolism

Laboratory investigations
Rapid fall in hemoglobin
Hypoxemia
Leucocytosis
Thrombocytopenia
Raised serum lipase
Fat globules in urine and sputum

ECG
Right axis deviation
Lead I Large S waves
Lead III Large Q waves

Radiological features
Mottled lung fields
Right ventricular dilation

Pathological features
Clinical incidence   5%- 10% } in injured
Autopsy Incidence 80%-100% }   patients
Fat embolism is direct cause of death in 5%-15%
  of severe cases

Lungs and brain
Vascular blockage from emboli and from
  vasoconstriction produced by platelet
  serotonin. Platelet adhesiveness and red cell
  aggregation increases in hyperlipemia
Local inflammatory changes increased by fatty
  acids formed from breakdown of fat

Lung
Fat emboli coated with platelets
Collapse of surrounding alveoli

Brain
Emboli produce 'ball and ring' infarcts which
  lead to focal necrosis.
Emboli must have passed through pulmonary
  circulation or an intra-cardiac defect

Removal of Emboli
Emulsification
Phagocytosis
Lipolysis
(Sevitt, 1962
Peltier, 1976)

Origin of fat Two theories:

1. Bone marrow
Intravasation of fat requires three conditions:
  Fat to be liquid
  Vessels to be torn
  Tissue pressure to force fat into veins

Points for: Fat embolism usually occurs after
      trauma
      Marrow emboli found in lungs at
        autopsy
      Fat emboli found after experimental
        fractures
      Fat stained in the fractured bone
        has been found in the lungs
Points   More fat is found in emboli than is
against: contained in fractured bone
      Cholesterol content of emboli is
        higher than marrow fat. (Armin,
  1951)

2. Changes in serum lipids
Points for: Fat emboli seen almost entirely in
      adults
      Diminished capillary fragility and
        hypoxemia indicates a
        generalised disorder
      Fat embolism is seen in uninjured
        patients but rarely seen in
        intramedullary nailing or hip
        arthroplasty when much marrow
        fat is disturbed
Points   Precise mechanism of change in
against: serum lipides has never been
        defined
      Volume of fat emboli may be more
        than volume of blood lipides
        (Lehman, 1927)

Hypoxemia
Occurs after most limb fractures but may not be
  clinically evident
Spontaneously corrects in 3-4 days
Probably due to pulmonary fat emboli causing
  intrapulmonary shunting of deoxygenated
  blood (Hassman, 1975 Wrobel, 1974)

Rare causes of fat embolism
Severe burns
Death from diabetes mellitus
Cardio-pulmonary bypass
Childbirth
Sickle cell crises
Post renal transplantation
Simulated high altitude flight

Treatment

Oxygen
Corrects hypoxemia
Usually given by mask
In coma, endotracheal intubation may be
  necessary with assisted ventilation
Aims:
  Rate 12/min
  Tidal Volume 1000 ml
  PO_2 50 mm
  P.E.E.P. : 10 cm. (Murray, 1974)

Steroids
Diminish inflammatory response
Hydrocortisone up to 1-2 g daily

Heparin
Clears lipemia, Activates pulmonary lipases 1000
  units/4 hourly

Sedation
Valium 5-10 mg/4 hourly
Chlorpromazine 25 mg/4 hourly

References:
Armin J, Grant R T 1957 Observations on gross pulmonary
  fat embolism in man and the rabbit. Clinical Science 10:
  441-469
Gurd A, Wilson R I 1974 The fat embolism syndrome.
  Journal of Bone and Joint Surgery 56b: 408-416, et seq
Hassman G C, Shauble J F 1975 Acute respiratory failure
  complicating multiple fractures in absence of fat embolism.
  Journal of Bone and Joint Surgery 57A: 188-195
Lehman E P, Moore R M 1927 Fat embolism, including
  experimental production without trauma. Archives of
  Surgery 14: 621-662
Murray D G, Racz G B 1974 Fat embolism syndrome
  (Respiratory Insufficiency Syndrome). Journal of Bone and
  Joint Surgery 56A: 1338-1349
Peltier L F 1969 Fat embolism, a current concept. Clinical
  Orthopaedics 66: 241-253
Sevitt S 1962 Fat embolism butterworth, London
Wrobel L J, Virgilio R W, Trimble C 1974 Inapparent
  hypoxaemia associated with skeletal injuries. Journal of
  Bone and Joint Surgery 56A: 346-357
Zenker F A 1862 Beitrage zu normalen und pathologischen
  anatomie die lunge. Dresden J. Braunsdorf

Venous thrombosis

General features
Nearly always in legs
Highest incidence after
hip
pelvic } surgery
abdominal

Clinical features
Pain, tenderness, increased heat in calf or thigh
Tenderness above inguinal ligament in
ilio-femoral thrombosis
Superficial venous engorgement
Small rise in pulse rate and temperature

Radiological features
1. Venography via
1. Long saphenous vein at ankle
2. Intra-osseous cannula
Good delineation of thrombi
But: Skilled technique for good results
Invasive method
Thrombi may be dislodged
2. Radio-isotope localisation (Flanc et al 1968)
^{125}I fibrinogen injected
Rapid and painless
But: Innaccurate in groin and pelvis
False positive over wounds and hematoma
3. Ultrasonic (Doppler) scan (Evans et al 1969)
Non-invasive and repeatable indefinitely
But some skill required, while false positives and
negatives are common

Pathological features
Virchow's Triad:
Stagnation of blood
Increased coagualability
Damage to vessel walls
Two principal sites:
Wide veins of soleus
Iliofemoral venous segment

Prophylaxis
Many varied methods will lessen the incidence
but none so far has been conclusively proved
superior
Pre-operative
Anticoagulants (Sharnoff et al 1976)
(Jennings et al 1976)
Bandaging of legs

Elastic stockings
Elevation of legs (Hartman et al 1970)

Per-operative
Pressure bags for legs (Hills et al 1972)
Dextran 70 infusions (Kline et al 1972)

Post operative
Electrical calf stimulation (Browse et al 1970)
Pressure stockings (Halford 1976)
Low dosage heparin
Passive exercise (Roberts et al 1971)
Active exercises

Treatment
Careful repeated examination of patient
Elevation of lower limbs

Superficial veins
No treatment apart from bandaging if
thrombosis is confined to this level

Calf veins
Anticoagulants
Heparin intravenous continuous infusion
(Kakkar 1972)
Subcutaneous bolus injections
Dicoumarol derivatives (Slow acting)
Under evaluation:
Viper venom preparations
Aspirin
Hydroxychloropine
Ilio-femoral veins
Anticoagulants
Thrombectomy (Mavor 1971)
Venograms required
Thrombectomy may need to be repeated
Local heparin infusion useful
Streptokinase infusions (Flute 1976)
Rapid action
Initial bolus to overcome streptokinase
antibodies
Induces allergy
Rarely repeatable

References:
Browse N L, Negus D 1970 Prevention of post operative leg
vein thrombosis by electrical stimulation. An evaluation
with ^{125}I-labelled fibrinogen. British Medical Journal 3:
615-618
Culver D, et al 1970 Venous thrombosis after fractures of the
upper end of the femur. A study of incidence and site.
Journal of Bone and Joint Surgery 52B: 61-69
Evans D S, Cockett F B 1969 Diagnosis of deep vein
thrombosis with an ultrasonic doppler technique. British
Medical Journal 2: 802-804

Flanc C, Kakkar V V, Clarke M B 1968 The detection of venous thrombosis of the legs using ^{125}I labelled fibrinogen. British Journal of Surgery 55: 742-747

Flute P T 1976 Thrombolytic therapy. British Journal of Hospital Medicine 16: 135-142

Harris W H, et al 1976 Cuff impedance phlebography and ^{125}I fibrinogen scanning versus roentgenographic phlebography for diagnosis of thrombophlebitis following hip surgery. A preliminary study. Journal of Bone and Joint Surgery 58A: 939-945

Hartman J T, Altner P C, Freeark R J 1970 The effect of limb elevation in preventing venous thrombosis. Journal of Bone and Joint Surgery 52B: 1618-1622

Hills N H, et al 1972 Prevention of deep vein thrombosis by intermittent pneumatic compression of the calf. British Medical Journal 1: 131-135

Holford C P 1976 Graded compression for preventing deep venous thrombosis British Medical Journal 2: 969-970

Kakkar V V 1977 Prevention of fatal post-operative pulmonary embolism by low doses of heparin. Lancet 1: 567-569

Kline A, et al 1975 Dextran 70 in prophylaxis of thrombo-embolic disease after surgery. A clinically orientated randomised double blind trial. British Medical Journal 2: 109-112

Mavor G E 1971 Surgery of deep vein thrombosis. British Journal of Hospital Medicine 6: 755-764

Roberts V C, et al 1971 Passive flexion and femoral vein flow. A study using a motorised foot mover. British Medical Journal 3: 78-81

Salman E W, Harris W H 1976 Prevention of venous thrombo-embolism in orthopaedic patients. Journal of Bone and Joint Surgery 58A: 903-913

Pulmonary embolism

General features
Much more common than is usually suspected
Is always a complication of phlebothrombosis elsewhere
Frequently misdiagnosed
Associated with previous:
1. Cardiac lesions
2. Surgery to abdomen pelvis chest
Wide spectrum of symptoms and signs from transient dyspnoea to sudden death.
Often provoked by defecation or exercise

Clinical features

Minor embolism
Sudden pleuritic pain.   R > L side
Base > Apex
Tachypnoea.   Tachycardia
Small rise in temperature and sedimentation rate
Pleural rub may be present
Hemoptysis later

Moderate embolism
Sudden dyspnoea.   Central chest pain
Hypotension
Venous engorgement
Hypoxemia
ECG changes – T wave inversion
  (variable)   Right axis deviation
          Bundle branch block
          Arrythmias

Major embolism
Collapse
Gasping respiration
Extreme hypotension
Death

Differential diagnosis
Pneumonia
Myocardial infarct, etc.

Radiological features
Radio isotope lung scans will show one or more areas of increased uptake
Pulmonary angiography will define site and size of embolus

Conventional films
1. Minor embolism:
      Wedge shaped peripheral opacity
      Elevation of diaphragm
      Intra pulmonary opacities
      Later: Pulmonary atelectasis
          Pleural effusion
2. Major embolism:
      Relative ischemia of whole or part of lung
      Dilation of right ventricle

Pathological features

Site of thrombosis	Risk of embolism
Superficial veins	Minimal
Calf veins	Minor (often multiple)
Iliofemoral veins	High (often single, massive fatal)

Signs, symptoms and effects are governed by size, position and progress of embolus
Minor multiple emboli may cause peripheral lung infarcts and late pulmonary hypertension
Major emboli may block once or both pulmonary arteries diminishing pulmonary venous flow to left side of heart. Emboli may **break up and pass more peripherally**
Pulmonary infarcts: Consist of alveoli which are airless, hemorrhagic and edematous. May lead to hemoptysis or lung abscess if infected

Raised
  sedimentation rate
  serum bilirubin
  lactic dehydrogenase
  fibrin degradation products in urine (FDP)

Treatment

All cases:
Analgesics (if required)
  Anticoagulants
  Antibiotics if infection is present or expected
  Physiotherapy for chest

Moderate embolism
Oxygen
Digoxin
Aminophylline

Recurrent embolism
Consider local treatment at site of origin if
  known
i.e. Thrombectomy
  Venous ligation
  Inferior vena caval plication

Major embolism
Intensive care
Consider Pulmonary embolectomy
  (Requires skilled cardiac bypass team)
Streptokinase infusion into pulmonary artery

References:

Editorial, 1973 Pulmonary embolism. British Medical Journal
  2: 1-2
Paraskos J A, et al 1973 Late prognosis of acute pulmonary
  embolism. New England Journal of Medicine 289: 55-58
Stein M, Moser K M 1973 (Editors) Pulmonary thrombo-
  embolism Chicago. Year Book Medical Publishers.

Air embolism

General features
Severe cases are infrequent
Minor episodes much more common

Mechanisms
Air injected under pressure
Artifical pneumothorax or pneumoperitoneum
Angiocardiography
Vaginal douching
Intra-arterial infusions
Air aspirated into low pressure veins
Neurosurgery in upright position
Cervical surgery
Cardio-pulmonary surgery
Drip lines: Running dry,
              Punctured, or leaking tubing

Clinical features
Deep gasping respiration

Venous
Cyanosis, unconsciousness
Hypotension
'Mill Wheel' splashing cardiac murmur
Right heart strain on E.C.G.
Ultrasonic probe easily detects bubbles in veins

Arterial
Pallor
Marbling } in skin area involved
Unconsciousness of very rapid onset if carotid
  arteries involved

Radiological features
Dilation of right ventricle
Pulmonary ischemia

Pathological features
8 ml/kg. of gas required to kill dogs

Venous embolism
Bubbles of gas foaming in right ventricle
Bubbles block pulmonary arterioles
Cessation of part of pulmonary circulation

Arterial embolism
May be rapidly fatal in cerebral circulation
Bubbles block part of peripheral tree
Venous embolism may become arterial if a patent
  foramen ovale exits

Prophylaxis
Avoid intra-arterial infusions
Provide intermittent jugular compression during
  operations in sitting position
Take care in cervical and thoracic surgery to
  avoid opening veins.
Give attention to drip lines

Treatment
Place patient head down
Right side uppermost
Give artificial respiration +/- cardiac massage
Aspirate right ventricle
Thoracotomy and aspiration under direct vision
  if time allows

References

Grace D M 1977 Air embolism with neurological complications. A potential hazard of central venous catheters. Canadian Journal of Surgery 20: 51-53

Lancet, 1976 Editorial: Brain operations in upright patients. Lancet 2: 352

Menkin M, Schwartzman R J 1977 Cerebral air embolism. Archives of Neurology 34: 168-170

Child abuse

Synonym
Battered child syndrome

General features
More common the more it is sought
Seen in all social classes
Sociopathic parent – usually mother
Parents often physically abused themselves as children
Usually an infant or young child involved
Stepchildren and adopted children have increased risk

Types
Physical:
    Fractures
    Bruises
    Burns
    Violent shaking – subdural hematomata
Sexual: Usually a girl
Nutritional: Water or calorie deprivation
Drugs: Administration or witholding of drugs
Emotional: Scapegoat syndrome

Clinical features
Stunted ill or injured child
Implausible history
Bizarre discrepancies
Delayed reporting or frequent attendance at emergency department
Lack of parental concern
Diagnosis:
    Full history
    Skeletal survey
    Blood clotting studies
    Serum biochemistry

Radiological features
Juxta epiphyseal fractures, often multiple
Skull fractures
Rib fractures
Subperiosteal hematomata and calcification

Differential diagnosis
Scurvy
Osteogenesis imperfecta
Coagulation disorders

Treatment
Appropriate to injury
Alert general practitioner
    Social Services
    Police (occasionally)
Retain child under long term supervision

References

Akbarnia B, et al 1974 Manifestations of the battered child syndrome. Journal of Bone and Joint Surgery 56A: 1159-1166

Cameron J M, Rae L J 1975 Atlas of the battered child syndrome. Churchill Livingstone, Edinburgh, London, New York

Helfer R E, Kempe C H (Editors) 1973 The battered child, 2nd Edition Chicago University Press

Jackson G 1972 Child abuse syndrome, The cases we miss. British Medical Journal 2: 756-757

Kempe C H 1971 Pediatric implications of the battered baby syndrome. Archives of Disease in Childhood 46: 28-37

Skeletal barotrauma

Synonyms
Caisson Disease, Aseptic necrosis of bone

General features
Occurs in those working under increased air pressure
    i.e. Tunnellers
        Divers
        Research workers
Subatmospheric pressures very rarely harmful in aircrew

Clinical features

Acute
Severe skeletal and soft tissue pains on too rapid decompression. (Bends) Short lasting

Chronic
Pain and stiffness around a major joint
    (Shoulder, hip, knee) Gradual onset, slowly worsening
Severe radiological changes may be symptomless

Radiological features

Indistinguishable from aseptic necrosis from
other causes.
Macroradiography useful for showing early
lesions.

Varieties
Dense areas with intact articular cortex
Spherical segmental opacities
Linear opacities
Structural failure:
    Translucent subcortical band
    Collapse of articular cortex
    Sequestration of part of cortex
Osteo-arthrosis

Situations
Head, neck and shaft of femur and humerus
    most often affected
Any other bone may be affected also

Radiological differential diagnosis
Bone necrosis:
    Gaucher's Disease
    Sickle cell anemia
    Steroid therapy
Bone islands
Osteochondritis Dissecans
Calcified enchondromata
Osteoblastic metastases

Pathological features

Incidence of lesions rises in proportion to
    Length of exposure to pressure
    High pressure exposure
    Incidence of attacks of bends
Uncertain how long a time is required to produce
    lesions
    i.e. 1 incident may produce a lesion
1600 compressions may not produce a lesion

Microscopy
Theory (no conclusive vidence yet available)
Nitrogen bubbles in intraosseous blood vessels
    lead to thrombosis and bone ischemia
Gravity leads to preponderance of lesions in
    heads of femora and humeri

Chronic lesions:
Areas of bone necrosis
Wider than radiological lesions
May be gradually revascularised
May lead to collapse of articular surface

Treatment
Prophylaxis
Prompt recompression if bends occur
No further compression work in those with
    radiological lesion

Conservative
Analgesics
Heat and exercises

Surgery
Drilling of necrotic area
Arthrodesis
Replacement arthroplasty

References
Chryssanthou C P 1978 Dysbaric osteonecrosis. Clinical
    Orthopaedics 130: 94-106, et seq.
MacCallum R E, Walder D N 1966 Bone lesions in
    compressed air workers. Journal of Bone and Joint Surgery
    48B: 207-235
Ohta Y, Matsunaga H 1974 Bone lesions in divers. Journal of
    Bone and Joint Surgery 56B: 3-16
Twyman G E 1888 A case of caisson disease. British Medical
    Journal 1: 190-191

Neonatal skeletal injuries

General features
Uncommon
Usually proximal segments of limbs involved in
    fractures
Chief cause is violent or unskilled delivery
Intra-uterine skeletal pathology is very rare

Clinical features
Infant is restless, irritable, feeding poorly
Minor pyrexia often present

Skull
Bruising or swelling over vault
    (cephalohematoma)
Depressed fracture may show as an indentation
    (see p. 62).

Limbs
Held immobile (pseudoparalysis)
Deformity may not be obvious at first
Bruising and swelling later
Characteristic position of upper brachial
    paralysis
(Waiter's tip position of arm)

Radiological features

Skull injuries
Fractures often indented or overlapped
Widened sutures from recent injury are unusual
Cephalohematomata may produce later
   pericranial calcification

Limb fractures
Epiphyseal displacements usually Salter Type I
Diaphyseal fractures often complete
Healing occurs with
   (1) profuse callus
   (2) remarkable remodelling

Pathological features

Intra-uterine skeletal abnormality is very rare
i.e. Fragilitas ossium
    Intra-uterine trauma

Mechanisms:
  Skull
  Faulty application of forceps
  Severe disproportion
  Precipitate delivery

Limbs
Malpresentation: Bringing down of arm(s) or
  leg(s)
Precipitate delivery
Brachial plexus lesions due to traction
  (See section on brachial plexus injuries)
  Erb's palsy, upper plexus, Klumpke's palsy,
  lower plexus

Treatment

Skull
Cephalohematoma
Overlapped sutures ⎫ Usually spontaneously
Depressed fractures ⎬   resolve
Asynclitism
(See section on depressed fractures of skull)

Limbs
Clavicle ⎫
Humerus ⎭ Bind arm to chest for 1-2 weeks
Femur   Binding legs together with padding
Tibia   or apply simple plastic or
         plaster splints for 2-3 weeks
Upper Brachial Plexus
Tie wrist to top of cot
Statue of Liberty splints difficult to apply
Passive movements to all joints

References

Behrman R E (Editor), 1977 Neonatal – Perinatal Medicine.
  2nd Edition Chapter 18 C. V. Mosby Co., St. Louis
Shulman B H, Terhune C B 1951 Epiphyseal injuries in
  breech delivery. Pediatrics 8: 693-700

Gangrene of the newborn

General features
Very rare
Visible at birth
Wide variety of possible causes

Clinical features
Area(s) of ischemia on trunk or limbs
Little systemic disturbance
Surrounding inflammation

Differential diagnosis
Infection
Emboli
Venepuncture mishaps

Radiological features
Nil unless local fractures or congenital heart
  disease are causative

Pathological features

Causes
Constriction syndromes:
   Congenital
   Umbilical Cord
   Wool threads
   Bandages
Emboli: Patent ductus arteriosus
         Other congenital cardiac defects
Venous or arterial puncture
Compression of infant against maternal pelvis

Associations
Long dry labour
Maternal diabetes
Rapid demarcation separation and healing
Joint contractures never follow

Treatment
Wait for demarcation +/- separation of slough
Surgery only
   if gross sepsis occurs
   if fascial decompression is required
Splintage to prevent contracture

Reference
Hensinger R M 1975 Gangrene of the newborn. Journal of
   Bone and Joint Surgery 57A: 121-123

Orthopaedic aspects of drug addiction

Infectious arthritis
Usually involves intravenous heroin
Unusual organisms cultured
   i.e. Pseudomonas
        Serratia marcescens
        Candida Albicans
(Gifford 1975, Ross 1974, Umber 1974)

Osteomyelitis
Can occur in any part of skeleton
Usually a sign of general debility
Pseudomonas vertebral infections not uncommon
(Weissman 1973)

Soft tissue necrosis
Caused by prolonged compression when the
   patient lies immobile for very long periods
Local ischemia from thrombosis of veins and
   arteries
(Howse et al 1966)

Puffy hands
Intravenous injections cause superficial cellulitis
   with venous and lymphatic blockage from local
   fibrosis
Early very radical surgery is required to give
   healing in quickest time before the patient
   defaults
(Neviaser 1972, Petrie et al 1973, McKay 1973)

References
Geelhoed G W, Joseph W L 1974 Surgical sequelae of drug
   abuse. Surgery Gynaecology and Obstetrics 139: 749-755
Gifford D B, Patzakism Ivler D, Swezey R L 1975 Septic
   arthritis due to pseudomonas in heroin addicts. Journal of
   Bone and Joint Surgery 57A: 631-635
Howse A J G, Seddon H 1966 Ischaemic contracture of
   muscle associated with carbon monoxide and barbiturate
   poisoning. British Medical Journal 1: 192-195
McKay D, Pascarelli E F, Eaton R G 1973 Infections and
   sloughs in the hands of drug addicts. Journal of Bone and
   Joint Surgery 55A: 741-746
Neviaser R J, Butterfield W C, Wieche D R 1972 The puffy
   hand of drug addiction. Journal of Bone and Joint Surgery
   54A: 629-633
Petrie P W R, Lamb D W 1973 Severe hand problems in
   drug addicts following self administered injections. The
   Hand 5: 130-134
Ross G N, Baraff L J, Quismorio F P 1974 Serratia arthritis
   in heroin users. Journal of Bone and Joint Surgery 57A:
   1158-1160
Umber J, Chapman M W, Drutz D J 1974 Candida
   pyarthrosis. Journal of Bone and Joint Surgery 56A: 1520-
   1524
Weissman G J, Wood V E, Kroll L L 1973 Pseudomonas
   vertebral osteomyelitis in heroin addicts. Journal of Bone
   and Joint Surgery 55A: 1416-1474

BURNS

With the assistance of I. F. K. Muir

Pathology of burns

Heat produces:
   inflammatory changes
   damage to cell membranes
   denaturation of proteins
   coagulation of protein
   vaporisation of cell water

Burn shock
Main cause is loss of plasma into burnt tissue
Increasing oligemia and rising hematocrit mostly
   due to loss of plasma water and
   disproportionate loss of sodium

Large burnt area leads to
exudation of body water
vaporisation of body water
increased heat loss
Burn toxins and antitoxins probably do not exist

Loss of red cells
Lost in burnt tissues
Sequestrated in partly burnt tissues
Shed into lacerations, fractures or hematomas if
   these occur at time of burn
Later may be lost in acute peptic ulceration
   (Curling's ulcer)

Tests
Blood film may show fragmented red cells
   (> 10% dangerous)
Sudden fall in hematocrit
Obvious loss – melena, hematemesis, jaundice,
   hemoglobinuria

Causes of fall in weight
Diminished intake of calories—anorexia
Lost meals – dressings
                  surgery
Increased catabolism
                  Repair processes
                  Infection of burn
Loss of ingested calories
                  Vomiting
                  Diarrhoea

References
Jackson D MacG. 1974 The psychological effects of burns.
   Burns 1: 70-74

Moyer C A, Butcher H R 1967 Burns, shock and plasma
   volume regulation. C. V. Mosby Co., St. Louis.
Sevitt S 1975 Burn wound healing – introduction. Burns I:
   189-191 et seq.

Classification of burns

Etiology
Dry heat   Flame
            Hot materials } Burn
Wet heat   Fluids }
            Steam }   Scald
Electricity
Chemicals

Depth

Partial thickness
Superficial: Heal within 14 days with good
                   quality skin
Deep: Heal slowly in 20-40 days with poor
                   quality skin and much scarring

Full thickness
Needs grafting

Discarded classifications

Hartford
A. Minor injury
   1. Epidermal   Heals within 14 days
   2. Superficial dermal Heals within 21 days
B. Major injury
   3. Intradermal Heals from base
                   within 120 days
   4. Subdermal   Heals only from margin
                   Requires skin grafting

Dupuytren
1st Degree: Blistering of skin
2nd Degree: Skin lost
3rd Degree: Fat damaged
4th Degree: Muscle damaged
5th Degree: Tendons and nerves damaged
6th Degree: Bone damaged

References
History of Burns and Treatment. Dupuytren G 1832 Lecons
   Orales de Clinique Chirgicale Vol. 1: 413. Germer-Balliere,
   Paris.
Moyer C A, Butcher H R 1967 Burns, shock and plasma
   regulation. Chapter 8. C. V. Mosby Co., St Louis.

Scheme of burns management

Initially
Estimate area burnt: 'Rule of Nines' or
                      'Rule of Fives'
Estimate weight: Known weight
                 Weighing bed
                 Age and height tables
Put up intravenous line:
Wide bore cannula into a major vein – arms or
  neck
Plan transfusion
  Use one of several plans
  All burns require i.v. fluid
    If over 20% in adults
    If over 10% in children
Suspect respiratory injury if hot gases or smoke
  inhaled
Nasogastric tube ⎫
Urinary catheter ⎭ For burns over 30%
Analgesics: Preferably intravenously
Oral fluids: 60-100 ml hourly if no nausea or
  vomiting

Secondarily
Prevent infection
Plan grafting procedures
Prevent weight loss. High calorie intake –
                      orally
                      intravenously

Severe burns
Require long term hospitalisation and major
  therapy
Those posing a continuing threat to life or
  livelihood
  1) Partial thickness > 30%
  2) Full thickness   >10%
  3) Burns complicated by:
      Respiratory tract burns
      Major soft tissue injury
      Fractures
  4) Electrical burns
  5) Full thickness burns of hands
      face
      feet

Moderate burns
Require hospitalisation for short periods
Minimal threat to life or livelihood
  Partial thickness > 30%
  Full thickness   > 10% excluding hands, face,
                           feet

Minor burns
Do not require hospitalisation
  Partial thickness > 10%

Assessment of adequacy of fluid replacement:
Restlessness
Color
Nausea, vomiting, large gastric aspirate
Blood pressure and pulse
Urine volume and specific gravity
  Volume: 25-50 ml/hour required
  S.G.   : Disturbed by glycosuria or
                    dextran leakage (if this is used)
Hematocrit
Re-assess frequently

Regimes of administration

A. 6 Ration Method (Muir and Barclay, 1974)
Plasma or dextran used
1. 1 Ration in ml.

$$\frac{\text{Total percentage body area burnt} \times \text{Weight in Kg}}{2}$$

    3 Rations in 1st 12 hours
    2 Rations in 2nd 12 hours
    1 Ration in 3rd 12 hours
2. *Severe deep burns* (> 10%)
    10% - 15% : 1 Ration replaced by blood
    15% - 25% : 2 Rations replaced by blood
    25% - 50% : 6 Rations replaced by blood

B. Lactated ringers solution method (Moyer,
  1965, Baxter, 1974)
Large volumes of lactated Ringers Solution
  (pH8-2) used
Volumes calculated from criteria (vide supra)
  and, particularly, hematocrit
Large extravascular sodium loss is replaced
Blood and colloid rarely required

C. Evans' formula (Evans, 1952)
  1st 24 hours:
    1 ml Plasma + 1 ml saline for every kg
      weight × every 1% burnt
    Plus 200 ml 5% dextrose.
  2nd 24 hours:
    Half previous volume of plasma and saline
      plus 200 ml 5% dextrose
See Figures 11, 12, 13, 14

Percentage surface area

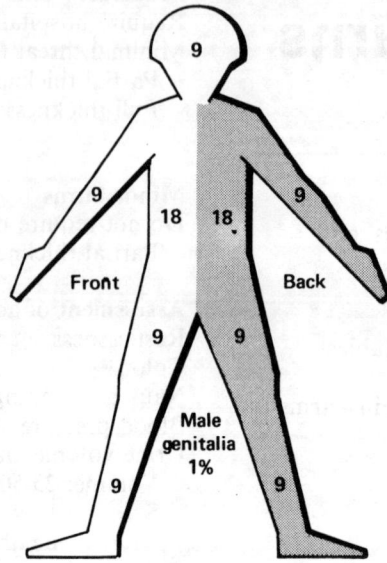

Fig. 11 Estimation of body surface area. Rule of nines.

Percentage surface area

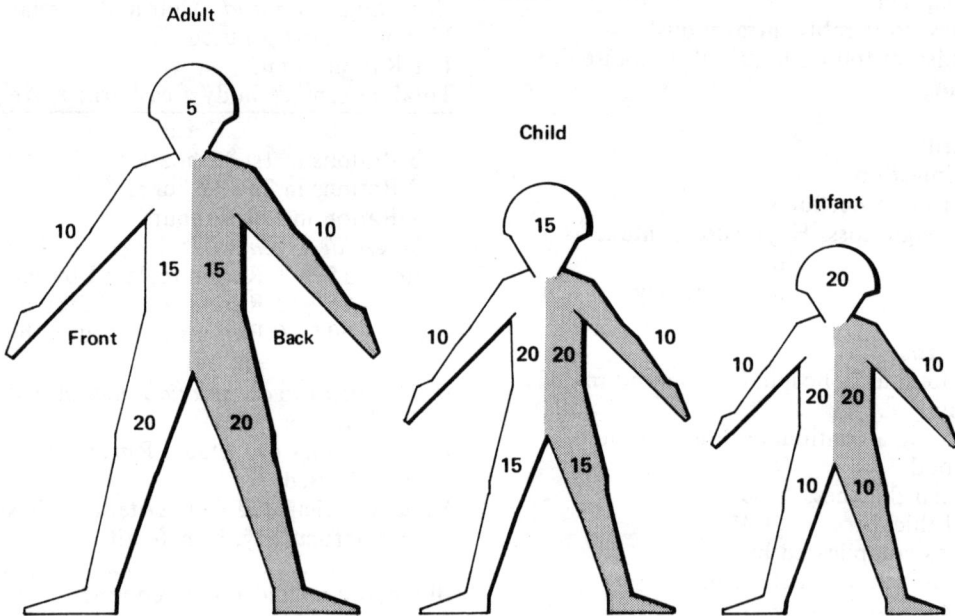

Fig. 12 Rule of fives.

FORESTERHILL AND ASSOCIATED HOSPITALS

BURN RECORD

Ages —
7½ years to Adult

Name .... Age .... Ward ....

Date of Observation ....

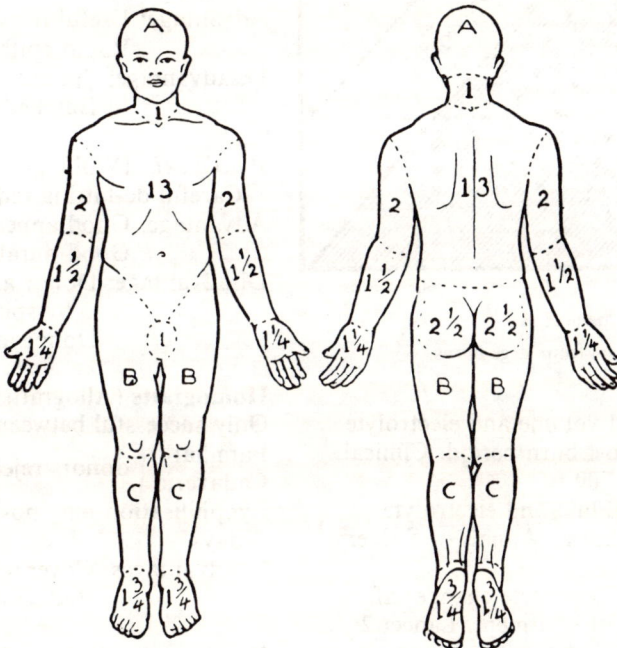

RELATIVE PERCENTAGES OF AREAS AFFECTED BY GROWTH

Area	Age	10	15	Adult
A = ½ of Head		5½	4½	3½
B = ½ of One Thigh		4¼	4½	4¾
C = ½ of One Leg		3	3¼	3½

% BURN BY AREAS

Probable 3rd° Burn	Head........... Neck........... Body........... Up Arm........... Forearm........... Hands.......					
	Genitals........... Buttocks........... Thighs........... Legs........... Feet...........					
Total Burn	Head...........Neck...........Body...........Up Arm...........Forearm...........Hands...........					
	Genitals........... Buttocks........... Thighs........... Legs........... Feet...........					
Sum of All Areas	Probably 3rd° .... Total Burn					

Fig. 13

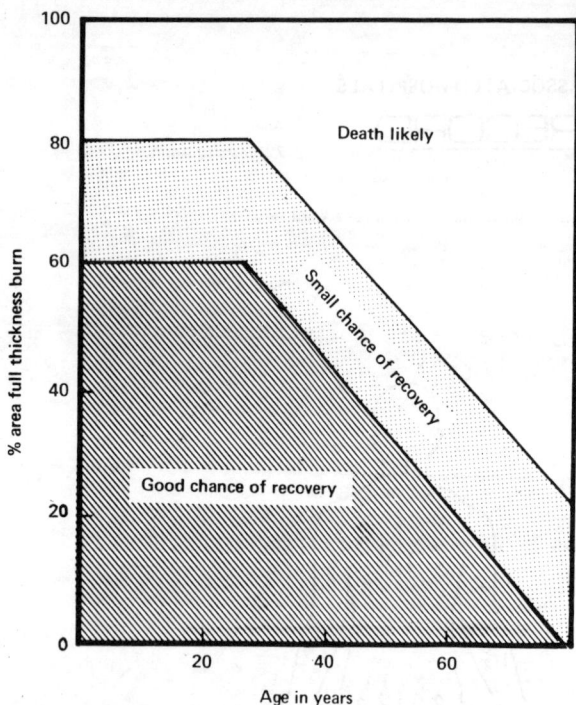

Fig. 14 Probability of survival from large burns.

References

Baxter C R 1974 Fluid volume and electrolyte changes of the early post burn period. Clinical Plastic Surgery 1: 693-709

Evans E I, et al. 1952 Fluid and electrolyte requirement in severe burns. Annals of Surgery 135: 804-817

Hinton P, et al. 1973 Electrolyte changes after burn injury and effect of treatment. Lancet 2: 218-221

Moyer C A, et al 1965 Treatment of large human burns with 0.5% silver nitrate solution. Archives of Surgery 90: 812-867

Muir I F K, Barclay T L 1974 Burns and their treatment. 2nd Edition. Chapter 2. Lloyd Luke, London

Skin grafting

Tools:

Humby knife, Campbell knife
  Adjustable depth of cut
Electric dermatome, Paget adhesive dermatome
  Excellent for large even grafts
  Blair knife, Razor blades
  Require more practice, only of historical interest

Autografts

Split skin (Thiersch grafts)
  0.008 - 0.010 in children
  0.012 - 0.105 in adults
Advantages: Large areas can be covered
        (Adjuvants: Meshing technique
                Postage stamp method)
      Donor areas can be cut again
        after 2-3 weeks
Disadvantage: Poor quality of skin
        Later contracture of graft
          thickness
Meshed grafts: 1→4 expansion of surface area
Advantage: Useful for very large burns
      Rapid epithelisation of raw gaps
Disadvantage: Special tool required
        Hatched appearance of graft

Whole skin (Wolfe grafts)
  Careful de-fatting required
Advantage: Good appearance – face
      Good durability – palm, sole
Disadvantage: Donor area has to be closed
        by split skin, etc.
      Donor areas cannot be used again

Homografts (Allografts)

Only successful between identical twins
Familial }
Cadaveric } donors rejected after 10-20 days
Lyophilisation may postpone rejection for 7-10 days
  Advantages: Coverage of very large areas
        Reducing exudate and infection

Heterografts (Xenografts)

Denatured pig skin and amniotic membrane under evaluation
May be useful as a biological dressing for very large burns for 1-3 weeks diminishing exudate and infection

Skin storage

+ 4° C = survival for 3 weeks
– 4° C = survival for 3 months
– 100° C = Dehydrated with glycerol – 3 years

References

Bose B 1979 Burn wound dressing with human amniotic membrane. Annals of Royal College of Surgeons of England 61: 444-447

Cochrane T 1968 The low temperature storage of skin. British Journal of Plastic Surgery 21: 118-125

Hobby J A E, Levick P L 1978 Clinical evaluation of porcine xenograft dressings. Burns 4: 188-192

Jackson D, et al. 1960 Primary excision and grafting of large burns. Annals of Surgery 152: 167-189

Mahler D, Hirschowitz B 1975 The use of xenografts in the treatment of burns. Burns 2: 44-46

Shepard G H 1972 The storage of split skin grafts on their donor sites. Plastic and Reconstructive Surgery 49: 115-122

Shuck J M 1975 The use of heteroplastic grafts. Burns 2: 47-53

Exposure treatment

Diminishes
fluid loss
bacterial growth

Depends on
Dryness
Coolness
Exposure to light

Particularly suitable for
Single surface burns of limbs or trunk
Burns of face
Burns of perineum
Extensive complicated burns

Disadvantages
Too rapid cooling of patient but environmental temperature at 28°-30° diminishes metabolic requirements of patient.
Requires relatively dry atmosphere
Unsuitable in highly contaminated atmospheres

Experimental techniques
Linear air flow rooms
Levitation air beds

References
Danielsson U, Arturson G, Wennberg L 1975 The elimination of hypermetabolism in burned patients. Burns 2: 110-114

Sanders R, Scales J T, Muir I F K 1970 Levitation in treatment of large area burns. Lancet 2: 677-681

Wallace A B 1951 The exposure treatment of burns. Lancet 1: 501-504

Infection in burns

Prophylaxis
Barrier nursing
Isolation of patients
Sterile air flow
Tetanus anti-serum
Penicillin 4-5 days in large burns
Later antibiotics according to wound culture
Convalescent serum discarded

Treatment
Exposure techniques
Removal of dead tissue
Early skin grafting
Early amputation if indicated
Topical antibiotics should be generally avoided
 – Ineffective
 – Promote bacterial resistance and sensitivity
Chemical dressings discarded except
 0.5% Silver Nitrate
 Silver sulfadiazine

Debridement techniques
1. Removal of eschar without analgesia as it separates:
    Prolonged, tedious
2. Repeated partial excision under general anesthetic
3. Tangential excision by skin grafting knife for deep partial thickness burns
4. Total excision under general anesthetic
    Large blood loss, i.e. Half blood volume in 10-20% burns
    Danger of worsening infection
5. Baths in saline or Locke's solution twice or thrice weekly to loosen eschar
6. Enzyme treatment experimental

Special infections
Tetanus
Gas gangrene

Pseudomonas pyocyanea
Commonly seen in large burns and in moist conditions
Large volumes of pus produced
Prevents grafts adhering
Bacteremia carries 60% mortality
Treatment:
 Systemic: Gentamicin
     Colistin
     Carbenicillin
 Topical: 0.5% Silver Nitrate (prophylactic)
     Sulfamylon Cream
 Hyper-immune serum in special bacteriocidal centres

Hemolytic Streptococci:
Much less serious since advent of penicillin
Must be eliminated from donor site before any grafting procedure

Bacterial enzymes strip off grafts and recently
regenerated epithelium
Treatment:
Systemic: Penicillin
Other appropriate antibiotics
Topical: Hypertonic saline
Hypochlorite solutions

References

Flick M R, Cluff L E 1976 Pseudomonas bacteremia.
American Journal of Medicine 60: 501-508
Pruitt B A, Curreri P W 1971 The burn wound and its care.
Archives of Surgery 103: 461-467

Chemical dressings

Objectives
Diminution of infection in burn wound
Elimination of specific pathogens

Discarded
Dermo- and hepato-toxic:
Phenol
Picric acid
Mercury salts
Tannic acid
Bacteriologically unsatisfactory:
Nitrofurazone
Dyes
Tribromophenol bismuth
Sulphonamides

Silver nitrate
0.5% solution bacteriostatic to all species except
Paracolon and Aerobacter
Non toxic
Easily obtainable
Stains patient's clothing and other materials
black
Leaches out chloride and patient may require
chloride supplements
Method
Gauze dressing applied daily to
eschar
grafts
raw areas
Kept wet by 3-4 hourly applications of 0.5%
silver nitrate
Overlying *dry* blanket or sheet (replaced when
wet) to prevent excess heat loss

Sulfamylon ('Mafenide')
Sulphonamide Derivative
Bacteriocidal to Pseudononas Aeruginosa and
other gram negative organisms relatively
ineffective against gram positive organisms
Applied as a cream daily to infected areas
Diffuses readily into tissues

Hypochlorite Solutions
Bacteriostatic but probably only for 20-30
minutes
Cheap, painless
Easy to apply
Efficacy lost if dressing is allowed to dry
Useful for separating dead tissue

Silver sulphadiazine
Bacteriocidal non-staining
Painless, applied as a cream

References

Bunyan J 1940 Envelope method of treating burns
proceedings of Royal Society of Medicine 34: 65-70
Fox C L 1968 Silver sulphadiazine – A new topical therapy
for pseudomonas in burns. Archives of Surgery 96: 184-188
Monafo W W et al. 1976 Cerium nitrate, a new topical
antiseptic for extensive burns. Surgery 80: 465-473
Moyer C A et al. 1965 Treatment of large human burns with
0.5% silver nitrate solution. Archives of Surgery 90: 812-867

Special problems

Extensive vascular thrombosis in electrical burns
Usually affects limb(s)
Results from prolonged contact with high
voltages
Vascular deficit usually obvious immediately
Risk of gas gangrene and tetanus

Treatment
Early amputation
If in doubt:
Elevation of limb
Anticoagulants
Infection prophylaxis
Decompressive fasciotomy
Later:
Total excision of dead tissue
Repair by pedicled flap

Circumferential burns

A. Limbs
Eschar may cause ischemia
Necrotic muscle may harbour gas gangrene or
   tetanus organism

Treatment:
   Early decompression of burn eschar
   Skeletal suspension of limb useful
      Allows exposure
              movement
              dressings
      Painless

B. Trunk
Surface on which patient lies becomes painful or
   moist
Dressings difficult to stablise and graft

Treatment
Exposure on net mattress
   or air flow bed
   or turning bed
   or skeletal suspension

Burns of skull
Necrosis often involves whole scalp thickness
If pericranium is burned, outer table of skull will
   be lost

Treatment
1. Excise soft tissue necrosis
   Allow outer table to dry
   Repair as much of soft tissues as possible
2. Secondary procedure
   Chip off necrotic outer table (and inner
      table if necessary)
   Allow to granulate
3. Tertiary procedure
   Apply grafts

Electrical burns of hands
Joints, bones and tendons frequently exposed
Rapid recovery of function essential to avoid
   stiffness and contractures

Treatment
Early excision
Early definitive repair for
   1) Low voltage contact injuries
   2) High voltage penetrating injuries
   3) Extensive high voltage injuries

Electrical burns around the mouth
Most often seen in children or infants
Caused by sucking a live wire

Treatment
Two schools of thought:
1. Conservative treatment
   Late reconstruction if necessary
2. Early complete excision
   Wedge resection usually enough
   Reconstructive procedures best left for six
 months,
      i.e. Tongue flap
          Cheek flap, etc. etc.

References:

Ho L C Y, Sykes P J, Bailey B N 1974 Extensive deep neck
   burns. Burns I: 149-159
Hunt J L, et al. 1974 Vascular lesions in acute electric burns.
   Journal of Trauma 14: 461-473
Hunt J L 1976 Electrical injuries of the upper extremity
   Major Problems. In: Clinical Surgery 19: 72-83
Jackson D 1975 Burns of bone: Can these bones live? Burns
   I: 342-374
Luce E A, Hoopes J E 1974 Electrical burn of the scalp and
   skull. Plastic and Reconstructive Surgery 54: 359-363
Muir I F K 1958 The treatment of electrical burns. British
   Journal of Plastic Surgery 10: 292-299
Oeconomopoulos C T 1962 Electrical burns in infancy and
   early childhood. American Journal of Diseases of Children
   103: 35-38
Peterson R A 1966 Electrical burns of the hand. Journal of
   Bone and Joint Surgery 48A: 407-424
Salisbury R E, McKeel D W, Mason A D 1974 Ischemic
   necrosis of the intrinsic muscles of the hand after thermal
   injuries. Journal of Bone and Joint Surgery 56A:, 1701-
   1707
Smith P J, Robinson P H 1976 Burns of the scalp involving
   bone, and alternative technique Burns 2: 254-260
Thomson M G, Juckes A W, Farmer A W 1965 Electric
   burns to the mouth in children. Plastic and Reconstructive
   Surgery 35: 466-477
Zarem H A, Greer D M 1974 Tongue flap for reconstruction
   of the lips after electrical burns. Plastic and Reconstructive
   Surgery 53: 310-312

Chemical burns

General features
Damage:
   Quality
   Quantity } of chemical agent
   Duration of contact
Local
Systemic } effects may result
Initial appearance may not reveal extent of
   damage

Prolonged pain with blistering or coagulation of protein
Mechanisms:
Spillage from containers
Splashing – deliberate
accidental
Swallowing – deliberate
accidental

Treatment
Wash very thoroughly
with water
or saline
or dilute specific antidote
Face and hands: expose to dry
Elsewhere: dry dressings appropriate
Surgery:
Injection of calcium gluconate 10% 0.5 ml/cm² to relieve pain of hydrofluoric acid
Excision of phosphorus or metallic sodium burns to remove remaining chemical
Excise and graft other burns when fully neutralised and defined
Esophagus:
Dilate strictures
Replacement of damaged segment

Specific chemicals

Oxidising agents
Chromic acid:
5-10g lethal. Coagulates protein, causing blistering and ulceration
Hypochlorites:
Release free chlorine. Only higher concentrations dangerous. Coagulate protein
Potassium permanganate:
Thick brown purple eschar of coagulated protein.
Crystals produce most damage. Earlier used as an abortifacient

Reducing agents
Alkyl mercuric agents:
5-50 mg/kg lethal dose
Blisters form and deepen if not evacuated
Hydrochloric acid ⎫ Water added to a
Nitric acid   ⎬ concentrated solution
                    ⎭ causes further ionisation
                      and additional damage

Corrosives
Phenol:
Rapidly absorbed. Gives a soft white coagulum. Sometimes drunk in suicide attempts

Phosphorus:
50-100 mg. is lethal. Burns more often seen in war injuries.
Particles fume and smoke as they oxidise in the tissues
Dichromates:
10g is lethal. Highly corrosive.
Soft yellow coagulum with deep ulcers
Alkalis   Cause liquefaction necrosis
Metallic sodium Soft brown friable tissue
                     destruction

Protoplasmic poisons
Salt formers:
Acetic Acid 5-50 mg/kg is lethal
Formic Acid Hard eschar formed
Metabolic competitors:
Oxalic Acid: 15-30g is lethal
White indolent ulcer formed
Hydrofluoric acid: 1.5g is lethal
Deep ulceration below tough coagulum
Persistently and severely painful

Dessicants
Sulphuric acid   Dilution in water is
                     exothermic
Hydrochloric acid Hard eschar formed with
                     indolent ulcer

Vesicants
Cantharides ⎫
D.M.S.O.   ⎬ cause edema and blistering
Mustard gas ⎬
Lewisite   ⎭

Treatment of chemical burns

Water lavage:
Chromic acid
Dichromate salts
Potassium permanganate
Alkalis
Hypochlorites
Phenol
Picric acid
Tannic acid
Trichloracetic acid
Acetic acid
Formic acid

Avoid water lavage:
Sodium metal
Sulphuric acid
Hydrochloric acid

Apply calcium salts:
    Oxalic acid
    Hydrofluoric acid

Cover with oil:
    Sodium metal
    Phenol
    Cresol
    White phosphorus
    Mustard gas

Special methods

Sodium metal: Excision
Alkalis: Weak acid lavage
Hydrofluoric acid: Boric acid or bicarbonate
    lavage
Chromic acid: Dilute sodium hyposulphite wash
Hypochlorites: Milk, egg white, starch paste or
    1% sodium thiosulphate
Phenol/cresol: Avoid alcohol. Use Polyethylene
    glycol or copious water
White phosphorus: 1/5000 Permanganate or
    Copper sulphate lavage
Dichromate salts: 2% Sodium hyposulphite wash
                7% 18% buffered diphosphate
                lavage
Alkyl mercury agents – Debride and remove
                          blister fluid
Sulphuric acid
Hydrochloric acid   Dilute alkali, or
                           magnesium hydroxide
                           wash

References

Ben-Hur N, Appelbaum J 1975 The phosphorus burn and its
    specific treatment. Burns I: 222-232
Jelenko C 1974 Chemicals that burn. Journal of Trauma 14:
    65-72
Orcutt T J, Pruitt B A 1976 Chemical injuries of the upper
    extremity. Major Problems in Clinical Surgery 19: 84-95
Pardoe R et al. 1977 Phenol burns. Burns 3: 29-41

Electrical burns

General features

Minor burns common
High voltage major burns are unusual
Unlimited variety of burn patterns
Shock of contact may cause:
    a fall
    +/- fracture(s)
    +/- internal injuries

Classification of injury

Low voltage usually 200-250 V
    1. Flash burn – superficial
    2. Contact burn – deep
High voltage usually 11,000+ V
    1. Flash – superficial
        Arc or contact:
            Punctate burn
            Extensive deep burn
            Extensive with vascular thombosis

Clinical features

Flash burns: Blackened skin–Volatalised metal
    Low voltages – partial thickness
    High voltages – full thickness
Contact burns: Central charring
    Areola of grey/white dead skin
    Peripheral areola of red coagulated skin
High voltage burns: May be circumferential
    May cause limb gangrene from major vessel
        thrombosis
Often little pain
Patient may be unconscious from brain injury
Shock is rare except in
    1. High voltage injuries
    2. Blood loss from other injuries

Radiological features

Early: Pathological fractures
        Periosteal new bone formation
Later: Osteoporosis
        Sequestrum formation

Pathology

Worst injury at points of contact and grounding
Very high temperatures may be produced by
    tissue resistance
Least resistance in blood vessels
Thus widespread thrombosis may occur in high
    voltage injuries of long duration when patient
    cannot release himself
Appearance:
    Central charred point of contact (grey-white,
        indrawn)
    Surrounding coagulation of skin (blood red)
Deepest damage under central point
Other injuries may be present apart from burns,
    i.e., fractures, intracranial, thoracic or
        abdominal injuries
Shock and fluid imbalance are rare

Factors influencing extent of damage

Voltage   } Major factors
Duration
Amperage
Resistance at point of contact

Resistance at point of grounding
Pathway of current through body
Type of current
Individual susceptibility

Treatment

Low voltage flash
Minor cleansing and debridement
Alternatives:
    Exposure
    Non-adherent dressings
    silver nitrate
Excision and graft rarely needed

Low voltage contact burns
Primary excision and split skin grafting
   (Caution with tendons, nerves, bones in hand
   or foot)
Secondary excision often required
   Skin grafting
   Pedicle flaps if bone or tendons exposed
Secondary or tertiary repair of excised structures
   i.e. Tendons, nerves, joints

High voltage flash burns
Difficult to evaluate initially
Often full thickness. Wait 3-5 days
Cleanse – minor debridement
Excise when defined
Graft as indicated

High voltage punctate burns
< 1 cm^2 – No treatment required
1-2 cm^2 – Initial excision
        Skin graft as indicated

Extensive high voltage burns
As patient's general condition allows:
   Primary excision
   Secondary excision
   Tertiary excision
Conserve important deep structures at first
   excision until certain of degree of damage
Delay repair procedures until all necrotic tissue
   has been excised

References

Barber J W 1971 Delayed bone and joint changes following electrical injury. Radiology 99: 49-53
Davies R M 1959 Burns caused by electricity. British Journal of Plastic Surgery 11: 288-299
Kragh L V, Erich J B 1961 Treatment of severe electric injuries. American Journal of Surgery 101: 419-427
Kay N R; Boswick J A 1973 The management of electrical injuries of the extremities. Surgical Clinics of North America 53: 1459-1468

Orthopedic complications of severe burns

Skeletal changes occur in a small percentage of large burns but may occur in regions remote from burnt tissue

Possible changes

Bone
Osteoporosis from:
   Immobilisation
   Local hyperemia
   Adrenal hyperplasia
Periosteal new bone formation
Diaphyseal exostoses
Pathological fractures
Tangential sequestra
Osteomyelitis
Premature closure of epiphyses

Joints
Septic arthritis
Spontaneous dissolution
Dislocation
Ankylosis
Scoliosis

Soft tissues
Pericapsular calcification
Heterotopic calcification
Muscle contractures

Treatment

Functional positioning of affected joints
   important
Early active exercises $+/-$ skeletal suspension
Early diagnosis and treatment of skeletal sepsis

References

Evans E B 1966 Orthopaedic measures in the treatment of severe burns. Journal of Bone and Joint Surgery 48A: 643-669
Franz C H, Delgado S 1966 Limb-Length discrepancy after third degree burns about foot and ankle. Journal of Bone and Joint Surgery 48A: 443-450
Jackson D 1975 Burns of bone: Can these bones live? Burns 1: 342-355 et seq.
Jackson D MacG. 1975 Burns into joints. Burns 2: 90-106

Pulmonary burns

General features
More commonly recognised with advent of
  intensive care units
Causes:
  Inhalation of hot gases, flame or steam
  toxic gases
  smoke
Associated with facial burns and other injuries

Clinical features
Three groups of patients:
1. Severe injury
   Pain in upper airway, stridor, dyspnoea within
   24 hours
2. Moderate injury
   Initially asymptomatic for 24 hours,
     thereafter:
   Cough
   Dyspnoea
   Tachypnoea
   Pyrexia
3. Minor injury
   Delayed onset of bronchopneumonia or
     embolism
Carbon Monoxide inhalation
  Masks cyanosis
  Diminishes consciousness

Radiological features
Soft tissue films may show narrowing of upper
  airways from edema
Chest films:
  Patchy opacities becoming confluent
  Later abscess formation

Pathological features
Thermal burns probably do not occur below
  trachea, because of efficient heat exchange
Chemical burns of lower airways and alveoli
  occur from smoke and toxic gases from
  burning synthetic materials
Carboxyhemoglobin produced by carbon
  monoxide
Laryngeal, tracheal, bronchial and bronchiolar
  obstruction from edema, causing stridor and
  dyspnoea
Alveolar edema from gases impairs gas exchange

$pO_2\downarrow$ $pCO_2\uparrow$ $pH\downarrow$

Treatment
Tracheostomy if airway is badly damaged
Monitor blood gases as aid to oxygen therapy
Intermittent positive pressure respiration (IPPR)
Positive expiratory end pressure (PEEP)
Bronchial dilators
Steroids
Antibiotics

References
Aub J C, Pittman H, Brues A M 1943 Pulmonary
  complications of burns. Annals of Surgery 117: 834-840 et
  seq.
McCardle C S, Finlay W E 1975 Pulmonary complications
  following smoke inhalation. British Journal of Anaesthesia
  47: 618-623
Mullins R B, Park S 1975 Respiratory complications of
  smoke inhalation in victims of fires. Journal of Pediatrics,
  87, 1-7
Munro A, Robertson G S 1975 Respiratory tract injury in
  burning accidents. Burns I: 285-290

Lightning injury

General features
Rare in temperate zones
Less rare in tropics
Produces electric effects
            blast effects   } on body

Clinical features
Cardiac and respiratory arrest
Flash and contact burns (clothing and flesh)
'Fern like' and 'feathery' skin patterns
Amnesia
Fracture may be present from violent muscular
  contraction and subsequent falls
Rupture of tympanic membrane
Cataract formation   } may occur

Pathological features
Electrical discharge may temporarily arrest
  cellular metabolism so allowing long survival
  of anoxia
Cerebral edema may result from electrical
  discharge or prolonged survival
No residual charge remains in patient
Magnetisation of metal objects on patient

Blast effects
Rupture of tympanic membrane
Contusion of lung
            myocardium } may occur
            intestines

Treatment
Cardiac-respiratory resuscitation
Must be prolonged as response may be long
 delayed
Fractures ⎫
Burns ⎭ Treated as required

References
Apfelberg D B Pathophysiology and treatment of lightning
 injuries. Journal of Trauma 14: 453-60
Bartholeme C W, Jacoby D, Ramchand S C 1975 Cutaneous
 manifestations of lightning injury. Archives of Dermatology
 111: 1466-1468
Hanson G C, McIlwrath G R 1973 Lightning Injury, Two
 case histories and a review of management. British Medical
 Journal 4: 271-274
Wright J W, Silk K L 1974 Acoustic and vestibular defects in
 lightning survivors. Laryngoscope 84: 1378-1387

Treatment
1. Rapid warming of trunk and unaffected limbs
 Exposure of frozen tissue in warm atmosphere
To improve tissue perfusion:
2. Systemic heparin
 Rheomacrodex intravenously
3. Wait for demarcation of dead tissue
 (Initial appearance worse than final result)
 Amputate gangrenous parts

References
Boswick J A 1976 Cold injuries. Major problems. In: Clinical
 Surgery 19: 96-106
Holm P C A, Vanggaard L 1974 Frostbite. Plastic and
 Reconstructive Surgery 54: 544-551
Kettelkamp D B, Bertvch C J, Ramsey P 1969 Radioisotope
 (I[131] RISA) evaluation of damage in frostbite. Journal of
 Bone and Joint Surgery 51A: 717-727

Frost bite

General features
Common in cold climates
Rare in temperate zones except for
 Military situations
 High altitude climbers
 Exposure with diminished consciousness

Clinical features
Fingers, toes, nose, ears, cheeks, first affected
Tissues become white, numb, stiff or hard,
 painless and functionless
Warming produces pain and hyperemia at
 margins of frozen tissue
Difficult initial assessment of final damage

Radiological features
None
Arteriography of no value in defining initial
 damage

Pathological features
Circulation slows on cooling
Arteriolar spasm
Arterio-venous shunting
Sludging of red cells
Tissue infarction is final result
Frozen tissue cells disrupted by ice crystals
Central tissues tendon and bone usually
 preserved
Experimental definition of damage by injection –
 Fluorescein
 Disulphine Blue
 Radio-isotope I[131] RISA

5

HEAD INJURIES

With the assistance of C. Blaiklock

Pathology of brain injuries

Blunt injuries
Most common in civilian life. Brain damage is
worst if head is free to move at moment of
impact – diffuse injuries from acceleration or
deceleration

Penetrating injuries
Most common in warfare. Local damage occurs
often without loss of consciousness

Crushing injuries
Rare and may cause extensive fractures without
brain damage or loss of consciousness

Primary brain damage
Uninfluenced by treatment
Diffuse neuronal damage
Shearing lesions
Contusion

Secondary brain damage
Effects mitigated by treatment
Swelling
Hemorrhage – Surface
            Intracerebral
Infection
Brain is incompressible but easily deformed
Rotatory or shearing stresses most likely to cause
damage at points of tethering of brain to its
ocverings and at interfaces of grey and white
matter.
Contusion is worst at summits of gyri and at
points where brain impinges on irregularities of
base of skull or dural folds

Brain swelling
Caused by edema
Venous obstruction
    Aggravated by: Head down posture
                Respiratory obstruction
                Injury or constriction of neck

Brain hemorrhage
May cause compression and distortion of brain
Intracerebral:
    Petechial
    Localised at grey-white matter interfaces

Subarachnoid:
    Tips of temporal lobes
    Inferior surfaces of frontal lobes
    Corpus callosum
Subdural: }
Extradural: }   can occur in various sites

Intracranial infection
Causes: Fractures into sinuses or ear
        Penetrating injuries

Causes of death in head injury
Widespread diffuse intracerebral injury
Injuries to medulla, midbrain and hypothalamus
Intracranial hematomas if not evacuated
Multiple injuries especially chest or abdomen
Pulmonary complications
Meningitis
Metabolic disorders:
    Cerebral fat embolism
    Unrelieved diabetes insipidus
    Adrenal failure
5% of adults reaching hospital alive with head
    injuries will die but only 0.5% of children

References

Strich S J 1961 Shearing of nerve fibres as a cause of brain
    damage due to head injury. Lancet 2: 443-448
Jennet W B 1977 An introduction to neurosurgery, 3rd
    Edition Chapter, 12. William Heinemann Medical Books
    Ltd. London

Initial management of head injuries

A common admission policy in many units

Admit
Any person concussed even momentarily
Patients with headaches, dizziness, visual
    visual disturbances
    Unequal pupils
    Vomiting
    Any neurological deficit
    Loss of CSF from nose or ear
    Fractured skull
Patients difficult to assess – children, drunkards
    etc.

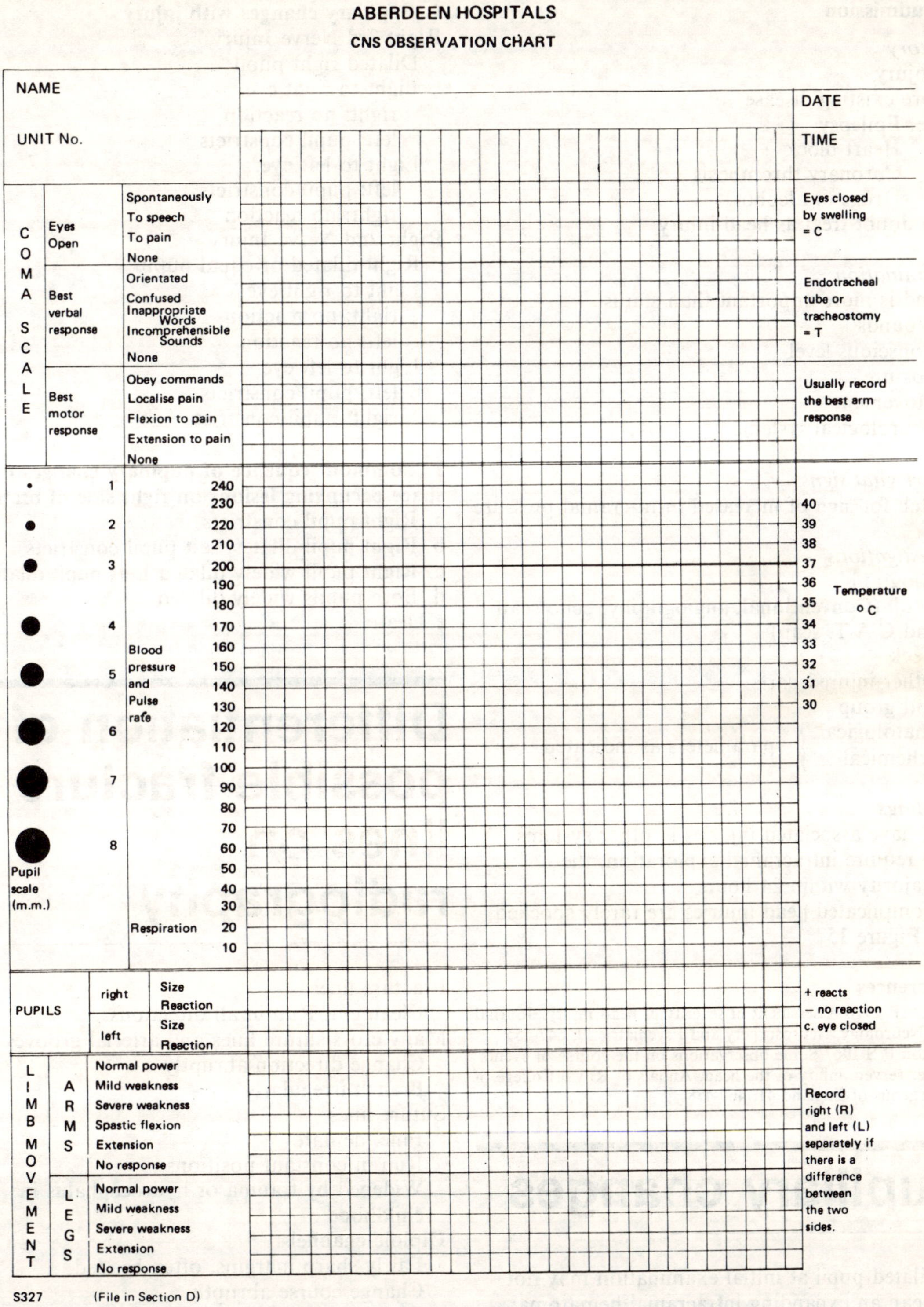

ABERDEEN HOSPITALS

CNS OBSERVATION CHART

NAME				DATE
UNIT No.				TIME

C O M A	Eyes Open	Spontaneously		Eyes closed by swelling = C
S C A L E		To speech		
		To pain		
		None		
	Best verbal response	Orientated		Endotracheal tube or tracheostomy = T
		Confused		
		Inappropriate Words		
		Incomprehensible Sounds		
		None		
	Best motor response	Obey commands		Usually record the best arm response
		Localise pain		
		Flexion to pain		
		Extension to pain		
		None		

Pupil scale (m.m.)
1
2
3
4
5
6
7
8

Blood pressure and Pulse rate
240
230
220
210
200
190
180
170
160
150
140
130
120
110
100
90
80
70
60
50
40
30

Respiration
20
10

Temperature °C
40
39
38
37
36
35
34
33
32
31
30

PUPILS	right	Size		+ reacts
		Reaction		− no reaction
	left	Size		c. eye closed
		Reaction		

L I M B M O V E M E N T	A R M S	Normal power		Record right (R) and left (L) separately if there is a difference between the two sides.
		Mild weakness		
		Severe weakness		
		Spastic flexion		
		Extension		
		No response		
	L E G S	Normal power		
		Mild weakness		
		Severe weakness		
		Extension		
		No response		

S327 (File in Section D)

Fig. 15

On admission

History
of injury
of pre existing disease
   i.e. Epilepsy
      Heart block
      Coronary thrombosis
      Drugs or alcohol
if in doubt treat as head injury

Examination
Trend is more important than status:
   Wounds
   Conscious level
   Posture
   Movement
   Neurological systems

Chart vital signs
Watch for sign of increased intra-cranial pressure

Investigations
Radiographic
   Skull (Conventional, angiography, echo scan
   and C.A.T. scan)
   Neck
   Other injured parts
Blood group
Hematological ⎫
Biochemical   ⎬ parameters as indicated

Findings
30% have associated injuries in other systems
 5% require intracranial exploration, the
   majority within 24 hours
Uncomplicated head injuries are rarely shocked
See Figure 15

References
Jennett B 1976 Assessment of severity of head injury. Journal of Neurology, Neurosurgery and Psychiatry 39: 647-655
London P S 1967 Some observations on the course of events after servere injury of the head. Annals of Royal College of Surgeons of England 41: 460-478

Pupillary changes

A dilated pupil at initial examination may not mean an expanding intracranial hematoma; orbital drainage may be responsible.

1. Pupillary changes with injury
Right 3rd Nerve Injury
   Dilated right pupil
   Light to right eye:
      right: no reaction
      left: pupil constricts
   Light to left eye:
      left: pupil constricts
      right: no reaction
Right 2nd Nerve Injury
   Right dilated or equal pupils
   Light to right eye:
      right: no reaction
      left: no reaction
   Light to left eye:
      left: pupil constricts
      right: pupil constricts

2. Common sequence of pupillary changes from space occupying lesions on right side of brain
a. Right pupil constricts
b. Right pupil dilates Left pupil constricts
c. Right pupil widely dilated Left pupil dilates
d. Both pupils widely dilated
e. Death

Differentiation of possible fracture lines on radiography

Fracture lines:
   Clean cut. Run in all directions
Many cross suture lines and arterial grooves
   Change direction abruptly
   Branch irregularly
Suture lines:
   Fine, dentate
   Run in constant positions
   Widened by trauma or hydrocephalus in childhood
Diploic channels:
   Fairly sharp margins, often beaded
   Change course abruptly
   Form irregular patterns
   Vary in width
   Often start near vertex of skull in diploic lakes

Meningeal grooves:
   Fairly sharp margins
   Run in known directions
   Branch dichotomously
   Reduce in size from below upwards

Reference
Rowbotham G T 1964 Acute injuries of the head. 4th Ed., p. 172, E. S. Livingstone, Edinburgh

Later management of head injuries

Chart
½ hourly for 6-12 hours
1 hourly for 24-48 hours. Longer if condition is slow to improve
1. Level of consciousness
      Eye response
      Speech response
      Limb responses
2. **Pupillary changes**
3. Pulse, Blood pressure, respiration, temperature
Watch airway and pulmonary changes
Protect pressure points on skin
Ensure adequate fluid balance.
   Intake: Intravenous line
                Nasogastric tube
   Output: Paul's tubing for men
                Catheter for women

Signs of cerebral compression
1. Reduction of conscious level as shown by eye, speech, limb, responses
2. Unilateral dilation of pupil followed by opposite pupil
3. Rising blood pressure, falling pulse rate
   Periodic or irregular respiration

Indicators of a bad prognosis
Total unresponsiveness
Fixed dilated pupils
Decerebrate rigidity

Measurement of severity of brain damage
Period of unconsciousness
Period of post traumatic amnesia

Cerebral irritation
All but the most trivial injuries pass through this phase

Duration α to severity of brain damage
This period is never remembered

Treatment
Protect patients' skin and limbs from injury
Protect other patients and staff from noise
Exclude a full bladder or late meningitis
Minor sedation particularly at night

Reference
Teasdale G, Jennett B 1974 Assessment of coma and impaired consciousness. Lancet 2: 81-83

Injuries of scalp

General features
Lacerations }
Abrasions   } very common
Avulsions }
Burns   } Uncommon

Clinical features

Lacerations
Profuse bleeding
Gaping only if galea is cut

Tears
Lift large flaps of tissue
Fractures and foreign bodies may lie underneath

Abrasions
Often difficult to shave because of multiple foreign bodies

Hematomata
Usually subaponeurotic
May be very large and fluctuant
Bruising later appears around margins of aponeurosis

Avulsions
Usually due to long hair
Usually major part of scalp torn off

Burns
Associated with unconsciousness or epilepsy
Often blackened and charred

Radiological features
Fracture of skull vault may be present
Foreign bodies may be seen under skin flaps

Pathological features

Scalp is very vascular

Tenuous pedicles will nourish large areas of scalp

Inefficient wound toilet will lead to cellulitis or
  osteomyelitis of skull

Avulsions: Usually galea aponeurotica is lost as
  well as skin and hair

Outer table of skull is exposed and will granulate
  if kept clean

Treatment

Hematomata Aspirate if fluctuant
              Often partially recur
              Evacuate if infected

Wounds
Thorough shaving and cleansing necessary

Lacerations and tears: Remove foreign bodies
                         Careful suture
                         Do not discard any
                         available skin flap

Avulsions
1. Pericranium intact:
     Shave scalp if available
     Replace as split skin grafts
2. Periosteum lost
     Remove outer table of skull
     Allow to granulate
     Cover with split skin grafts

Burns Excise when demarcated
        Allow to granulate
        Graft when clean

References

Gillies M 1944 Note on scalp closure. Lancet 2: 310-311
Kazanjian V H, and Converse J M 1959 The surgical
  treatment of facial injuries. 2nd Edition Chap. 20. Williams
  and Wilkins, Baltimore.

C.S.F. otorrhoea

(See section on facial injuries for C.S.F.
  rhinorrhoea) p. 93

General features
Rare
Due to fracture of base of skull
Occurs in 20% of middle ear injuries
            30% of inner ear injuries

Clinical features
Fluid issuing from ear
Rarely profuse
50% immediately apparent
50% visible after some days
Deafness (conductive or neural or both)
Tinnitus vertigo and nystagmus common
Rupture of tympanic membrane frequently
  present

Radiological features
Fracture of temporal bone, either longitudinal or
  transverse
Intra-cranial aerocoele may be visible

Pathological features
Track:
  Rupture of dura mater over petrous temporal
    bone
  Fracture leading into middle ear or external
    meatus
Drainage:
  Via Eustachian tube if membrane is intact
  Via external meatus otherwise
Intra-cranial aerocoele may arise from sneezing,
  etc.
(See section on injuries to inner ear)

Treatment:
Raise head
Loosely plug external meatus with sterile wool or
  cover with sterile gauze
Antibiotics

Complications
20% Meningitis: Antibiotics, etc.
 5% Persistence after 3 weeks
Craniotomy in middle and/or posterior cranial
  fossa.
Fascial graft to defect.

References

Albert P W R M, Dawes J D K 1961 Cerebrospinal
  otorrhoea in chronic ear disease. Journal of Laryngology
  and Otology 75: 123-135
Karnik P P et al 1975 Otoneurological problems in head
  injuries and their management. International Surgery 60:
  466-469
Skolnik E M, Ferrer J L 1959 Cerebrospinal otorrhoea.
  Archives of Otolaryngology 70: 795-799

Extra dural hematomata

General features
Most rapidly fatal complication of head injury
M > F

Clinical features

Immediate effects
Patient unconscious, condition worsening, signs
of intracranial pressure

Delayed effects
Patient stunned, lucid interval
Deepening unconsciousness
Signs of raised intracranial pressure

Late effects
Injury may or may not produce unconsciousness
    (20-25% not unconscious)
Long lucid interval – several days
Gradual onset of coma
    signs of raised intracranial pressure

Signs of raised intra cranial pressure
Bradycardia
Hypertension
Pupillary changes
Papilledema after some hours

Symptoms
Headache }
Blurred vision } if conscious
Vomiting: irregular respiration

Radiological features
No fracture may be present 2-5%
More frequently a fracture of squamous temporal
    bone is present crossing the middle meningeal
    artery groove
Midline shift on echo-scan, angiography or
    C.A.T. scan

Pathological features
83% Middle meningeal artery or branches are
    damaged
17% Diploe veins or dural sinuses damaged
20-30% Mortality even in best centres
50% if patient is stuporose when first seen

Extra dural hematomata usually rapidly increase
    in size. Usually temporal, rarely posterior or
    para-sagittal
Ipsilateral pupil affected first, then contralateral
    pupil
Death follows from coning of brain stem

Treatment
Rapid surgical decompression
Sometimes difficult to decide which side to
    explore first if C.A.T. scan is unavailable
Scheme:
Explore the side of scalp bruising
If no bruising: Temporal fossa on side of fracture
If no fracture: Side of more dilated pupil
If both pupils equal: side opposite the more
    spastic limbs
If no neurological or radiological clues: Prepare
    to explore both sides of skull
Osteoplastic flaps slightly longer but gives better
    access

References

Galbraith S 1976 Misdiagnosis and delayed diagnosis in
    traumatic intracranial haematoma. British Medical Journal
    I: 1438-1439
Jamieson K G, Yelland J D N 1968 Extradural haematoma.
    Report of 167 cases. Journal of Neurosurgery 29: 13-23
McKissock W. et al 1960 Extradural haematoma.
    Observations on 125 cases. Lancet 2: 167-172

Subdural hematomata

General features
Part of the spectrum of intracranial hematomata
    i.e. Subaponeurotic
        Extra-dural
        Sub-dural
        Intra-cerebral
        Intra-ventricular
Common in the elderly and in infants
May develop after a minor injury
x3 frequency of extra dural hematoma

Clinical features
Presentation and features can be grouped

Immediate
Signs of increasing cerebral compression

Delayed
Lucid interval before deterioration sets in
Indistinguishable from an extra dural hematoma

Late
Apparently normal for days or weeks after injury
Gradual onset of:
   Headaches   ⎫
   Dizziness
   Disturbed vision   ⎬ In variable
   Personality changes   patterns
   Fluctuating consciousness ⎭

Radiological features
Conventional films may show a fracture of skull
Echo-scan   ⎫ Will show midline shift
Angiography ⎬ and/or space occupying
Brain Scan   ⎭ lesion

Pathological features
Bleeding occurs from damaged cerebral
   tributaries to venous sinuses
Low pressure – slow collection
Cerebral atrophy in elderly predisposes to venous
   injury from minor trauma
Vomiting, coughing, sneezing, straining, will raise
   intra cranial venous pressure and promote
   bleeding
Hematomata often bilateral
Tributaries of superior sagittal sinus most often
   affected
   Petrosal sinuses less often
Large volumes can collect in the elderly
Clotting often long delayed
Hygroma is formed eventually before complete
   resolutions

Treatment
Localisation
Burr holes – series all over skull required if
   localisation uncertain
Removal of hematoma; hemostasis
Drainage

References
McKissock W, Richardson A, Bloom W M 1960 Subdural
   haematoma – A review of 389 cases. Lancet 1: 1365-1370
McLaurin R L, Timperman A 1972 Management of post-
   traumatic subdural hematoma in infancy. Clinical
   Neurosurgery 19: 271-280.
Editorial 1979 Chronic subdural haematoma. British Medical
   Journal 1: 433-434

Indented and depressed fractures of skull

General features
Babies' skulls indent easily in birth trauma
Children's skulls indent with moderate trauma
   and usually fracture
Adults' skulls require major localised force and
   always fracture

Clinical features
Often minimal disturbance in babies
Very variable clinical picture in children and
   adults
Depression may be concealed in hair
Fractures may be open or closed

Neurological changes
Sometimes none
Loss of consciousness variable
Local neurological deficit uncommon

Radiological features
Best seen on tangential views
No fractures in babies
Only inner table may split in children
Inner table often splintered and displaced
   inwards in adults
A whole bone may shift at its suture lines
   without other fracture
C.A.T-scan   ⎫
Angiography ⎬ May show a midline shift
Intracranial aerocoele
                ⎫ Rare in civilian
Intracranial foriegn bodies ⎭ life

Pathological features
Focal neurological deficit may be present if
   certain cerebral regions are injured

Complications
Infection
Intracranial hematoma
Venous sinus involvement
Post-traumatic epilepsy
Penetration of brain by bone fragment(s)

Treatment
Consider every case individually

Indentation
Indications for surgical elevation
At birth:
A large indentation with signs of cerebral
compression
At 3 months:
Disfiguring indentations outside the hair line
Any indentation over motor cortex
Indentations associated with epilepsy
At 3 years:
Any indentation > 3 cm. diameter

Depression
No action:
Small lesion less depressed than 1 skull
thickness
No neurological deficit
Consider action:
Larger lesion
No neurological deficit
Patient < 30 years
Fracture overlying major sinus
Certain action:
Cerebral compression
Localising neurological deficit
Bone fragment likely to have pierced dura
Gross cosmetic defect

References
Jennett B 1977 An introduction to neurosurgery, 3rd Edition,
Chapter 14. William Heinemann Medical Books Ltd.,
London.
Miller J D, Jennett W B 1968 Complications of depressed
skull fractures. Lancet 2: 991-995
Rowbottom G F 1964 Acute injuries to the head. 4th Ed., p.
279 et seq. E. S. Livingstone, Edinburgh.

Open fractures of the skull

General features
Due to localised severe trauma (road accidents)
or to gun shot wounds
Types of injury:
1. Wounds with linear fracture of skull
2. Compound depressed fractures with dura
intact
3. Compound depressed fractures with dura
damaged
4. Wounds with indriven fragments and
missiles
5. Wounds with fractures of mastoid region or
frontal sinuses (See separate section) p. 92

Clinical features
Wound is usually obvious
Large blood loss – scalp laceration or damaged
venous sinuses
Most patients are conscious: this may mean
1. Minor fracture without cerebral damage or
2. a major fracture with 'a silent' area of the
brain injured
Localised neurological deficit may be present

Radiological features
Fracture lines usually easily visible
Depressed fractures best seen on tangential or
oblique views
Inner table may be splintered
Intra-cranial aerocoele may be present
Foreign bodies usually present in gun shot
wounds
Echoscan
Angiography } May show a mid line shift

Pathological features
All grades of brain damage may be present
Some bullet wounds may pass through the skull
from side to side
Orbital roof is at risk in children falling on sharp
objects

Complications
Infection:
Osteomyelitis of skull
Extra dural or intradural abscesses
High risk if frontal or mastoid regions are
damaged
Brain fungus
Extrusion of brain tissue:
Very rare nowadays
Due to combinations of:
High intracranial pressure
Infection
Edema
Poor scalp closure

Treatment
Resuscitative measures
Shave scalp
Gentle wound debridement with lavage
Ensure absolute hemostasis. Postoperative
monitoring of intra-ventricular pressure
Remove easily accessible foreign bodies only
Close carefully. Antibiotics

Infection of skull
Remove sutures or make fresh incision
Drainage
Antibiotics

Brain fungus
Never amputate protruding brain
Eliminate intracranial sepsis
Control local infection
Lower C.S.F. pressure
Apply split skin grafts.

References

Coates J B, Meirowsky A M 1965 Neurological surgery of trauma. Office of the Surgeon General, Department of the Army, Washington D. C.
Guthkelch A N 1960 Apparently trivial wounds of the eyelids with intra-cranial damage. British Medical Journal 2: 842-844
Meirowsky A M 1966 Penetrating cranio-cerebral trauma. Clinical Neurosurgery 12: 253-265

Osteomyelitis of skull

General features
Rarely seen
Causes:
    Infected hematoma
    Sinusitis
    Infected scalp wound
    Hematogenous spread

Clinical features
Pain, swelling, redness, tenderness
Increased heat
Symptoms and signs of previous injury or sinusitis may be present

Later
Localised abscess formation (Pott's Puffy Tumour) or multiple discharging sinuses

Radiological features
Fractures
Foreign bodies   }
Surgical trephine holes } May be visible
Opaque sinuses   }

Later
Superficial erosion of cranial vault
Irregular rarefaction and density
Thickening of cranial vault

Pathological features
Direct spread of infection from extracranial source through diploic venous channels
Hematogenous infection also centres in the diploë minimal localisation
Phlebothrombosis promotes spread of infection
Chronicity of infection may be due to
    Sequestra
    Hemopoetic diseases
    Mistaken diagnosis,
        i.e. Tuberculosis
            Syphilis
            Metastatic tumour

Treatment

Local infection
Wide drainage
Appropriate antibiotics
Allow to granulate

Generalised or chronic osteitis
Vertical parallel incisions in scalp
Remove sequestra and outer table of skull

Complications
Extra dural abscess
Meningitis
Cerebral thrombophlebitis
Encephalitis
Cerebral Abscess

References

Burry U F, Hellerstein S 1966 Septicaemia and subperiosteal hematomas. Journal of Pediatrics 66: 1133-1135
Falconer M A, Latham G R W 1964 Spreading frontal osteomyelitis. Report of two cases cured by sequestrectomy and frontal sinus exenterations. Journal of Laryngology · and Otology 78: 937-951
Miles J, Hughes B 1970 Tuberculous osteitis of the skull. British Journal of Surgery 57: 673-679
Wilensky A O 1933 Osteomyelitis of skull. Archives of Surgery 27: 83-158

Diagnosis of brain death

Unresponsive patients with severe brain damage on artificial respiration are now common
Many continue to be kept alive with
Emotional trauma to relatives
Big demands on nursing staff

Criteria of brain death
1. Patient deeply comatose
Not due to
drugs
hypothermia
metabolic disturbance
2. Patient on ventilation because of failure of spontaneous respiration
Not due to
neuromuscular blocking agents
other drugs
3. No doubt about severe irremediable brain damage

Timing of decision
Rapid:
Severe head injury
Spontaneous intracranial hemorrhage
After neurosurgery
Delayed:
After cardiac arrest
circulatory insufficiency
cerebral air embolism
cerebral fat embolism

Tests
1. Absent brain stem reflexes
Fixed dilated pupils
Absent corneal reflex
Absent vestibulo-ocular reflexes
2. No motor responses in cranial nerves from stimulation of any somatic area
3. No gag reflex to bronchial suction
4. No respiratory movements after disconnection from ventilation and $P\,CO_2$ over 6.7 kPa

Other factors
Tests should be repeated to avoid error over a period of 12-24 hours
Spinal reflexes may be retained
E.E.G. recordings not necessary
Body temperature must be over $35°\,C$

Two experienced clinicians should agree on removal of ventilator

References
Diagnosis of Brain Death 1976 Statement issued by the honorary secretary of the Conference of Medical Royal Colleges. British Medical Journal 2: 1187-1188
A definition of irreversible coma, 1968 Report of the Ad Hoc Committee of the Harvard Medical School to Examine the Definitions of Brain Death. Journal of American Medical Association 205: 337-340

Sequelae of head injury

Glasgow Outcome Scale (Jennett et al 1976)
1. Dead
2. Vegetable State: Sleep/wake but not sentient
3. Severely Disabled: Conscious but dependent
4. Moderately Disabled: Independent but disabled
5. Good recovery: May have minor sequelae
Children recover better than young adults who recover better than older adults.
Mental and physical disability go together but one or other may predominate
Little change in state after six months although minor adaptions to disability may take place

Early local neurological deficits
Spasticity Hemiplegic
Quadriplegic
Aphasia
Hemianopia
Hydrocephalus
Cranial nerve paralyses

		of severe head injuries
1st 10%	6th 1.5%	
2nd 3%	7th 4.5%	
3rd 1.5%	8th 3%	
4th 1.5%	9th-12th rarely damaged	
5th 0.3%		

Rare early complications
Hypothermia
Diabetes insipidus
Hypernatraemia/hyponatraemia
Hypersomnia
Pulsating exophthalamos
Peptic ulceration

Later problems
Headache
Epilepsy (Jennett, 1962)
Dizziness
Intellectual impairment (Schuman, 1972)
Emotional liability
Anxiety and neurosis (Miller, 1961)
Dysphasia

Rehabilitation (Lewin, 1968) (Evans et al, 1977)
May require to recapitulate the learning of first
    five years of life in 3-6 months
Splintage of limbs may be required for short or
    long periods
Specialist treatment required for specific
    disabilities
Employment prospects very poor for those who
    have been unconscious for long periods
Unconsciousness for over 48 hours always results
    in some cerebral defect which may be apparent
    only to the immediate family of the patient

References
Evans C D, et al 1977 Rehabilitation of the brain damaged
    survivor. Injury 8: 80, 97
Jennett B 1975 Epilepsy after non-missile head injuries.
    Heinneman, London
Jennett B, et al 1976 Predicting outsome in individual
    patients after severe head injury. Lancet I: 1031-1034
Lewin W 1968 Rehabilitation after head injury. British
    Medical Journal 1: 465-470
Miller H 1961 Accident neurosis Lecture I. British Medical
    Journal 1: 919-925 Accident neurosis Lecture II. British
    Medical Journal 1: 992-998
Schulman K 1972 Late complications of head injuries in
    children. Clinical Neurosurgery 19: 371-380
Teasdale G, Jennett B 1974 Assessment of coma and
    impaired consciousness. Lancet 2: 81-83

EAR AND THROAT INJURIES

With the assistance of L. C. Wills

Injuries of external ear

General features
Minor injuries very common
Major injuries rare
Chief effect is cosmetic
Major deformities can be hidden by hair

Clinical features

Lacerations
Profuse bleeding
Little pain
Deformity from loss of substance

Contusions
(Cauliflower ear, Otohematoma, Hematoma
    auris)
Severe pain
Increasing swelling and tenderness

Avulsion
Tearing or biting
Relatively painless later
Little blood loss

Thermal injury
Frostbite:
    Affects tips and lobes of ear first
    Painless when frozen
    Painful swelling when thawing
    Later gangrene of periphery of auricle
Burns:
    Very varied extent
    Death of tissues: Painless
    1st and 2nd degree burns: Painful swelling

Treatment
Lacerations:
    Surgical repair
Contusion:
    Marginal incision to drain hematoma
    Moulded soft pressure dressing
    Later excision of thickened cartilage
Loss of lateral margin:
    Fine tubed pedicle graft from base of neck
Loss of cartilage:
    Soft tissue flap fashioned to contain
        autogenous cartilage grafts

Loss of auricle:
    Multiple reconstructive procedures (after age
        of 10 when adequate costal cartilage is
        available for grafts)
    or prosthesis (adults only)
    or different hair style

References
Davis P K 1971 An operation for haematoma auris. British
    Journal of Plastic Surgery 24: 277-279
Kazanjian V H, Conuerse J M 1959 The surgical Treatment
    of Facial Injuries. 2nd Edition. Chapter 28. William &
    Williams Co, Baltimore.
Potsic W P, Naunton R F 1974 Reimplantation of an
    amputated pinna. Archives of Ototaryngology 100: 73-75
Tauzer R C 1959 Total reconstruction of the external ear.
    Plastic and Reconstructive Surgery 23: 1-15

Injuries of external auditory meatus

General features
Usually due to introduction of foreign bodies
Mental defective + children: Self inflicted, often
                                repeated
Normal adults   : Other accidents

Clinical features
Pain
Bleeding – may be profuse
Unilateral deafness from blood clot if meatus is
    completely occluded
Conductive type

Radiological features
Radio-opaque foreign body may occasionally be
    present

Pathological features

Abrasions
May lead to infection, acute or chronic (otitis
    externa)

Lacerations
Bleed freely
If repeated, periosteal new bone may partly
    occlude external meatus

Foreign bodies
Animal, vegetable or mineral
May cause chronic sepsis and deafness if not
    removed

Treatment

Lacerations
Expectant
Gentle toilet to meatus
   24 to 36 hours after bleeding stops

Foreign bodies
Hook out object under otoscopic vision

Failure
Open meatus by a post-auricular incision
Insects or vegetable foreign bodies may be
   floated out by injecting oil gently into deepest
   part of meatus.
Insects should first be killed with drops of
   alcohol

Injuries of tympanic membrane

General features
Commonly due to trauma
Less commonly due to middle ear sepsis
   nowadays

Clinical features
Pain, tinnitus and vertigo (all usually transient)
Conductive deafness
Minor blood loss
Otoscopy:
   Rupture usually in the postero-superior
      segment
   Blast injuries always affect pars tensa

Radiological features
None, per se.
Fracture of temporal bone may be visible

Pathological features
Damage occurs from
   Foreign bodies in external meatus
   Blast Injuries
   Barotrauma (High or Low pressure)
   Fracture of middle cranial fossa

Treatment
No wound toilet of external meatus
Sterile plug of cotton wool

Raise head. No nose blowing
Antibiotics if infection is likely
Spontaneous healing in a normal membrane in
   two months
Persistent rupture with conductive deafness and
   otherwise normal ear: Skin graft to membrane

References
Edmonds S C 1973 Otological aspects of diving. Australian
   Medical Publishing Co. Ltd., Glebe, New South Wales.
Kerr A G, Byrne J E T 1975 Concussive effects of bomb blast
   on the ear. Journal of Laryngology and Otology 89: 131-
   143
Kerr A G, Byrne J E T 1975 Blast injuries of the ear. British
   Medical Journal 1: 559-561
Willis R 1970 Tympanoplasty, The Posterior Wall; The
   preservation of the posterior skin wall. Journal of the
   Otolaryngological Society of Australia 3: 31-34

Investigation of injuries of middle and inner ear

Investigation
History
Examination
Neurological examination
Otoscopy
Hearing tests:
   Bone conduction Usually impractical for some
   Air conduction   time after serious head injury
Electronystagmography
Radiography of Temporal Bone

Later
Audiometry (air and bone conduction,
   impedance, tympanometry)
Vestibular Tests
Strength – Duration curves of facial nerve
   (lacrimation, salivation and taste tests)

Reference
Cawthorne T 1953 The surgery of the temporal bone. Journal
   of Laryngology and Otology 67: 437-448

Injuries of middle ear

General features
Usually occurs from violent trauma, often unilateral
Damaged in 5-8% of skull fractures
Neurological and other injuries may be present

Clinical features
Pain
Conductive Deafness
Bleeding from external meatus
Tinnitus: Often low pitched and pulsatile
Facial Palsy

Otoscopy
Hematotympanum or a ruptured tympanum may be present.
These are the most likely causes of unilateral deafness after head injury.
C.S.F. otorrhoea (50% Immediate)
(50% Delayed)
in 20% of cases

Radiological features
Fracture of temporal bone
Usually present, 30% longitudinal in axis of petrous bone
Tomography may show ossicular disruption

Pathological features
Causes
Blast injury
Forceful insertion of foreign body
Fracture of base of skull

Effects
Rupture of tympanic membrane
Disruption of auditory ossicles
(Incudostapedial joint most often damaged)
Damage to tensor tympani

Treatment
Rest
Elevation of head
Antibiotics
No toilet of external meatus
Later: Ossicular surgery may be feasible

References
Holler F C, Greenberg L M 1972 Incudostapedial joint disarticulation. Archives of Otolaryngology 95: 182-184
Hough J V D 1969 Restoration of hearing loss after head trauma. Annals of Otology, Rhinology and Laryngology 78: 210-225 et seq.
Messervy M 1972 Unilateral ossicular disruption following blast exposure. Laryngoscope 82: 372-375
Tos M 1971 Prognosis of hearing loss in temporal bone fractures. Journal of Laryngology and Otology 85: 1147-1159

Injuries of inner ear

General features
Due to violent trauma to skull
Occurs in 1-3% of head injuries
Long term injury may be caused by industrial noise

Clinical features
Neural deafness
May be absolute
or high tone only
Tinnitus, high pitched, constant
C.S.F. otorrhoea is common
Facial nerve paralysis in 50%
Vertigo and nystagmus (rotational and positional)
Tympanic membrane may be ruptured

Radiological features
Transverse fracture of temporal bone is common
Tomography may show
(1) fracture passing through the cochlea and/or vestibule
(2) middle ear ossicular disruption

Pathological features
Disruption of 8th nerve
Hemorrhage into cochlea and vestibule

Treatment
Nerve deafness: No treatment
Nystagmus: Treat other causes if any are found to be operative
Vertigo: Sedation, anti-emetics
Reassurance
Positional exercises (Cooksey-Cawthorne exercises)

C.S.F. otorrhoea: Raise head
  Antibiotics
  Sterile plug for external
  meatus
  No nose blowing
If persistent after 3 weeks: Fascial graft to dura
Facial nerve paralysis: Early decompression if
  no sign of recovery
  ⅔ patients have residual
  symptoms
Disrupted ossicular chain: Surgical repair

References

Arora M M L, Bhattacharya T, Mehra Y N 1971 Facial paralysis by direct transtympanal trauma. Journal of Laryngology and Otology 85: 983-984

Barber H O 1972 The diagnosis and treatment of auditory and vestibular disorders after head injury. Clinical Neurosurgery 19: 355-371

Campbell E D R et al. 1962 Value of nerve-excitability measurements in prognosis of facial palsy. British Medical Journal 2: 7-10

Freeman P, Edmonds C 1972 Inner ear barotrauma. Archives of Otolaryngology 95: 556-563

Hough J V D 1969 Fractures of the temporal bone and associated middle and inner ear trauma. Proceedings of Royal Society of Medicine 63: 245-256

Skolnik E M, Ferrer J L 1959 Cerebrospinal otorrhoea. Archives of Otolaryngology 70: 795-799

Fractures of temporal bone

1. Longitudinal

Blows on side of head
Fracture crosses floor of middle cranial fossa
  Extends into squamous temporal and mastoid
  air cells
  Often involves tympanic ring

Otological features
Bleeding from ear
C.S.F. otorrhoea is rare
Tear in postero-superior tympanic membrane
Possible damage to ossicles
Some damage to inner ear
VII nerve paralysis rare

2. Transverse

Blows on occiput
Fractures passes through inner ear

Otological features
C.S.F. otorrhoea
Bleeding from ear unusual
Hematympanum present
Middle ear damage is rare
VIII nerve total loss
VII nerve paralysis in 50%

Reference

Barber H O 1972 The diagnosis and treatment of auditory and vestibular disturbances after head injury. Clinical Neurosurgery 19: 355-370

Types of deafness

Table 1 Types of deafness

	Conductive	Perceptive
Site of lesion	External or middle ear	Inner ear or VIII nerve
Degree	May be severe but never complete	May be complete
Associated symptoms	Tinnitus and vertigo in some cases	Tinnitus and vertigo more common
Otoscopy	Almost always some abnormality	Often no abnormality
Tuning fork	Heard better by bone conduction	Heard better by air conduction
Prognosis	Fair in untreated cases	Poor except in milder case
Treatment	Surgery often of value	No effective treatment other than hearing aid

Reference

Brain D J 1967 A practical guide to the care of the injured. Chapter 27. E & S Livingstone, Edinburgh.

Differences between central and peripheral causes of vertigo and nystagmus

Table 2 Differences between central and peripheral causes of vertigo and nystagmus

Peripheral	Central
Vertigo and nystagmus only occur when the head is in one critical position usually with the damaged ear lowermost	There are often several and sometimes variable critical head positions
Symptoms occur after a short latent period	No latent period
Vertigo and nystagmus quickly pass off usually within 15 seconds	Mystagmus (and sometimes the vertigo) persists as long as the head is kept in the critical position
Fatigue is noticed when the head is repeatedly placed in the critical position	No fatigue

Reference

Brain D J A practical guide to the care of the injured. Chapter 27. E & S Livingstone, Edinburgh.

Laryngeal injuries

General features

Increasingly common
Causes:
Gun shot wound
Lacerations
Blow on front of neck
Throttling
Inhalation of
foreign bodies
Corrosives
Burns
Associated esophageal and jugulo-carotid injuries

Clinical features

Open wound
Air leak
Bubbling blood loss
Hemoptysis
Surgical emphysema

Closed wound
Swelling, bruising,
Dysphagia
Hemoptysis
Surgical emphysema } If mucosa is torn

Radiographic features

Fractures of hyoid, thyroid and cricoid may be visible
Less often seen:
Subcutaneous emphysema
Fractures of cervical spine
Will define injuries to larynx if time allows:
Tomography
Ultrasonic scan

Pathological features

Both calcified and non-calcified laryngeal cartilages may be fractured
Fracture or cornu of hoid is characteristic of throttling injuries
Fibrous union of cartilages will give adequate function if undisplaced

Permanent change in voice from:
Change in length or position of cords
Laryngeal stenosis
Damage to inferior or superior laryngeal nerves
Fibrosis in crico-arytenoid joints

Laryngeal stenosis may occur from:
Unreduced fractures
Impaction of a foreign body
Too high a tracheostomy
Burns and scalds are associated with oral and pharyngeal damage – rapid onset of dangerous edema occluding the airway.

Diagnosis

Secure airway
Then: Laryngoscopy
Bronchoscopy
Esophagoscopy

Treatment

Trauma
Immediate repair gives best results
For all but minor injuries:
   Tracheostomy
   Nasogastric intubation
   Wound toilet
   Laryngeal fractures reduced and fixed by wires
   Cartilage deficiencies filled by rib cartilage
   Cords, cartilages, skin grafts held by laryngeal
     stent or polyvinyl mould
   Delto-pectoral skin flap for major skin loss

Foreign body
Remove as soon as it is localised by
   laryngoscopy or bronchoscopy
Thoracotomy for peripheral bronchial impaction
   of small objects

Burns
Tracheostomy
Steroids, antibiotics, analgesics
Intermittent positive pressure respiration may be
   necessary (Anaesthesiological help mandatory)

References

Cohn A M, Larson D L 1976 Laryngeal injury. A critical
  review. Archives of Otolaryngology 102: 166-170
Fieselman J F, Zavala D C, Keim L W 1977 Removal of
  foreign bodies (two teeth) by fibre-optic bronchoscopy.
  Chest 72: 241-243 et seq.
Krekorian E A 1975 Laryngo-pharyngeal injuries.
  Laryngoscope 85: 2069-2086
Shumrick D A 1967 Trauma of the larynx. Archives of
  Otolaryngology 86: 691-696

EYE INJURIES

With the assistance of F. M. Bennett

Investigation of eye injuries

History

Examination
Inspection
Records of visual acuity
Fluorescein straining
Evertion of eyelids
Ophthalmoscopy
Visual field charts

Special testing
Slit lamp inspection
Tonometry ⎫ Glaucoma tests
Tonography ⎬ (to be avoided if
Gonioscopy ⎭ globe rupture is suspected)
Transillumination of globe

Radiography
Conventional films
Tomography
Stereoradiography
'Bone free' films
Ultrasonic scan
Computer assisted tomographic scan

Reference
Duke-Elder S (Editor) 1972 System of Ophthalmology, XIV, Part 1. Henry Kimpton, London.

Contusion of the eye

General features
Very common, often self inflicted accidentally
Wide spectrum of damage
L > R
M > F
Affects every age group

Clinical features
Pain
Blurred or lost vision
Swollen bruised lids and/or periorbital tissues
Sub-conjunctival hemorrhage

Possible serious findings
Corneal abrasion or edema progressing to variable opacities (traumatic keratopathy)
Hyphema
Traumatic mydriasis from ciliary detachment
Dislocation of lens (variable position) with tremulous iris
Later rosette cataract formation
Vitreous hemorrhage
Retinal edema (Berlin's edema)
Detachment of retina
Rupture of globe
Rupture of optic nerve
'Blow-out' fracture of orbit

Radiological features
Ultrasonic scan will show disturbances of anatomy of eye
Views of facial skeleton and tomography will define orbital fractures
(*See* p. 87 on blow-out fractures)

Pathological features
Any but the most trivial injuries may permanently damage vision
Secondary glaucoma arises from:
  ciliary body damage
  hyphema
  some disturbances of lens
Hyphema may stain cornea permanently
  10% bleed a second time with worse prognosis
Choroidal tears give permanent visual field defects

Treatment
Examine every patient with care
Refer all but trivial injuries to ophthalmologist
See appropriate section for each injured structure

Orbital hematoma
Eye pad
Conjunctival antibiotic
Fibrinolytic and hyaluronidase preparations of doubtful value

Hyphema (Nurse sitting up (blood sinks to bottom of anterior chamber))
Bed rest initially
Anti-fibrinolytics on trial
Sedative. No mydriatics
Occular pressure lowered by
  Hypotensives
  Acetazolamide
  Mannitol

Surgery: (Microscopic)
  Irrigation of anterior chamber
  Lysis of clot by urokinase

References

Read J E, Goldberg M F 1974 Comparison of medical treatment for traumatic hyphema. Transactions of American Academy of Ophthalmologists and Otolaryngologists 78: 799-815

Read J E, Goldberg M F 1974 Blunt ocular trauma and hyphema. International Ophthalmology Clinics 14: 57-97

Injuries of eyelids

General features

Lacerations frequent – may involve levator palpebris superioris (LPS)
Loss of lid substance uncommon
  May be due to
    explosions
    road accidents
    assaults
Often accompanied by other injuries to the eye

Clinical features

Lacerations
Profuse bleeding
Rapid development of edema, ptosis if levator affected
Damage to infra or supra-orbital nerves
Medial lacerations may cut lacriminal ducts

Avulsions
Lower > Upper lid
Corneal and scleral damage
Lacrimal ducts often avulsed

Radiological features

In more severe injuries, fractures of orbital margins or anterior cranial fossa may be present

Pathological features

Exceptionally good blood supply
An exposed cornea may become dry, abraded, infected and opaque
Scarring and contraction may lead to ectropion or entropion
A vertical scar causes notched lid edge
Scarring of lacrimal ducts leads to epiphora

Treatment

Lacerations of skin and LPS: Careful suturing
Tears of tarsal plate: Replacement and suturing in layers – knots outside
Lacrimal ducts: Identify and oppose cut ends over micro-catheters or nylon thread under microscope
Loss of Tissue: Upper lid: Tarsorraphy and split skin graft over a dental mould
Lower lid: Cheek flap to reconstitute the skin of lid
Upper lid tarsal plate: Cartilage autograft

References

Fox S A 1972 Ophthalmic plastic surgery 4th Edition. Greene and Stratton, New York and London.

Kazanjian V H and Converse J M 1959 The surgical treatment of facial injuries. 2nd Ed., Chap. 21, Williams and Wilkins, Baltimore.

Injuries of conjunctiva

General features

Trauma common
Chemicals } relatively uncommon
Burns

Clinical features

Pain
Hemorrhage
Blepharospasm
Lacrimation
Examine carefully for perforations, lacerations or foreign bodies
Tears are associated with damage to eyelids

Radiological features

None per se
Foreign body may be present in perforating injuries

Pathological features

Conjunctiva heals very rapidly
Cornea and/or sclera is/are often damaged simultaneously with conjunctiva
Epithelium rapidly regenerates if stripped

Later effects
1. Infection
2. Exuberant granulations around retained foreign body leading to a traumatic implantative cyst
3. Symblepharon (Lid/globe adhesions) often after chemical damage

If injury is at all severe, refer to opthalmogist

Treatment

Abrasions
1. Apply local antibiotic
2. Eye patch
3. Local anaesthesia and wash out eye thoroughly with saline if foreign material involved

Tears
Repair eyelid damage
Conjuctival flaps may be sutured

Chemicals
Wash out repeatedly with saline or dilute solution of chemical antidote if known or available
Apply local antibiotics
Eye patch

Injuries of cornea

General features
Very common and painful
May rapidly threaten the vision of the eye

Clinical features
Pain
Lacrimation
Photophobia
Blepharospasm
Lesion may be visible by
    naked eye
    fluorescein staining
    magnification
Iris may be trapped in a perforating wound
Hyphema may be present
Ophthalmoscopy: Damage to lens, choroid, and retina may be present

Radiological features
None per se
Foreign bodies may be present in the globe or orbit in perforating wounds

Pathological features

Causes of Injury
Trauma: Abrasion
            Peforation
            Concussion
Foreign bodies: Retained under lids
                    Adherent to cornea
                    Present in globe
Chemicals: Crystals
            Alkalis
            Acids
Infection:

Effects
Abrasions → Infection → Perforation →
    → Infection → Hypopyon →
    Endophthalmitis →
Opacification, loss of globe or sight.

Treatment
Consider every lesion as threatening vision

Foreign bodies
Remove under local anesthesia with hypodermic needle
Instil local antibiotic
Mydriatic if iris may be involved
Eye patch

Laceration
Should be sutured by ophthalmologist
Abscise prolapsed iris
Local antibiotic
Eye patch

Abrasions
Instil local antibiotics
Eye patch

Chemicals
Wash out eye repeatedly with diluted solution of chemical antidote if available (or saline otherwise)
Intense blepharospasm may indicate a general anesthetic
Mydriatic
Local antibiotics
Watch for corneal perforation, eyelid adhesions

Opacification of cornea
Consider surgery when healed and dense
Corneal grafting

References

Fox S A 1972 Lid surgery, Chapter 24 Graeme and Stratton, New York

Rabb M F 1972 Acute corneal injuries, classification and management. Surgical Clinics of North America 52: 107-113

Yasuna E 1974 Management of traumatic hyphema. Archives of Ophthalmology (Chicago) 91: 190-191

Rupture of globe of eye

General features
(Rare injury.) Left eye most commonly affected
Causes:
    Blow to orbit forcing globe to upper inner angle
    Shock wave of high velocity missile
    Impingment of a sharp object

Clinical features
Swollen painful lids
Loss of vision (not complete)
Loss of tension of globe – DO NOT MEASURE THIS
Iris drawn towards rupture
May be a traumatic mydriasis
Tear may be visible on transillumination
Rupture concealed by subconjunctival hemorrhage

Ophthalmoscopy
Lens often dislocated
Intra-occular hemorrhage may be present

Radiological features
Orbital fracture(s) seldom present

Pathological features
Myopic or glaucomatous eyes are at risk
Tear usually occurs 5mm. behind and parallel to cornea in naso-superior quadrant
Uveal prolapse and intra-vitreous hemorrhage
Loss of vitreous: retinal damage
Healing may occur spontaneously
Sympathetic ophthalmia may occur if neglected

Treatment
All ruptured globes are sutured
Cryotherapy to re-attach retina
Abscission of uveal prolapses
Suture of sclera
Disrupted globes: Enucleated

Reference
Cherry P M H 1972 Rupture of the globe. Archives of Ophthalmology (Chicago) 88: 498-507

Perforation of eye

General features
Common but very variable severity
Often due to
    hammering
    industrial accidents
    explosions
Patient may be unaware of penetration

Clinical features
If cornea or conjunctiva is lacerated:
    Pain
    Blepharospasm
    Lacrimation
    Hyphema if iris is injured
    Intra-vitreous hemorrhage
    Foreign bodies may be visible

Radiological features
Most foreign bodies can be seen on tomographic views or ultrasonic scans if not first noted on conventional films
Localisation to within 1 mm. is required

Means
Stereoradiography
"Bone free" radiography
Lead marked contact glass or limbal ring

Pathological features
75% of foreign bodies are metal fragments

1. Types
Vegetable matter may become encapsulated
Glass plastic stone – often minimal reaction
Iron will cause siderosis of globe
Copper will cause chalcosis

2. Situation
Any part of the globe
Several fragments may be present
May become entangled in ciliary body or iris

3. Early effects
Corneal, lental, retinal damage) singly or in
Hyphema, vitreous hemorrhage) combination

4. Late effects
Corneal opacity and distortion
Cataract formation (many varied types)
Occlusion of pupil
Retinal detachment
Sympathetic ophthalmia

Treatment
Very accurate localisation is mandatory
Consider each case individually
Ferrous fragments removed by magnet
Other fragments can be removed by surgery
Lacerations to coats of eye sutured accordingly
   Release uveal prolapses
   Remove opaque lenses
   Cryosurgery for retinal detachments
Enucleation:
   For very large wounds with loss of vitreous
   Multiple foreign bodies
   Infection of globe
   Severe siderosis
   Sympathetic ophthalmia

References
Fox S A 1972 Ophthalmic plastic surgery, Chapter 22. Graeme and Stratton, New York.
Gilbert H D, Smith R E 1976 Traumatic hyphema. Treatment of secondary haemorrhage with cyclodiathermy. Ophthalmic Surgery 7: 31-35
Kurz G H, Henkind P 1965 Siderosis lentis produced by an intralenticular foreign body. Archives of Ophthalmology 73: 200-201
Rosen E 1949 Copper within the eye. American Journal of Ophthalmology 32: 248-252
Ross W H, Tasman W S 1975 The management of magnetic intraocular foreign bodies. Canadian Journal of Ophthalmology 10: 168-173

Injury to lens of eye

General features
Usually due to contusion or rupture of the globe
Less often due to perforation by foreign body
Rarely due to pre-traumatic congenital
   abnormality

Clinical features
Impaired vision +/- Diplopia
Pain ⎫
Hyphema ⎬ from associated injuries
Variations in depth of anterior chamber

Dislocation alone:
   Causes astigmatism
   Tremulous iris
Foreign body or perforation track may be visible
   with a slit lamp

Radiological features
Conventional films may show a foreign body
Ultrasonic scan will show lens damage or foreign
   body

Pathological features
Lens itself is avascular and devoid of nerves
Damage to suspensory ligament leads to partial
   or total dislocation
Common displacement is into the anterior
   chamber
Lens may rupture into the anterior chamber
   causing increased intraocular pressure
Cataract formation
   From perforation of lens capsule
   From prescence of foreign body
   From concussion effects (punctate or rosette
      shaped)

Treatment
Removal if totally dislocated
Forward dislocation:
   Avoid miotics
   Phako-emulsification if
      1. Causing symptoms
      2. Lens is flocculent
      3. Patient is over 35 years
Posterior dislocation:
   Remove if possible
   or suitable spectacles
   or iridectomy.

References
Chandler P A 1964 Choice of treatment in dislocation of the lens. Archives of Ophthalmology (Chicago) 71: 765-786
Hiles D A, Wallar P H, Biglan A W 1976 The surgery and results following traumatic cataracts in children. Journal of Pediatric Ophthalmology 13: 319-325
Jarrett W H 1967 Dislocation of the lens. Archives of Ophthalmology (Chicago) 78: 289-296

Detachment of retina

General Features
Myopic eyes most at risk
May occur
1. spontaneously
2. from trivial violence

Clinical features
Initially: Flashes of light and/or floating spots
Later: Partial or even complete loss of vision in one eye

Ophthalmoscopy
Early:
    Grey background
    Loss of light reflex
    Peripheral balloon may overhang normal retina
    Vessels appear tortuous and dark

Retinal tear
Bright red appearance
(Often at bifurcation of vessels)

Radiological features
An orbital fracture may be present if major trauma has occurred

Pathological features
Formation of edema is a concussion effect ('Berlin's edema')
In myopic eyes, peripheral retina is degenerate
Choroid is more easily ruptured than a healthy retina
Either a tear or a detachment may be seen first followed by the other
Exudate fills region of tear
Subretinal fluid collects

Treatment
Possible methods
1. Adhesions promoted by
    Diathermy or cryosurgery
    Photo coagulation or laser therapy
2. Scleral plication by silicone plombes or bands
3. Replacement promoted by vitreous air or gaseous injection

References
Freeman H M 1973 Vitreous surgery. Current status of vitreous surgery in cases of phlegmatogenous retinal detachment. Transaction of American Academy of Ophthalmologists and Otolaryngolists 77: 202-217
Hilton G F et al 1969 Retinal detachment surgery. A comparison of diathermy and cryosurgery. Bibliotheca Ophthalmologica 79: 440-448
Tulloch C G 1968 Trauma in retinal detachment. British Journal of Ophthalmology 52: 317-321

Injuries of optic nerve

General features
Rarely due to penetrating wounds of orbit
More often due to a blow at upper outer angle of the orbit
Often first discovered by the patient

Clinical features
Blind eye
Pupil responds to consensual stimulation only
Edema
Subconjunctival hemorrhage } usually present
Ophthalmoscopy initially normal
Optic pallor appears after 1-2 weeks

Radiological features
Fracture line may pass through optic canal
Variety of other orbital fractures may be present
Sometimes no fracture is present
Tomography elucidates doubtful cases

Pathological features
Optic nerve may be
    torn – (soft tissue displacement)
    or compressed by bone fragments
Retinal Artery may be
    torn
    compressed
    thrombosed
Damage to nerve or artery will obliterate vision
Only a minimal recovery is to be expected

Treatment
If recognised within 12-24 hours –
Constriction of optic foramen·
    Operative decompression
Retinal artery thrombosis:
    Anticoagulation

References
Hillman J S, Myska V, Nissim S 1975 Complete avulsion of the optic nerve. British Journal of Ophthalmology 59: 503-509
Levy J, Chatfield R K 1969 Optic atrophy following eyelid injury. British Journal of Ophthalmology 53: 49-52
Weisz G M, Hemli I, Kraus J J 1975 Transient blindness following minor head injuries. Injury 6: 348-350

Sympathetic ophthalmia

General features
Caused by a perforating wound of eye
Children very susceptible
Occurs within 4-8 weeks of injury but rarely 5 days up to 40 years after.
Rarer with good treatment

Clinical features

Normal Eye
Headaches
Photophobia
Lacrimation
Defective vision
Tenderness of globe

Slit lamp
Keratitic precipitates
Cells and fluid in anterior chamber
Ring synechiae and secondary glaucoma

Exciting Eye
Return of irritation
Iridocyclitis
Keratitic precipitates
Eventually a shrunken globe with defective vision

Pathological features
Uncertain causation
Theories:
  Viral infection
  Allergy to uveal tissue
Exciting eye usually has an injured ciliary body but rarely an infection
Prophylaxis:
  Remove injured eye as soon as possible if no useful vision remains

Treatment
Careful consideration of each individual
Systemic steroids + immunosuppressive drugs, local steroids + mydriatics
Exciting eye:
  Poor vision—Remove early
  Useful vision—Retain, give local steroids and mydriatics.
Reacting eye:
  Subconjunctival injection of steroids and mydriatics.

References:
Allen J C 1969 Sympathetic ophthalmia, a disappearing disease. Journal of American Medical Association 209: 1090
Brauminger G E, Polack F M 1971 Sympathetic ophthalmitis. American Journal of Ophthalmology 72: 967-968
Marak G E 1976 Immunopathology of sympathetic ophthalmia. Modern Problems in Ophthalmology 16: 102-105

8

FACIAL INJURIES

With the assistance of P. B. Clarke

Injuries to soft tissues of face

General features
Very common. All grades of severity.
Major injuries appear worse at first sight.
Skin and tissue loss is rare in civilian life.

Clinical features
Profuse bleeding.
Distortion of soft tissues in major lesions
Consider: Damage to
  orbit
  nose
  mouth (including tongue)
  teeth
Definition of loss of tissue often difficult
Suspect underlying facial fractures
Glass, gravel and other foreign bodies may be
  present

Radiological features
Facial fractures frequently found
  (See sections on facial fractures)
Foreign bodies may be visualised

Pathological features
Excellent blood supply
Rapid onset of edema
Ingrained dirt may remain as a tattoo
Post traumatic infection unusual if wound toilet
  and repair is efficient
Scarring   } May distort final
Keloid formation } appearance

Treatment
Very careful debridement
Scrub dirt from abrasions
Meticulous suturing with fine material
Suture skin to mucosa if tissue is lost from
  around mouth and cheeks
Cover bare bone ends when tissue loss exists
Refer to an expert for facial reconstruction

References
Kazanjian U H, Converse J M 1959 The surgical treatment of
  injuries of the face. 2nd Edition. Williams and Wilkins
  Company, Battimore.
Rowe N L, Killey H C 1968 Fractures of the facial skeleton.
  2nd Edition. E & S Livingstone Ltd, Edinburgh and
  London.

Gunshot wounds of face

General features
Common in warfare
Unusual in civilian life –
  suicide attempts
  shot gun accidents

Clinical features
Shrapnel and bullet wounds of high or low
  velocity
1. Through and through injuries
  Small entry wound
  Large exit wound
2. Shotgun injuries
  Blasting effect with destruction of tissues
  Shot and packing in the wound
  Burning and tattooing of skin edges in close
    discharge injuries
  Patient may not lose consciousness and may
    be able to walk

Radiological features
Loss of bone with comminution } are common
Foreign bodies present   } features

Pathological features
Orbital and cranial injuries are frequent
Loss of whole or part of mandible causes loss of
  tongue control
Gross distortion of facial features may occur,
  aggravated by edema
In high velocity injuries, bone fragments become
  secondary missiles causing further tissue
  damage
Life threatening hemorrhage is unusual

Treatment

Transport
Walking or sitting with head held forward
Lying ¾ prone

Primary
Preservation of life and airways:
                (oro-pharyngeal
  Plastic airway { naso-pharyngeal
                (naso-tracheal

  Tongue traction
  Tracheostomy

Prevention of infection
  Local: Skin to mucosa sutures
  Intracranial: Antibiotics
  Pulmonary: Secure air way with adequate toilet
    Naso/oro-bronchial tube
    Nasopharyngeal airway
Elimination of pain, but not with respiratory
  depressants
  Observation for:
    Increased intracranial pressure
    Abdominal injuries
    Thoracic injuries

Intermediate
Wound debridement
Search for foreign bodies and secondary missiles
Immobilise fractures
Watch for secondary hemorrhage
Oral hygiene
Saliva shield if necessary

Reconstruction
Restoration of lost soft tissue and bone
Enlargement of microstomia
Establishment of foundations for prostheses
Jaw exercising appliances if trismus persists

Reference
Rowe N L, Killey H C 1968 Fractures of the facial skeleton.
  2nd Edition, Chapter 25. E. & S. Livingstone, Edinburgh
  and London.

Fractures of nasal bones

General features
Very common
Not often compound
Frequently associated with other facial fractures
  as in Le Fort II and III and central ring (nose,
  frontal process of maxilla and ethmoids)

Clinical features
Pain, swelling, brusing ± peri-orbital hematoma
  and subconjunctional hemorrhage
Epistaxis and occlusion of airway
Deformity and telecanthus may be present
C.S.F. rhinorrhoea indicates fracture of anterior
  cranial fossa

Radiological features
Fractures well shown on
  AP view of skull (deviation of nasal septum)
  15°-30° occipito mental views
  Underexposed lateral views

Pathological features:
Depression of nasal bridge or lateral deviation
  disturb appearance and rarely visual fields
Deviation of septum will occlude an airway
Fractures readily unite
C.S.F. rhinorrhoea due to damage to
  ethmoid/frontal area
Occlusion of lacrimal ducts produces epiphora

Treatment
1. Minor deformity }
   Undisplaced fractures } No treatment
2. Minor deviation or depression:
     Manipulation by forceps
     Packing of nasal airway – best avoided if
     C.S.F. rhinorrhoea presents
     Splintage by plaster
3. Severe depression:
     Manipulation by forceps
     Splintage by wires and plaster headcap
   or: open reduction and compression plates
4. Compound fracture:
     Wound toilet
     Manipulation and splintage as indicated
   or: open reduction and direct wiring
5. Septal deviation:
     Immediate replacement in groove
   or: Later resection

References
Crawford B S 1963 The treatment of malunited fractures of
  the nose with lateral deviation. British Journal of Plastic
  Surgery 16: 231-233
Fry H J H 1967 Nasal skeletal trauma and the interlocked
  stresses of the nasal septal cartilage. British Journal of
  Plastic Surgery 20: 146-158

Fractures of frontal sinuses

General features
Common in any series of head injuries
Often compound
Associated with facial and orbital injuries
Frontal sinuses are occasionally absent

Clinical features

Periorbital hematoma +/- subconjunctival
   hemorrhage
Supra-orbital anesthesia
Varied lacerations ⎫
C.S.F. rhinorrhoea ⎭ may be present

Radiological features

Essential films
Lateral skull
Antero-posterior
Occipito-mental

Useful films
Rotated occipito-mental
Oblique orbital views

Damage to dura mater is likely if
1. Wide gap in posterior wall of sinus
2. Fracture in base of sinus passes across full
   width of anterior cranial fossa
3. Sharp bone fragment projects posteriorly
4. Fracture line widens as it descends posterior
   wall into ethmoid sinuses
5. Medial displacement of zygomatic process of
   frontal bone with tilting of crista galli
6. Intracranial aerococle

Pathological features:

Types of fracture
1. Not involving anterior cranial fossa
      Simple linear fracture
      Simple depressed fracture
      Compound linear fracture
      Compound depressed fracture
      Compound comminuted fracture
2. Involving anterior cranial fossa and posterior
   wall of sinus
      Simple linear fracture
      Compound linear fracture
      Compound and/or comminuted depressed
         fracture

Infection is likely
In children
In compound fractures
In tears of sinus mucosa
Meningitis is possible in posterior wall fractures
   especially with C.S.F. rhinorrhoea

Treatment

Prophylactic sulphonamide and antibiotic
1. Principles
Avoid infection

Restore normal sinus drainage
Repair cosmetic defect

2. No fracture of anterior cranial fossa
Simple undisplaced fracture:
   No surgery
   Antibiotics
Simple depressed fracture:
   Elevate via supra-orbital incision
Compound fractures:
   Wound toilet. Preserve mucosa – if possible
   Elevation of depressed fragments
   Antibiotics
   Otherwise, obliterate sinus and mucosa and
      pack with bone chips

3. Fractures involving anterior cranial fossa
Closed fractures:
   Controversial – surgery or no surgery
   Increased death rate by waiting too long
Certain indication for surgery – C.S.F.
   rhinorrhoea
Compound fractures:
   Wound toilet
   Repair dural defect
   Remove mucosa
   Antibiotics

4. Neglected fractures
   Elevate depression
   Reconstruct fronto-nasal duct
   OR
   Obliterate sinus and mucosa and pack with
      bone chips

References

Lewin W 1954 Cerebrospinal fluid rhinorrhoea in closed head
   injuries. British Journal of Surgery 42: 1-18
Rowe N L, Killey H C 1968 Fractures of the facial skeleton,
   2nd Edition Chapter 16, p 251-275 E & S Livingstone,
   Edinburgh and London 1968.

C.S.F. rhinorrhoea

General features

Dural tear usually in region of
   cribriform plate
   or ethmoid sinuses
Always suspect in any fracture of upper ⅔ of
   face
Occurs in 2% of head injuries

Clinical features

Persistent dripping fluid from nose
Worse on sitting up
   bending forwards
   coughing
   straining
   jugular compression (dangerous)
Most stop within a few days

Radiological features

Presumptive evidence
Wide split in posterior wall of frontal sinus
Basal fracture crossing whole width of anterior
   cranial fossa
Fracture line widening as it approaches ethmoids
Intracranial aerocoele
Any facial fracture passing through the high mid-
   face

Pathological features

Diagnosis difficult because of other causes
Differentiations:
   Blood clot serum: Protein present
   Saliva   : Amylase present
   Nasal secretions: Mucin   No sugar
   C.S.F.   : Low protein, no amylase
                : Some sugar present
Danger of meningitis by contamination from
   nasal passages
Healing occurs by dural fibrosis, but a large gap
   may not be closed naturally leading to
   persistent leakage
Injection of radio-isotope(s) into C.S.F. may help
   to identify the precise point of leakage

Treatment

1. Reduce any facial or skull fractures
2. Antibiotics Sulphatriad 1 g. six hourly
               Penicillin 500 mg. six hourly
   Continued for 5 days after cessation of
     drainage
   No nose blowing or straining
3. Persistence:
   Seek neurosurgical opinion
   Continue antibiotics
   Surgical repair:
     Dural flap
     Fascial flap
     Muscle flap

References

Crow H J, Keogh C, Northfield D W C 1956 The localisation
   of cerebrospinal fluid fistulae. Lancet 2: 325-327
Jamieson K G, Yelland J D N 1973 Surgical repair of the
   anterior fossa because of rhinorrhoea aerocoele or
   meningitis. Journal of Neurosurgery 39: 328-331
Jefferson A T, Reilly G 1972 Fractures of the floor of the
   anterior cranial fossa. The selection of patients for dural
   repair. British Journal of Surgery 59: 585-592
Lewin W 1954 Cerebrospinal fluid rhinorrhoea in closed head
   injuries. British Journal of Surgery 42: 1-18
Schneider R C, Thompson J M 1957 Chronic and delayed
   traumatic cerebrospinal rhinorrhoea as a source of
   recurrent attacks of meningitis. Annals of Surgery 145: 517-
   529

Blow-out fractures of the orbit

Synonym

Fractures of the orbital floor

General features

Caused by a blow on the globe of the eye,
   injuring soft tissues of orbit
Orbital rim usually not damaged

Clinical features

1. Pain, subconjunctival hemorrhage
2. Bruising, edema
3. Enophthalmos
4. Infra-orbital anesthesia
5. Diplopia
6. Restricted elevation of the eye. Positive muscle
   traction test.
7. Nerve palsies
8. Intraocular damage
9. Blindness

Radiological features

Tomography essential to show fractures in
   orbital walls

Pathological features

Thin bone of orbital floor gives way under
   increased pressure
Inferior oblique and inferior rectus muscles may
   herniate with some periorbital fat

Treatment

Best performed within 48 hours of injury
1. Free incarcerated muscles
2. Elevate orbital floor by packing maxillary
   antrum or inflating a catheter balloon
3. Graft orbital floor.
   Bone
   Cartilage
   Silastic implant

References

Evans J N G, Fenton P J 1971 Blow out fractures of the orbit. Journal of Laryngology and Otology 85: 1127-1145

Sveinsson E 1973 Pure blowout fractures of the orbital floor. Journal of Laryngology and Otology 87: 465-474

Lang W 1889 Traumatic enophthalmos with retention of perfect acuity of vision. Transactions of Ophthalmic society of United Kingdom 9: 41-45

Hotte H A 1970 Orbital fractures. Von Gorum Co. Assen.

Superior orbital fissure syndrome

General features
Rare
Recognised more frequently in recent decades

Clinical features
Facial/orbital injury
Diplopia, retro-orbital pain
Numbness around orbit and forehead
Opthalmoplegia, ptosis, proptosis
Fixed dilated pupil

Radiological features
Fracture into superior orbital fissure identified on tomography
Other facial fractures usually present, particularly the zygomatic complex

Pathological features
(May occur also from infection or neoplasia)
Hematoma or aneurysm formation
Within the fissure causes loss of function in:
   1. 3rd, 4th, 6th cranial nerves
   2. Vth (ophthalmic divison)
   3. Orbital sympathetic nerve fibres
   Proptosis due to paralysis of extra ocular muscles
   Prognosis is fair

Treatment
Rest with head elevated
Definitive surgery rarely required –
   Removal of fragments impinging in fissure

Reference
Banks P 1967 Superior orbital fissure syndrome. Oral Surgery 24: 455-458

Hirschfeld L 1858 Epanchement de sang dans le sinus caverneux du cote gauche diagnostique pendant la vie. Compte Rende Societe Biologie, 138-140.

Fractures of mandibular rami

General features
Common in adults, less common in children
Often associated with other facial fractures
Consider all fractures in tooth bearing area to be compound
External compounding less common

Clinical features
Pain, swelling, deformity
Acute tenderness on light touch over fracture site
Intra-oral lacerations frequently present
Loss of function, crepitus on movement
Malocclusion of teeth, some loosened
Difficulty in speaking and swallowing
Mouth usually held open with tongue protruding slightly
Mental anesthesia if fracture damages inferior dental nerve

Radiological features:
Important to visualise whole of mandible
Double fractures (contre-coup injuries) often present
Lateral, oblique and P-A mandibular views
30° Fronto-occipital view for condyles and symphysis
Occlusal views for alveoli and midline symphyseal region

Pathological features
High rate of union if splinted
Fractures through pathological areas may result in delayed, or non-union
Established infection may occur from external compounding or presence of foreign bodies (usually a dead tooth in the fracture line)
Tetanus, gas gangrene or actinomycosis are rare possibilities
Little re-modelling of malunion in adults
Fractures may be vertically or horizontally favourable or unfavourable
Muscle action may distract, close, or displace the fracture line
Dissimilar metallic fixation must not provoke electrolytic reaction

Classification of mandibular fractures

A. Comprehensive
1. Aveolar fractures
2. Single unilateral fractures
   Condyle:Intracapsular
           Not displaced
           Displaced
         Extracapsular
           Deviated
           Dislocated
   Coronoid: Displaced
           Undisplaced
   Ramus: Linear fractures
           Comminuted fractures
   Angle and body: Horizontal
             Favourable
             Unfavourable
           Vertical
             Favourable
             Unfavourable
   Symphysis: Midline fracture
           Paramedian fracture   May be very
                                  oblique
3. Double Unilateral fractures
4. Bilateral fractures: Fracture dislocations of
                   condyles
                Horizontally unfavourable
                   fractures at angles
                Canine regions
5. Common combinations:
       Condyle and opposite angle
       Condyle and opposite premolar region
       Premolar region and opposite angle
       Bilateral angle
       Bilateral premolar regions

B. Fractures of rami only
Class I   Teeth on both fragments
Class II Teeth on one fragment only
Class III Edentulous mandible

Treatment

Class I Fractures: (Teeth on all fragments)
Adequate teeth:
    Interdental eyelet wiring (At least one pair of
        eyelets on stable teeth on either side of the
        fracture)
Inadequate teeth:
    Arch bars or
    Cast metal cap splints

Class II Fractures: (Teeth on one fragment only)
1. Short edentulous posterior fragment
     (a) Favourable fracture line
         Interdental wiring or
         cap splints or
         arch bars with or without-
         Bone wiring upper border (intra-orally)
           or lower border (extra-orally)
     (b) Unfavourable fracture line
         Closed fractures:
           Transosseous wires or
           Bone plate
           Transfixion Kirschner wires
         Compound fractures: External pin
fixation to Halo frame
2. Long edentulous posterior fragment
     (a) Treat as above or
     (b) Consider wiring in place of the patient's
         own dentures if available or
         Gunning splints made from the dentures
     (c) Extra-periosteal bone plate
     Beware: Excess periosteal stripping
            Thin edentulous elderly mandible

Class III Fractures: (Edentulous mandible)
Single or compound fractures within denture
    area
1. Without severe displacement:
       Gunning splints with peralveolar or
         circumferential wires
2. With severe displacement:
       Transosseous wiring and immobilisation
         to maxilla
3. Compound fracture with gross displacement
       External pin fixation to Halo frame or
       Extra periosteal bone plating

Notes on treatment methods

1. Upper or lower border wiring
Indications:
    Compound fractures
    Comminuted fractures
    2 fractures on same side of mandible
    If intermaxillary fixation is undesirable

2. Extra-oral skeletal fixation:
Indications:
    Edentulous posterior fragment with gross
      displacement
    Severe infection at fracture site
    Control of edentulous fragments after bone
      grafting
Disadvantages:
    Absolute fixation is impossible
    Awkward unsightly apparatus

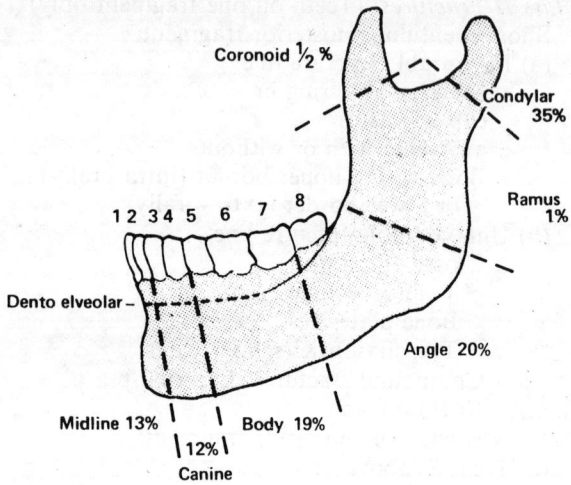

Fig. 16 Incidence of sites of fracture of mandible.

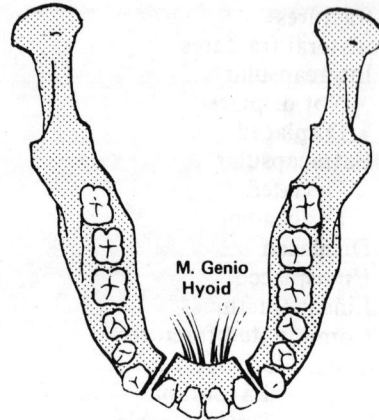

Downward and posterior displacement of central section of mandible

Fig. 18 Bilateral fracture of mandible distal to canine.

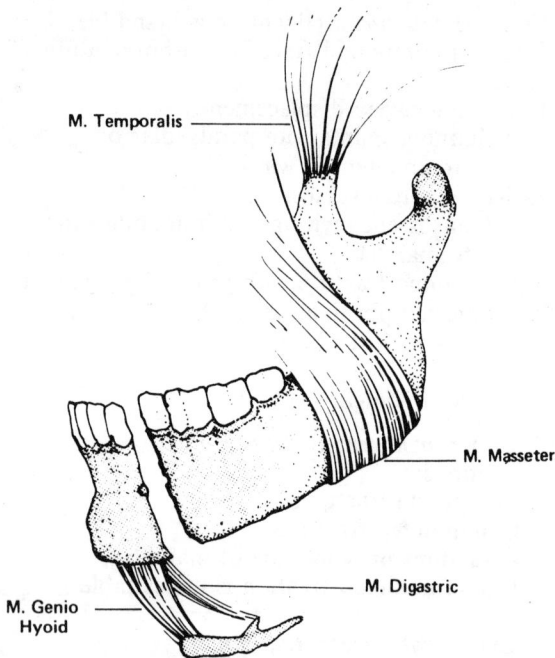

Fig. 17 Horizontally unfavourable line of fracture in left premolar region of mandible.

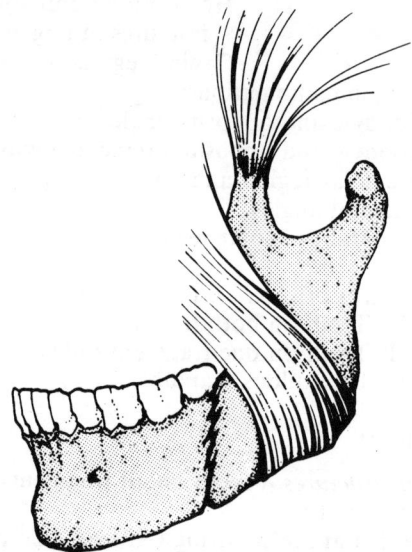

Fig. 19 Horizontally favourable line of fracture at angle of mandible.

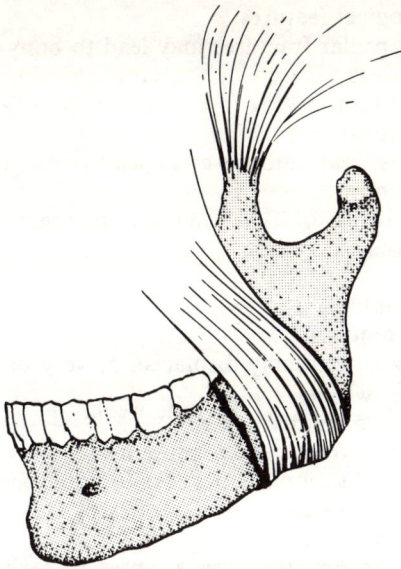

Fig. 20 Horizontally unfavourable line of fracture at angle of mandible.

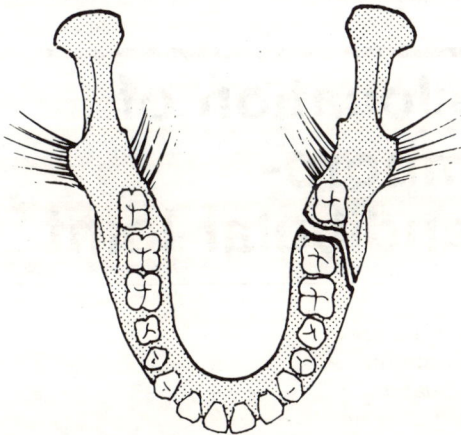

Fig. 21 Vertically favourable line of fracture through left angle of mandible.

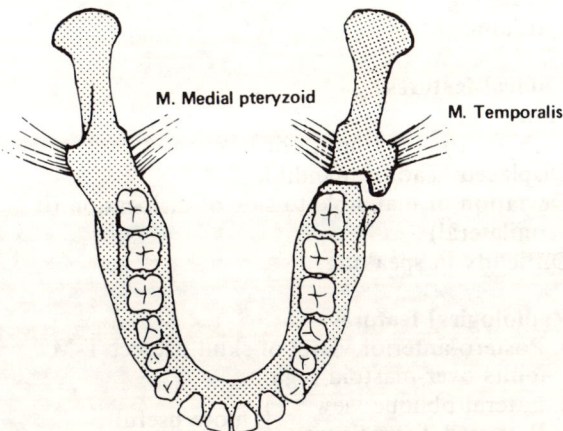

M. Medial pteryzoid

M. Temporalis

Fig. 22 Vertically unfavourable line of fracture through left angle of mandible.

Complications:
Infection and loosening of pins
Inferior dental neuritis
Partial facial palsy
Salivary fistula
See Figures 16-22

References

Dingman R O, Natvig P 1964 Surgery of facial fractures. Chapter 6. W. B. Saunders Company, Philadelphia and London

Killey H C 1971 Fractures of the mandible. John Wright and Sons, Ltd., Bristol

Rowe N L, Killey H C 1968 Fractures of the facial skeleton. 2nd Edition, Part I. E & S Livingstone, Edinburgh & London

Fractures of mandible in children

General features
Rare. 1-2% of adult cases
Children less likely to suffer major trauma

Clinical features
As in adults
Multiple fractures very uncommon
Variable patterns of deciduous and permanent teeth

Radiological features
Standard views required as in adults
Multiplicity of teeth may obscure a fracture

Pathological features
Children's mandibles are elastic
High osteogenic potential
Rapid alveolar bone growth
Large capacity for remodelling to accommodate mal-occlusions
Fragility and shape of deciduous teeth make them unsuitable for fixation purposes

Treatment
Retain as many teeth as possible

0-2 years:
Acrylic splints and circumferential wires

2-5 years:
As for 0-2 year group
Possible alternatives –
  Interdental eyelet wiring
  Arch bars
  Cap splints

5-11 years:
As for 2-5 year group
If insufficient teeth are available
  Pyriform fossa wires
  Circumzygomatic wires may be used

References

Maclennan W D 1957 Injuries involving the teeth and jaws in young children. Archives of Disease in Childhood 32: 492-494

Thomson H G, Farmer A W, Lindsay W K 1964 Condylar neck fractures of the mandible in children. Plastic and Reconstructive Surgery 34: 452-463

Fractures of mandibular condyle

General features
Common
Often associated with other fractures of
  1. Mandibular body
  2. Facial skeleton

Clinical features
Pain on movement
Local tenderness and swelling
Head of mandible may be displaced
If unilateral the mandible will be deviated to the side of the injury
Gagging on side of injury on last molars (if present)
Anterior open bite if bilateral fractures are present

Radiological features
1. Postero-anterior view of skull project T-M joints over mastoid regions
   Fractured condyle apparently widened on this view
2. Lateral oblique view
   Reversed Towne's view } More useful

Pathological features:
Intra-capsular fractures may lead to bony ankylosis
Marked remodelling in children with perfect function
In adults, mal-union is compatible with good function
Hemarthrosis of T-M joint may be present
Pyarthrosis very rare

Treatment:
Rarely required
If laterally markedly displaced, or very painful—
  Eyelet wiring
  Gunning splints } for one week
If bilateral fractures are present—
  Immobilisation for 6 weeks in good occlusion with interdental eyelet wires or Gunning Splints, etc.
If intracapsular fractures are present early active movements
  Jaw exercises

Dislocation of temporo-mandibular joint

General features
Very common
Often bilateral
May occur from
  yawning
  chewing
  laughing
  trauma

Clinical features
Pain
Inability to close mouth or to chew
Displaced head of mandible
Deviation of mandible to side of dislocation (if unilateral)
Difficulty in speaking

Radiological features
1. Postero-anterior views of skull project T-M joints over mastoid regions
2. Lateral oblique view
   Reversed Towne's view } more useful

Pathological features

Anterior displacement most common, often becomes recurrent

Rarieties:

Other types of displacement
Fracture of glenoid fossa
(Damage to tympanic plate
Bleeding from external auditory meatus)

Treatment

Acute:

Closed reduction by manipulation

Recurrent:

Closed reduction
Open reduction rarely required
Correct malocclusion
Correct over closure (provide dentures if necessary)
Plicate capsule
Remove meniscus

References

Editorial (1975) Temporo-mandibular joint syndrome. Lancet 2: 859-860
Freedus M S, Ziter W D, Doyle P K 1975 Principles of treatment for temporo-manidibular joint ankylosis. Journal of Oral Surgery 33: 757-765
Sanders B, Newman R 1975 Surgical treatment for recurrent dislocation or chronic subluxation of the temporo-mandibular joint. International Journal of Oral Surgery 4: 179-183

Fractures of middle third of face

Synonym

Dish face, stove-in face

General features

More common with advent of motor vehicles
Rarely seen in children
Associated with other cranial and trunk injuries

Clinical features

Flattening of facial features
+/- Lacerations, contusions, abrasions
Rapid onset of massive bilateral edema
Traumatic telecanthus

Malocclusion
CSF rhinorrhoea not uncommon
Nasal and pharyngeal hemorrhage
Subconjunctival hemorrhage
Infra-orbital anesthesia common
Facial paralysis and surgical emphysema are rare complications

Radiological features

(See section on radiography of facial skeleton)

Lateral views   ) show backward
30° Occipito-mental views) displacement

10° Occipito-mental view shows downward displacement and antral and orbital margins
Antero-posterior tomography will elucidate fractures of orbital floor, etc. etc.

Pathological features

Fractures readily unite
CSF rhinorrhoea common in high level fractures
Wide variety of fracture combinations

Classification of fractures

Le Fort I:
Horizontal low level fracture through maxillae and septum
Le Fort II:
Fracture line passes through the infra-orbital rim, orbital floors, root of nose, and pterygoid plates
Le Fort III:
Fracture line passes higher through the lateral orbital rim, zygomatic arches, root of nose and high in pterygoid plates

Fractures of palatal unit

Horizontal fracture +/- open bite deformity (Le Fort I)
Vertical separation of maxillae (often with mid-line separation)
Palatal-alveolar fractures usually with an ipselateral frctured zygoma

Principle of treatment

Reduce the injured to the injured part and fix as necessary

Methods of treatment

No fixation:
Minimal displacement or mobility
Elerly edentulous poor risk patients
Intra-oral fixation only
Alveolar fractures
Fracture of one maxilla only

External fixation:
Cranio-maxillary   ) via halo frame or plaster
Cranio mandibular) head cap with rods
                            and intra-osseous pins

Internal fixation
1. Transosseous wiring:
        Zygomatico-frontal
    or: Zygomatico-maxillary
    or: Palatal processes
    or: Fronto-nasal
2. Direct wiring suspension:
        Pyriform fossa
    or: Zygomatic buttress
    or: Zygomatic arch
    or: Inferior orbital rim
    or: Zygomatic process of frontal
3. Transfixion:
        Steinman pins *or* Kirshner wires
        Zygoma to zygoma
    or: Zygoma to opposite maxilla
        (Crossed pins require care with
            nasotracheal tube)

Stages of treatment

Primary
Secure airway, tube or tracheostomy
Stop hemorrhage. Nasal and pharyngeal packs
  Care if C.S.F. leak is present
Obtain good radiographs
Plan definitive treatment
Discuss anesthetic problems

Secondary
A. Order of procedures:
Prepare halo framework or plaster head cap
Reduce and fix mandibular fractures
Mobilise depressed or displaced zygoma(s)
Reduce maxillary-dento-alveolar fracture
Check occlusion of teeth
Fix maxillar to head cap
Fix zygoma to reduced maxilla
Reduce and fix nasal fractures
Pack antrum if necessary to elevate orbital floor

B. Specific problems:
1. Alveolar fractures: Acrylic dental splint or arch
   bar
2. Fracture of one maxilla:
   Teeth on both maxillae:
       Complete interdental wiring or cap splints
   Teeth on unfractured maxilla: Manipulate only
       and splint

Displaced edentulous maxilla:
    Repair mucosa after reduction
    May need halo splintage
    Check nasal septum
Edentulous undisplaced maxilla: No treatment
    required
Teeth on fractured maxilla only:
    External splintage to halo frame
Both maxillae edentulous: Manipulate and
    repair mucosa
3. Bilateral fractured maxillae: No midline
    separation
Teeth in upper and lower jaws:
    Cap splints
    External fixation to halo frame
Maxillae edentulous:
Mandible bearing teeth:
    Gunning splint
    Circumzygomatic wiring
Teeth in maxillae: Manipulation, cap splints
Mandible bearing teeth: External fixation to
    halo frame
Both maxillae and mandible edentulous:
    Gunning splint with
        circumzygomatic or
        cranio-mandibular fixation
4. Bilateral fractured maxillae with midline
    separation
Teeth present on each maxilla:
    Disimpact, Reduce
    Cap splints, locking bar
    External fixation to halo frame
Teeth on one maxilla: Manipulation
Other maxilla edentulous:
    Mandibular splint
    External fixation to halo frame
Both maxillae edentulous:
    Manipulate
    Pyriform fossa wiring
5. Neglected middle third fractures:
    Best manipulated within 10 days
    Manipulation impossible after 21 days
    Thereafter re-fracture is necessary
    Methods: Traction via maxillary splint.
                Balkan beam and weights.
                Elastic traction from framework

                attached to halo frame or
                plaster head cap
Later: Extraction of teeth and/or alveolectomy
        Surgical refracture of maxilla

Post-operative care
Maintenance of airway
   Tracheostomy rarely required
   Naso-pharyngeal airway
   Wire cutters at patient's bedside
Oral hygiene
Protection of lips, tongue, larynx
Prevention of sepsis, oral and pulmonary
Maintenance of weight:
   Semi-solid diet
   Tubing or feeder cup behind molar teeth

Complications of middle third fractures
Infection
Residual dish face deformity

Cranial
Headaches
Anosmia
Diplopia or squint (Nerve damage or blindness
   or globe displacement)
Personality defects
Epilepsy

Dental
Mal-occlusion
Oro-nasal or oro-antral fistulae

Nasal
Depressed nasal bridge
Nasal blockage
Epiphora
(*See* Fig. 23)

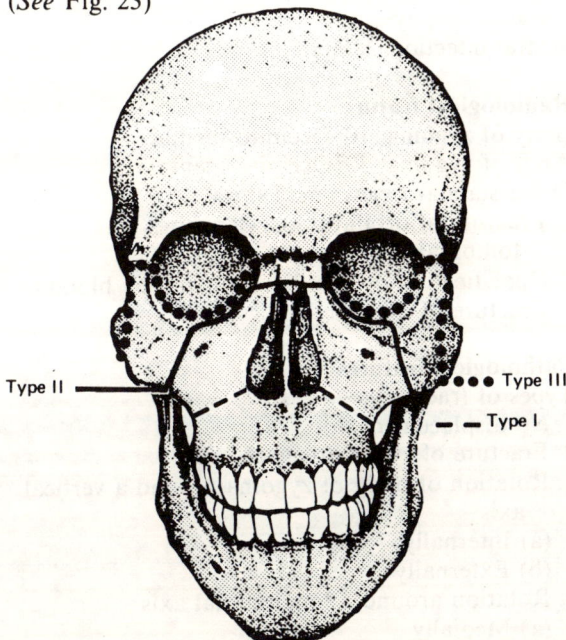

Fig. 23 Le Fort classification of maxillary fractures

References
Geddes D A M 1963 Diet for patients with maxillo-facial injuries. British Dental Journal 115, 235, 237.
Killey H C 1977 Fractures of the middle third of the facial skeleton. 3rd Edition John Wright and Sons, Ltd., Bristol

Fractures of the middle third of the face in children

General features
Rare – 0.2% of facial fractures

Clinical features
Fractures less likely because of elastic tissues and
   incomplete ossification
Otherwise symptoms and signs as for adults
Exclude
   Cranial fractures
   C.S.F. rhinorrhoea
   Damage to teeth

Radiological features
Fracture lines often difficult to detect because
1. Incomplete ossification
2. Overlapping shadows of teeth
Tomography valuable

Pathological features
Le Fort II & III uncommon in younger children
Classification of damage to teeth
1. Fracture of crown of tooth
   Fracture of enamel only
   Fracture of enamel and dentine
   Fracture of enamel and dentine and
exposure of pulp
2. Fracture of root of tooth
   Apical third of root
   Gingival third of root
3. Displacement of root from its socket
   Subluxation
   Dislocation
4. Intrusion into alveolus (usually incisors)

Treatment
Factors in Selection of Methods, etc.
  Nature of injury and time since occurrence
  Presence or absence of pain
  Firmness of tooth in its socket
  Extent and nature of damage to crown of
    tooth
  Presence or absence of root fracture
  Vitality of pulp

A. Teeth:
Splint loose teeth for six weeks—arch bar, or
  acrylic or metal splints
1. Exposed dentine: Cover with Zinc-Oxide-
  Eugenol paste
2. Fracture of crown involving pulp
    Open apex, vital tooth: Partial pulpectomy
    Closed apex, vital tooth: Removal of pulp
3. Fracture of root
    Dead pulp apical third fracture:
      Removal of pulp
      Removal of apical fragment
    Dead pulp, gingival third fracture: Removal of
    tooth
4. Displacement of tooth:
  i) In socket: Manipulate and reduce
    subluxation (Finger pressure)
  ii) Displaced tooth:
    a) Within 6 hours
      Wash tooth in saline penicillin
      Remove pulp. Ream out root canal
      Syringe out socket with penicillin
      Replace tooth and splint for 6 weeks
      Poor prognosis
    b) Over 6 hours
      Discard tooth
  iii) Intruded teeth:
    Leave alone
    Most re-erupt

B. Maxilla
Select simple methods as for adults
Preserve teeth
Minimal apparatus. Plaster head caps tend to
  slip.
  Halo frames give better fixation
Internal fixation often appropriate

References

Bennett D T 1963 Traumatised anterior teeth British Dental
  Journal 115: 309-311
McCoy F T, Chandler R A, Crow M L 1966 Facial fractures
  in children. Plastic and Reconstructive Surgery 37: 209-215

Fractures of the zygomatic-maxillary complex

General features
Due to blow on cheek
Zygoma and/or zygomatic arch may be broken
Other facial fractures often present
Not often compound

Clinical features
Flattening of cheek
Pain, swelling, bruising
Bleeding from nostril
Infra orbital anesthesia

Visual
Subconjunctional hemorrhage
Diplopia (or even blindness)
Irregularity of orbital rim

Dental
Disturbed occlusion sometimes found from
  associated alveolar fracture
Trismus – due to restricted coronoid movement

Unusual
Surgical emphysema
Antral infection (later)

Radiological features
Body of zygoma: 10° Occipito-mental
Arch of zygoma: 30° Occipito-mental
Other standard views may show
  Fracture of orbital floor. (Requires
    tomography)
  Opacification of maxillary antrum by blood
  Fracture of maxilla

Pathological features
Types of fracture –
1. No displacement
2. Fracture of zygomatic arch only
3. Rotation of body of zygoma around a vertical
  axis
  (a) Internally
  (b) Externally
4. Rotation around a longitudinal axis
  (a) Medially
  (b) Laterally

5. Displacement of zygomatic complex
   (a) Medially
   (b) Inferiorly
   (c) Laterally
6. Displacement of orbito-antral partition
   (a) Superiorly
   (b) Inferiorly
7. Displacement of segments of orbital rim
8. Complex comminuted fractures
9. Fractures involving adjacent tooth bearing part
   of maxilla
   Stable fractures: 1, 2, 3, 4,a
Unstable fractures: 4b, 5, 6, 7, 8, 9
Displacement of orbital floor causes visual
   disturbance.
   If severe, optic nerve or retinal artery may be
   damaged
Depression of arch obstructs movement of
   coronoid process of mandible
Fractures unite readily

Treatment
No displacement: No treatment
Displacement/Depression: Elevation (via
   temporal approach if possible)

Instability
Internal fixation.
   Packing of antrum (or balloon catheter)
   Intra-osseous wires
External fixation. Via halo frame or plaster head
   cap

Compound fractures
   Wound toilet with pin fixation
   Careful closure of soft tissues
   Packing of antrum via oral or nasal approach

Neglected fractures:
Cosmesis: Elevate fragments
            (Osteotomy if necessary)
Onlays to restore contours
   (Cartilage)
   (Bone)
   (Silastic)
Diplopia: Often due to orbital Hematoma
            Majority recover spontaneously
            Elevate orbital floor and
            Splint by reconstructing floor.
Alternative approaches to depressed fragments –
   Intra-oral
   Intra-nasal
   Antro-oral
   Direct extra oral

References
Killey H C 1977 Fractures of the middle third of the facial
   skeleton. 3rd Edition. John Wright and Sons, Bristol.
Knight J S, North J F 1961 The classification of malar
   fractures. An analysis of displacement as a guide to
   treatment. British Journal of Plastic Surgery 13: 325-339
McCoy F J et al 1962 An analysis of facial fractures and
   their complications. Plastic and Reconstructive Surgery 29:
   381-391
Rowe N L, Killey H C 1968 Fractures of the facial skeleton.
   2nd Edition. Chapter 17. E & S Livingstone, Ltd.,
   Edinburgh and London.

Radiography for facial injuries

Mandible
Lateral oblique views:
   Good for ramus
   No overlap of left and right rami
Intra oral dental films for individual teeth
   10° for angle
   15° for molars
   30° for premolars
   45° for canines
   60° for incisors
Occipito-frontal view: Good for condyles and
   rami
Rotated occipito-frontal view: Good for condyle
   of opposite side
Rotated fronto-occipital view: Less satisfactory.
   Used when patient cannot turn face down
30° Fronto-occipital view: Good for condyles
   and symphysis
Occlusal views: Good for midline symphyseal
   region and alveolar processes
Pan-mandibular views, may obscure some
   fractures by overlapping teeth

Temporo-mandibular Joints
Affected joint laid on film
Central ray passes through this joint avoiding
   upper joint
Do not overlook fractures on opposite side of
   mandible
Tomography may be helpful

Maxilla
10° and 35° occipito-mental view: Good for
   orbital margins and antrum
Rotated occipito-mental view: Good for plan
   view of zygoma

Submental vertical view: Good for outline of
  zygomatic arch
Occlusal views: Good for alveolar fractures
Lateral views: Good for backward displacements
Soft film (lateral): Good for nasal displacements

References
Blackman A A 1954 Radiography of the mandible and
  adjacent structures. Radiography 18: 103-116
Blackman S 1963 Radiography of the temporo-mandibular
  joint. British Journal of Oral Surgery 1: 132-146
Ingham H W 1950 A technique on facial maxillary injuries.
  Radiography 16: 166-167
Shenton J 1952 Radiography of the mandible and maxilla to
  demonstrate fractures. Radiography 18: 78-81

9

BLOOD VESSEL INJURIES

With the assistance of J. Engeset

Injuries of carotid and jugular vessels

General features
High death rate, often before reaching hospital
Causes: Gun shot wounds
        Lacerations
        Stab wounds etc.
Associated damage frequently seen in
        Brachial plexus
        Trachea
        Esophagus

Clinical features
Very variable—sometimes silent
Pulses absent distal to lesion
External wound—often initial massive
  hemorrhage
Sometimes:
  Horner syndrome: damage to cervical
    sympathetic chain
  Hemiplegia—loss of cerebral circulation
  Paralysed arm—brachial plexus injury

Radiological features
Associated fractures are rare
Angiography (arch aortogram) will show site of
  lesion but is usually superfluous

Pathological features
Effects on cerebral function depend on potency
  of circle of Willis with flow from contralateral
  carotid vessels
Arterial lacerations usually retract and clot
Damage to jugular vein may lead to air
  embolism
Initial massive blood loss may have ceased by
  admission to hospital

Treatment
Resuscitation (Intravenous line must not be distal
  to venous lesion)
Wound dressing
Very early exploration
  Wide exposure required, i.e. Resection of
    medial clavicle, division of sterno-mastoid,
    etc.
Lacerations: Suture

Loss of vessel length:
  Tie off external carotid artery if necessary
  Reversed vein grafts to internal carotid artery
    and/or internal jugular vein
  Reconstruction with arterial prosthesis

References
Flint L M et al 1973 Management of major vascular injuries
  in the base of the neck. Archives of Surgery, 106: 407-413
Fordham S D 1976 Bullet embolism. International Surgery
  (Chicago), 61: 481-483
Penn I 1973 Penetrating injuries of the neck. Surgical Clinics
  of North America, 53: 1469-1478
Schneider R C et al 1972 Blood vessel trauma following head
  and neck injuries. Clinical Neurosurgery, 19: 312-354
Thavendran A et al Penetrating injuries of the neck. Injury 7:
  58-60

Injuries of subclavian vessels

General Features
Uncommon in civilian life
Closed injuries are rare
Usual causes:
  Gun shot wounds
  Stabbing
  Compound fractures of clavicle and/or upper
    ribs
Associated injuries frequently seen –
  Mediastinal lesions
  Brachial plexus damage

Clinical features
Absent pulses in arm
Pain, numbness, weakness in arm
External wound: May be some distance away
Closed injury :
  Local swelling
  Venous engorgement
  Dyspnoea ⎫
  Dysphagia ⎭ may occur
Hemo/pneumothorax
Cardiac tamponade

Radiological features
Fractures may be present:
  Clavicle
  Upper ribs
  Sternum
Hemo/pneumothorax
Widened mediastinum

Arch aortograms (if time allows)
  show site and nature of lesion
  will indicate best approach

Pathological features
Vessels may avulsed at origin from aorta
  Lacerated
  Transected } at any point
  Thrombosed
Veins and Arteries usually damaged together
Arm rarely becomes gangrenous because of
  shoulder arterial anastomosis

Treatment
Resuscitation (Intravenous line must not be distal
  to venous lesion)

Wide exposure
Supraclavicular or
Resection of clavicle or
Median Sternotomy

Lacerations
Repair

Loss of vessel length
Reversed vein graft
Prosthetic graft often unsatisfactory
Tie off rarely indicated

References
Chan R M W, Duffield R G M 1975 Subclavian artery
  rupture (an unusual seat belt injury). Injury, 7: 29-32
Flint L M et al 1973 Management of major vascular injuries
  in the base of the neck. Archives of Surgery, 106: 407-413
Heath R D 1972 The subclavian steal syndrome. Journal of
  Bone and Joint Surgery, 54A: 1033-1039
Rich N M et al 1973 Subclavian artery trauma. Journal of
  Trauma, 13: 485-495
Sturm J T et al 1974 Blunt trauma to the subclavian artery.
  Surgery, Gynaecology and Obstetrics, 138: 915-918

Vascular injuries in upper limb

General features
Multiplicity of causes, i.e.,
  Gun shot wounds and compound fractures
  Lacerations
  Closed injuries
    Fractures   Supracondylar humerus
                 Humeral shaft
    Dislocations: Shoulder
                 Elbow

Clinical features
Pain, hemorrhage/swelling
Loss of distal pulses
Variable loss of power and/or sensation

Radiological features
Fracture of dislocation may be present
Angiography will show site (and sometimes
  nature) of vascular lesion

Pathological features
Good collateral circulation makes peripheral
  gangrene unusual
Nature of injury may be
  Avulsion
  Laceration
  Internal tear of intima
  Compression from external hematoma or
    displaced bone
  Thrombosis

Treatment
Reduction of dislocation or fracture
If pulse does not return
  Explore site of blockage. Operative
    arteriography may be helpful
  Decompress neurovascular bundle
  Avulsion: Suture +/- reversed vein graft
  Laceration: Repair or excise with
    reanastomosis
  Intimal tear: Repair +/- reversed vein graft
  Tie off smaller peripheral vessels unless
    patentcy is vital—
    Repair with microscopy

References
Debakey M E, Simeone F A 1946 Battle injuries of the
  arteries in World War II. Annals of Surgery 123: 534-579
Green D P 1973 True and false traumatic aneurysms in the
  hand. Journal of Bone and Joint Surgery 55A: 120-128
Louis D S, Ricciardi J E, Spengler D M 1974 Arterial injury:
  a complication of posterior elbow dislocation. Journal of
  Bone and Joint Surgery 56A: 1631-1636
Louis D S, Simon M A 1974 Traumatic false aneurysms of
  the upper extremity. Journal of Bone and Joint Surgery
  56A: 176-179
Shaw R S 1959 Reconstructive arterial surgery in upper
  extremity injuries. Journal of Bone and Joint Surgery 41A:
  665-673
Smyth E H J 1969 Major arterial injury in closed fracture of
  the neck of the humerus. Journal of Bone and Joint
  Surgery 51B: 508-570
Tsuge K 1975 Treatment of established Volkman's
  contracture. Journal of Bone and Joint Surgery 57A: 925-
  929

Axillary vein thrombosis

Synonym
Paget-Schrotter Syndrome

General features
Uncommon
20-40 age group
M > F
R > L
Very rarely bilateral

Clinical features
Often begin during or after strenuous effort
Develop over 12-48 hours
Aching, swollen arm
Distended veins, unrelieved by elevation
Tenderness in axilla in line of vein
Spontaneous recovery in 1-2 months
Rarely persistent or recurrent

Radiological features
No skeletal abnormality
Venography will demonstrate blockage in
    axillary-subclavian segment

Pathological features
Cause is uncertain. Several theories:
1. Minor anatomical variations at thoracic inlet
    may compress axillary vein
    i.e. Insertion of M. Scalemus Anterior
        Abnormal phrenic nerve roots
2. Forced expiration may compress axillary vein
    against M. sublcavius and the costocoracoid
    ligament
Pulmonary embolism is very rare

Treatment
Elevation of arm
Analgesics
Anti-coagulants

Surgery
Rarely necessary
Indications:
    Embolisation
    Abnormal thoracic inlet anatomy

Procedures:
    Thrombectomy
    Axillary-Internal jugular graft
    Division of M. scalemus anterior insertion
        when abnormal anatomy is found

References
Adams J T, Deweese, J A 1971 Effort thrombosis of the
    axillary and subclavian veins. Journal of Trauma 11: 923-
Kleinsasser L J 1949 Effort thrombosis of the axillary and
    subclavian veins. Archives of Surgery 59: 258-274
Weathersby H T 1956 Valves of the axillary vein. Anatomical
    Record, 124: 379-380

Injuries to major vessels in abdomen

General features
Uncommon
May be rapidly fatal
Due to penetrating wounds (gunshot, stabbing)
    Blunt trauma (Seat belts, Kicks)
    Iatrogenic = Vascular catheterisation
                Discectomy

Clinical features
Hypovolemic shock
Abdominal pain and distension
Shifting dullness
Blood on paracentesis
Diminution of blood flow to legs

Delayed
Enlarging and/or pulsatile swelling
Bruit
High out-put cardiac failure if arterio-venous
    fistula is present

Radiological features
Abdominal film may show a pre-existing aortic
    aneurysm

Contrast studies
Arteriography for arterial injuries
Venography for great vein injuries
Time may not allow if clinical situation is critical

Pathological features
Hepatic veins associated with liver injury

Portal vein	Bowel
	Pancreas
Iliac veins	Fractures of pelvis

Aorta	Tear	Devitalisation of
	Rupture	gut and legs
	False aneurysm	

Iliac arteries	Fractures of pelvis
	discectomy

Treatment
Restoration of blood volume if possible
Laparotomy: this may be part of resuscitation
  Tie off non-essential vessels
  Primary repair of essential vessels
    End-to-end, end-to-side anastomosis
  or Vein graft
  or Synthetic grafts

References
Albo D et al 1969 Massive liver trauma involving the superarenal vena cava. American Journal of Surgery 118: 960-963
Allen T W et al Surgical management of aortic trauma. Journal of Trauma 12: 862-868
Bricker D L et al 1971 Surgical management of injuries to the vena cava. Changing patterns of injury and newer techniques of repair. Journal of Trauma 11: 725-735
Horton R E, Hamilton S G I 1968 Ligature of the internal iliac artery for massive haemorrhage complicating fracture of the pelvis. Journal of Bone and Joint Surgery 50B: 376-379
Hunt T K et al 1971 Arterio-venous fistulas of major vessels in the abdomen. Journal of Trauma 11: 483-493
Lim R C, Glickman M G, Hunt T K 1972 Angiography in patients with blunt trauma to the chest and abdomen. Surgical Clinics of North America 52: 551-565
Mattox K L et al 1974 Management of upper abdominal vascular trauma. American Journal of Surgery 128: 823-828
Shirkey A L, Quast D C, Jordan G L 1967 Superior mesenteric artery division and intestinal function. Journal of Trauma 7: 7-24

Injuries of femoral artery

General features
Not uncommon
M > F
Closed injuries > open injuries
Rapid death from hemorrhage in many open injuries

Clinical features
1. Variable external wound – Minute to massive Rapid exsanguination
2. No external wound
  Large painful swelling of rapid onset
  Fracture(s) may be present

All cases
Diminution of sensation and power in leg
Distal pallor of limb
Loss of distal pulses

Radiological features
Fracture of femur may be present
Soft tissue swelling outlined
Angiography may be diagnostic of level of lesion and nature of lesion

Pathological features
Avulsion and transverse lacerations retract to give spontaneous cessation of hemorrhage
Oblique lacerations especially in old vessels continue to bleed until death
Injuries proximal to profunda femoris artery usually lead to gangrene of lower leg if untreated

Treatment
Exploration of wound
(Most difficult at origin of profunda femoris vessels)
Internal fixation of fracture (if present)
Lacerations: Suture
Internal damage } Vein graft
Loss of segment }
Separate careful suture of femoral veins

Complications
Thrombosis of injured segment }
Hemorrhage } Common to all
Peripheral gangrene } vascular surgery
Arterio-venous aneurysm }

References
Abraham E, Pankoulch A M, Jansey F 1975 False aneurysm of the profunda femoris artery resulting from intertrochanteric fracture. Journal of Bone and Joint Surgery 57A: 871-872
Brown R et al 1968 Arterial obstruction of the femoral artery secondary to femoral osteotomy. Journal of Bone and Joint Surgery 50A: 1444-1446
Dameron T B 1964 False aneurysm of profunda femoris artery resulting from internal fixation device (Screw). Journal of Bone and Joint Surgery 46A: 577-580
Dorr L D et al 1974 False aneurysm of the femoral artery following total hip surgery. Journal of Bone and Joint Surgery 56A: 1059-1062

Hegarty M M et al 1975 Traumatic arteriovenous fistulae. Injury 7: 20-28

Isaacson J, Louis D S, Costenbader J M 1975 Arterial injury associated with closed femoral shaft fracture. Journal of Bone and Joint Surgery 57A: 1147-1150

Klingensmith W, Oles P, Martinez H 1965 Arterial injuries associated with dislocation of the knee or fracture of the lower femur. Surgery, Gynaecology and Obstetrics 120: 961-964

Koostra G et al 1976 Femoral shaft fracture with injury of the superficial femoral artery in civilian accidents. Surgery, Gynaecology and Obstetrics. 142: 399-403

Miller J W et al 1974 Gluteal artery aneurysm. Journal of Bone and Joint Surgery 56A: 620-622

Neviaser R J, Adams J P, May G I 1976 Complications of arterial puncture in anti-coagulated patients. Journal of Bone and Joint Surgery 58A: 218-220

Injuries of popliteal artery

General features
Causes:
   Gunshot wounds
   Popliteal hematoma
   Dislocation of knee
   Supracondylar fracture of femur
   Fracture of upper tibia

Clinical features

Open injury
External wound with hemorrhage

Closed injury
Pain, swelling

Both types
Distal palor
Loss of pulses
Diminution of power and sensation in feet

Radiological features
Fracture(s) or dislocation may be present
Femoral angiography:
   Blockage of or leakage from popliteal vessels

Pathological features
Poor collateral circulation around knee
Unrelieved popliteal blockage often causes
   gangrene of lower leg
Popliteal artery and vein usually both damaged
   together

Treatment
Immediate exploration of popliteal space
Laceration of vessels:
   Suture
Avulsion or crushing:
   Excision of damaged segment
   Insertion of reversed vein graft(s)
Thereafter:
   Internal fixation of fracture
   Wide fasciotomy of lower leg (anterior and
   posterior compartments)

Reference
Connolly J F, Whittaker D, Williams E 1971 Femoral and tibial fractures combined with injuries to the femoral or popliteal artery. Journal of Bone and Joint Surgery 53A: 56-68

10

CHEST INJURIES

With the assistance of A. V. Foote

Fractures of ribs and sternum
Open wounds of thorax
Hemothorax
Pneumothorax
Flail chest
Cardiac contusion
Cardiac rupture
Aortic rupture
Esophageal trauma
Diaphragmatic rupture
Pulmonary contusion
Inhalation lung
Traumatic asphyxia
Oxygen toxicity

Fractures of ribs and sternum

General features
Very common
Persistently painful
May be trivial or serious
Caused by direct blow on chest wall
  (Rarely from muscle contractions)
Compound fractures are rare in civilian life
Fractures of sternum may be associated with
  fractures of thoracic spine

Clinical features
Pain: on local pressure
      respiration
      movement
Local bruising if several ribs are broken or if
  patient is thin
Crepitus
Surgical emphysema } May be present

Complications
May occur singly or in combination
Flail segment
Pneumo thorax
Hemothorax
Massive emphysema
Ruptured diaphragm ⎫
    Liver   ⎪
    Spleen   ⎬ Steering wheel injuries
    Aorta   ⎪
    Esophagus ⎭

Radiological features
P-A films should be taken with patient erect
  (Supine films conceal hemo/pneumothorax)
Oblique films show middle/anterior parts of ribs
Anterior ends of ribs difficult to visualise
Lateral films essential for sternum
Only 50% of rib fractures are visualised (Post-
  mortem evidence)

Pathological features
Upper ribs may break from muscle contraction
  or may be indicative of major injury at root of
  neck
Fractures will all unite unless previously diseased
Hemo/pneumothorax ⎫ May occur from a single
                ⎬ fracture, but more
Surgical emphysema ⎭   commonly from
                     multiple fractures

Pneumonia   ⎫ May occur in the elderly or
Respiratory failure ⎬ in those with pre-existing
              ⎭ lung disease

Pathological fractures of ribs:
  Carcinomatosis
  Osteomalacia
  Osteopetrosis
  Fragilitas ossium etc.

Treatment
1. Single rib:
    No treatment
2. Several ribs:
    Strapping of minimal benefit
    Long acting local anesthetic
3. Severe pain +/- chronic bronchitis
              +/- Acute infection
    Premixed nitrous oxide/oxygen
  or Epidural anesthesia
  or Repeated local anesthesia
  or Big analgesic injection before vigorous
    physiotherapy

Treatment
3. Compound fractures:
    Occlusive dressings as first aid to prevent
      a) further lung collapse
      b) paradoxical respiration
    Thoracotomy and wound toilet for all but
      most trivial wounds
4. Fractured Sternum:
    Internal fixation
      If displaced,
        Very mobile, or painful
5. Respiratory Infection:
    Culture sputum
    Appropriate antibiotics
    Intensive physiotherapy
6. Flail segment ± respiratory failure ⎫
7. Hemothorax   ⎪
8. Pneumothorax   See
9. Intra-abdominal injury   ⎬ appro-
10. Ruptured diaphragm   ⎪ priate
11. Ruptured aorta   section
12. Ruptured oesophagus   ⎭

References
Conn F H et al 1963 Thoracic trauma. Analysis of 1022 cases. Journal of Trauma 3: 22-40
Joshi S G, Parulkar G B, Sen P K 1965 Bilateral fracture of the first rib. Journal of Bone and Joint Surgery 47B: 283-285
Richardson J D, McElvein R B, Trinkle J K 1975 First rib fracture, a hallmark of severe trauma. Annals of Surgery 181: 251-254

Open wounds of thorax

General features
Caused by
   bullets or shrapnel
   explosions
   stab wounds
Often associated with other injuries

Clinical features
Depend on
   size of wound
   site of wound
   direction of wound
   nature of damage/causative agent
Pain, Dyspnoea, Tachypnoea
Hemorrhage. Hypovolemic chock
Paradoxical respiration with large wounds (i.e.
   Sucking wound)

Radiological features
Fractures of ribs or spine may be present
Hemo/Pneumothorax ⎫
Hemopericardium   ⎪
Enlarged mediastinum ⎬ May be visible
Surgical emphysema   ⎪
Ruptured diaphragm   ⎪
Foreign bodies   ⎭

Pathological features
Infinite variety of damage and complications may
   occur
Abdominal → Thoracic wounds more dangerous
   than the reverse
Foreign bodies.
   May move widely within thorax
   May embolise the great vessels or heart
Retained metal fragments may cause hemoptysis
Damage to mediastinal structures may be life
   threatening
   i.e. Great vessels: Immediately
      Thoracic duct: After long interval
         (chylothorax)

Treatment
First Aid: Block large wounds with occlusive
   dressing
Very minor wounds: Drain chest and watch
   carefully

All others:
   Thoracotomy:
      Hemostasis: Tetanus Toxoid/Antibiotics
      Remove foreign bodies easily accessible
      Suture damaged tissues
         (Conservation with lung)
      Drain chest
   Mediastinal Damage:
      Major blood replacement
      Cardiac bypass occasionally required
      Drain pericardium
      Drain chest
   Chest wall defects:
      Close with skin/muscle flap
      Rib grafts
      Acrylic patches (not infected cases)

References
Beall A C et al 1961 Penetrating wounds of the heart.
   Journal of Trauma 1: 195-207
Conn J H et al 1963 Thoracic trauma. Analysis of 1022 cases.
   Journal of Trauma 3: 22-40
Dillard B M, Staple T W 1969 Bullet embolism from the
   aortic arch to the popliteal artery. Archives of Surgery 98:
   326-328
Laaveg S J, Sprague B L 1978 Traumatic chylothorax. A
   complication of fracture-dislocation of the spine. Journal of
   Bone and Joint Surgery 60A: 708-709
Le Roux B T 1964 Maintenance of chest wall stability.
   Thorax 19: 397-405
Naclerio E Z 1964 Penetrating wounds of the heart diseases
   of the chest. 46: 1-22
Patterson L T, Schmitt H J, Armstrong R G 1968
   Intermediate care of war wounds of the chest. Journal of
   Thoracic and Cardiovascular Surgery 55: 16-23
Roy P H, Carr D T, Payne W S, 1967 The problem of
   chylothorax. Proceedings of the Mayo Clinic 42-457-467.
Salzstein E C, Freeeark R J 1962 Bullet embolism to the
   right axillary artery following gunshot wound of the heart.
   Annals of Surgery 158: 65-69
Vogt-Moykoff I, Krumhaar D 1966 Treatment of intra
   pulmonary shell fragments. Surgery Gynaecology and
   obstetrics 123: 1233-1236

Hemothorax

General features
Usually due to trauma to chest wall
Rarely due to other causes
   i.e. carcinoma
      torn adhesion in spontaneous
         pneumothorax
Usually rib fracture(s) are present

Clinical features

From injury
Pain worse on respiration and movement
Local tenderness and bruising

From hemothorax
Tachypnoea
Shoulder tip pain

From hypovolaemia
Pallor
Rising pulse
Falling blood pressure

Radiological features
Supine chest film:
  Diffuse haziness in lung fields
  Maximal at costo-vertebral margin
Erect chest film:
  Diffuse opacity in lower lung fields rising
    towards axilla
  Blurring of costo-phrenic angle
  Flattening of diaphragm
  Fluid level if pneumothorax is also present
Rib fractures visible in most cases

Pathological changes
Blood remains liquid for long periods:
  loculation may occur
Large volumes may collect with pulmonary
  atelectasis and collapse
If untreated fibrinous masses form covering ribs
  diaphragm and lung
Infection may occur in
  open injuries
  associated lung damage/infection

Treatment
Aspiration
Drainage via underwater seal or valve
Correction of hemorrhagic disease
Infection: Drainage of empyema: antibiotics:
  decortication if chronic

References
Beall A C, Crawford H W, Debakey M E 1966
  Considerations in the management of acute traumatic
  haemothorax. Journal of Thoracic and Cardiovascular
  Surgery 52: 351-360

Pneumothorax

General features
Common
Usually occurs from rib fractures
Non-traumatic cases occur from rupture of
  pulmonary bullae
Always present if surgical emphysema occurs

Clinical features

Common features
Breathlessness
Diminished breath sounds } Locally
Increased resonance

Bilateral
Severe dyspnoea and tachypnoea
Cyanosis
Bilaterally diminished breath sounds and
  increased resonance
Central mediastinum

Tension
Usually unilateral
Steadily increasing symptoms and signs
Tracheal deviation away from pneumothorax
Shift of cardiac dullness
Increased central venous pressure
Bulging intercostal spaces in thin subjects
Catastrophic worsening if given positive pressure
  ventilation with massive surgical emphysema
  likely

Radiological features
Pulmonary edge visible. Erect films always
  required
Absent lung markings at periphery of thorax
  (surgical emphysema may obscure both)
Mediastinal shift

Tension
Total pulmonary collapse
Marked mediastinal shift
Flattened diaphragm

Pathological features

Non-traumatic
Bulla(e) on pulmonary surface
Small pleural effusion

Traumatic
Rib fracture(s)
Small pulmonary perforation or tear
Hemothorax

Rarely
Major pulmonary rupture
Bronchial or tracheal tear

Treatment

Conservative
Very few small unilateral pneumothoracies
Chest films required 4-6 hourly for 24 hours,
   even if no clinical change

Active
Chest drainage with valve or underwater seal
(Upper anterior chest wall)
Continued for 48-72 hours
Daily chest radiograph
Full expansion: Clamp drainage tube for 24
   hours
If no further leakage:
   Remove tube
   Chest radiographs at 24 and 48 hours

Problems
1) Persistent leakage:
      Continue drainage up to 3 weeks
      Loculations may require multiple tubes
2) Repeated or long continued pneumothorax:
      Thoracotomy
      Staple or suture site of leakage
3) Bronchial or tracheal tear:
   a) Minor leak chest drainage and observe
   b) Major leak (or persistence)
         Endotracheal tube and chest drainage
         Positive pressure respiration
      Bronchogram
         Thoracotomy
         Suture site of drainage.

References

Guest J L, Anderson J N 1977 Major airway trauma in
   closed chest trauma. Chest 72: 63-66
Relland J Y M, Miller D M, Carberry D M 1973 Traumatic
   rupture of the tracheo-bronchial tree. New York State
   Journal of Medicine 73: 1292-1295

Flail chest

Synonym
Stove in Chest

General features
Becoming more common. Due to massive blunt
   trauma
Usually
   1. Due to road accidents
   2. Anterior chest wall involved
   3. Other injuries and facial lacerations are
      present
Particularly dangerous in
   1. The elderly
   2. Those with pretrauma lung disease

Clinical features
Pain on respiration and movement
Local tenderness, abrasions, crepitus over broken
   ribs
Tachypnoea
Cyanosis
Paradoxical respiration
      i.e. Injured chest wall drawn in at inspiration

Radiological features
Double fractures of a series of ribs on one or
   both sides of thorax
Fractures of costochondral junctions difficult to
   visualise
Sternum and scapula may also be fractured
Patchy opacities in underlying lung (lung
   contusion/atelectasis)
Hemo/Pneumo-thorax }
Surgical emphysema   } May be present

Pathological features

Lungs
   Diminished tidal volume
   Shunting of gas from one lung to the other
   Due to paradoxical respiration
Blood gases altered
   Hypoxemia
   Hyper carbia
   Respiratory Acidosis

Heart
Shift of mediastinum if flail segment is unilateral
Diminished venous return
Diminished cardiac output

Ribs
Common patterns of injury
   Sternum with anterior rib segments
   Anterior ribs on one side of thorax
   Upper ribs on one side (splinted by scapula
     and shoulder)

Treatment
   Drainage of hemo/pneumo thorax
   Careful bronchial toilet
   Prevent paradoxical respiration
   If respiratory failure threatens or develops
   By 1) Intermittent positive pressure respiration
      (I.P.P.R.)
   or 2) Costal traction (inefficient)
   or 3) internal fixation of ribs
   or 4) Carapace dressing (restricts breathing)
Problems of I.P.P.R.
   Endotracheal tube may ulcerate cords or
     trachea
   Pulmonary infection
   Diminution of venous return to heart

References
Cullen P et al 1975 Treatment of flail chest. Archives of
   Surgery 110: 1099-1103
Le Roux B T 1964 Maintenance of chest wall stability.
   Thorax 19: 397-405
Prys-Roberts C 1974 Respiratory problems of the seriously
   injured patient. Injury 5: 67-78

Cardiac contusion

General features
Usually
   due to massive blunt trauma to trunk
   due to road accidents
   associated with major thoracic fractures

Clinical features
Anginal pain (Differentiate from pretrauma
   myocardial ischemia)
Dyspnoea
Hypotension
Arrythmias and palpitations

Radiological features
Slight cardiac enlargment
Cardiac catheterisation) May show mural
Coronary angiography) thickening

Pathological features
Minor Injury:
   Small petechiae or ecchymoses
Major Injury:
   Hematoma of whole thickness of wall from
     torn coronary artery or vein
Mechanisms:
   Compression between sternum and vertebrae
   Violent increase in intra-thoracic pressure
Later Effects:
   Cardiac tamponade
   Pericarditis
   Cardiac tupture (aneurysm)
E.C.G. Changes:
   Non specific usually i.e.
     Atrial or ventricular extrasystoles
     Degrees of A/V Block
     ST elevation
   Cardiac enzymes may indicate major/minor
     infarction

Treatment
Rest
Serial E.C.Gs/enzymes
Anti-arrythmic drugs as indicated
   Lignocaine, Propranolol, Quinidine
Digitalis used cautiously
No anti-coagulants or vaso-dilators

References:
Demuth W E, Baue A E, Odom J A 1967 Contusions of the
   heart. Journal of Trauma 7: 443-455
Naclerio E A 1964 Penetrating wounds of the heart. Diseases
   of the Chest, 46: 1-22
Symbas P N 1972 Traumatic injuries of heart and great
   vessels. Thomas, Springfield.

Traumatic cardiac rupture

General features
Rare
Due to massive blunt trauma to trunk
Usually occurs in road accidents
Rarely occurs from stabbing incidents
Few reach hospital alive
Frequent association with other injuries

Clinical features
Symptoms and signs often obscured by those of other injuries

1. Cardiac tamponade: Ruptured ventricle or atrium
Reduced pulse rate
Reduced blood pressure
Venous distension of face and neck
Muffled heart sounds

2. Congestive cardiac failure: Rupture of a valve, septum or papillary muscle
Dyspnoea
Edema
Venous distension
Abnormal heart sounds

Radiological features
Enlarged heart shadow. Pulmonary venous congestion/Edema
Fractured ribs
Hemothorax
Cardiac catheterisation may show intra-pericardial abnormalities
Ultrasonic scan may be abnormal

Pathological features

Causes
Puncture by a rib
Compression between ribs and vertebrae
Sudden increase in intra-thoracic pressure at full diastole

Types
Rupture of wall leads to hemopericardium occurs immediately after injury
    Later after an infarct
Rupture of valve, septum, papilla
    Leads to congestive failure
    Delayed symptoms and signs

Investigations
Abnormal E.C.Gs.
Pressure studies, etc. usually precluded by urgency of treatment in mural rupture

Treatment

Mural rupture
Immediate thoracotomy
Repair of rent
Drain chest/pericardium

Valve or septal damage
Supportive measures
Accurate diagnosis
Cardiac bypass
Operative repair

References
Geiran O, Solkheim K 1974 Acute rupture of the heart after blunt trauma. Report of a successful operation. Injury 5: 54-58
Symbas P N 1972 Traumatic injuries of heart and great vessels. Thomas, Springfield.

Rupture of aorta

General features
Due to massive blunt trauma to trunk
Usually due to road accidents
Only 10-20% reach hospital alive
Features are often masked by other major injuries

Clinical features
Chest or back pain
Dyspnoea
Frequent inability to feel or move legs
Increased pulse amplitude and blood pressure in arms
Decrease pulse amplitude and blood pressure in legs

Radiological features
Widening of mediastinum (may be minimal or confused by portable X-ray)
Fractures of thoracic cage are frequent
Aortography will confirm rupture

Pathological features
Rupture usually occurs just distal to ligamentum arteriosum
More rarely in ascending or descending aorta
Incomplete rupture may cause a slowly enlarging aneurysm with possible delay in diagnosis

Treatment
As soon as diagnosed
(Cardiac bypass may be required if ascending aorta)
Thoractomy
Repair of rupture
Dacron prosthesis may be required
Prognosis bad if over 40

References
Sevitt S 1976 Traumatic ruptures of the aorta. A clinico-pathological study. Injury 8: 159-173
Symbas P N et al 1973 Traumatic rupture of the aorta. American Journal of Surgery 178: 6-11

Esophageal trauma

General features
Rarely due to external trauma, blunt or penetrating
Rarely due to forceful vomiting
More often iatrogenic –
  foreign bodies
  esophagoscopy

Clinical features
Pain:
  Increasingly severe in injuries to mid and lower thirds.
  Worsened on swallowing
Surgical emphysema at root of neck
External wound may be present in penetrating injuries

Radiological features
Mediastinal widening and emphysema
Cervical soft tissue emphysema
Pleural effusion
Hydro-pneumothorax
Gastrografin swallow. Leakage of dye into tissues or into pleural cavity

Pathological features
Cervical lesions
From penetrating external trauma
  Esophagoscopy

Mid thoracic lesions
From Esophagoscopy
  Swallowed foreign bodies

Lower thoracic lesions
From blunt external trauma
  Previous thoracic surgery
  Esophagoscopy

Supradiaphragmatic lesions
From vomiting
Previous abdominal or diaphragmatic surgery

Pre-existing esophageal disease
may lead to injury
and complicate treatment

Treatment
Consider an esophageal obstruction below the lesion

Cervical lesion:
Often suitable for conservative care
  i.e. Naso gastric tube
    Drainage of site of lesion
    Antibiotics

Thoracic lesions:
Rarely suitable for conservative care
Thoracotomy
  Bypass obstruction
  Repair lesion
  Drain chest

References
Popovsky J, Lee Y C, Berk J L 1976 Gunshot wounds of the esophagus. Journal of Thoracic and Cardiovascular Surgery 72: 609-612
Spenler C W, Benfield J R 1976 Esophageal disruption from blunt and penetrating external trauma. Archives of Surgery 111: 663-667
Triggiani E, Belsey R 1977 Esophageal trauma, incidence, diagnosis, management. Thorax 32: 241-249

Rupture of diaphragm

General features
Becoming more common from road accidents
Caused by massive blunt trauma to trunk
Mainly in young men
Associated with pelvic and thoracic fractures and visceral injuries

Clinical features
Specific features may be obscured by signs and symptoms of other injuries.
Diagnosis may be immediate or delayed

Acute
Pain on respiration
Dyspnoea, Tachypnoea, Cyanosis

Acute and delayed
Basal dullness. Occasionally mediastinal shift
Intestinal sounds in thorax

Radiological features
Elevated diaphragm
Intestinal gas shadows in thorax with fluid levels
Absence of diaphragmatic movement on
    screening
Contrast studies may show stomach above the
    diaphragm

Pathological features
Left dome of diaphragm injured more frequently
Rupture may occur through regions of weakness
    i.e. Esophageal hiatus
        Foramen of Bochdalek

Left dome
Damage to spleen
Fractures of left ribs
Herniation of stomach
    +/- Spleen
    +/- Small intestine or Large intestine

Right dome
Damage to liver
Fractures of right ribs
Herniation of liver
Herniation of other viscera is rare
Herniated bowel may be obstructed or
    strangulated – extreme urgency

Treatment
Resuscitation
Full preoperative diagnosis, nasogastric tube
Surgical repair. Thoracolaparotomy usually
    required
Resect strangulated bowel

References
Childress M E, Grimes O F 1961 Immediate and remote
    sequelae in traumatic diaphragmatic hernia. Surgery,
    Gynecology and Obstetrics 113: 573-584
Gourin A, Garzon A A 1974 Diagnostic problems in
    traumatic diaphragmatic hernia. Journal of Trauma 14: 20-
    31
Griswold F W, Warden H E, Gardner R J 1972 Acute
    diaphragmatic rupture caused by blunt trauma. American
    Journal of Medicine 124: 359-362
Marchand P 1962 Traumatic hiatus hernia. British Medical
    Journal 1: 754-759

Pulmonary contusion

Synonym
Bruised lung, wet lung, traumatic pneumonia

General features
Due to major blunt thoracic injury
In civilian life most often due to road accidents
Usually associated with thoracic fractures
In children may be severe even without fractures

Clinical features
Increasing restlessness
    dyspnoea
    tachypnoea
    cyanosis
    pulse rate
    temperature } Rising
Local pain, tenderness, bruising around point of
    impact on chest wall
Possible crepitus from rib fractures
Cough. Frothy blood stained sputum
Rising pCO_2, Falling pO_2, Acidosis
Progresses over 5-10 days
Regresses over 14-21 days

Differential diagnosis
Head injury
Fat Embolism
Drug withdrawal syndrome
Hemo/Pneumothorax
Pulmonary atelectasis

Radiological features
Initial irregular pulmonary opacities
Becoming confluent in a few days
Intra-pulmonary fluid level may appear
Abscess formation
Gradual resolution over 21-28 days

Pathological features
Intrapulmonary hematoma leading to
    Filling of alveoli
    Small airway collapse more frequently in
elderly
        Localised consolidation
Later, necrosis of lung tissue with infection

Gas exchange
Pulmonary compliance reduced
Shunting of blood through unaerated lung
Diminished alveolar/capillary gas exchange
Some permanent loss of respiratory reserve in
  every person who survives

Treatment
Sit the patient up
Monitor blood gases
Administer Oxygen/Air mixture
Antibiotics
Diuretics
Steroids
Respiratory Physiotherapy

Severe Cases
Tracheostomy
Bronchial toilet
Intermittent positive pressure ventilation
(± Positive expiratory end pressure)

References
Burford T H, Burbank B 1945 Traumatic wet lung. Journal
  of Thoracic Surgery 14: 415-424
Caseby N G, Porter M F 1976 Blast injuries to the lungs.
  Clinical presentation management and course. Injury 8: 1-
  12
Prys-Roberts C 1974 Respiratory problems of the seriously
  injured patient. Injury 5: 67-78

Inhalation lung

Synonym
Mendelson's Syndrome, Aspiration Lung

General features
Due to depressed consciousness
  or depressed pharyngeal and laryngeal reflexes

Acute
Rapid onset of dangerous illness with high
  mortality rate
Head injury, drunkenness, anesthesia

Chronic
Repeated minor episodes with progressive
  damage to lung
(Nasogastric tubes, tracheostomies, hiatus hernia,
  megaesophagus)
Acidic gastric contents inhaled into lung

Clinical features

Acute
Sudden onset of tachypnoea, cyanosis,
  hypotension
Bronchospasm
Pink frothy sputum coughed up
Pyrexia. Hypoxemia
Patient becomes dangerously ill in 2-12 hours
  from aspiration

Chronic
Repeated episodes of bronchopneumonia

Radiological features
Irregular opacification of lung
Becoming confluent
Areas of atelectasis or lobular collapse
Foreign bodies may be visualised in bronchi

Pathological features
Acidic gastric contents (pH 2-5) will cause a
  chemical burn of air passages
Loss of epithelium
Rapid onset of edema
Exudate blocks alveoli and bronchioles
Food particles may add to blockage
Early onset of infection with local abscess
  formation
Right lower lobe most often affected

Treatment
Aspiration of air passages via bronchoscope
Bronchial lavage with saline

Drugs
Bronchodilators
Steroids
Antibiotics
Respiratory physiotherapy – vigorous and
  aggressive

Severe cases
Assisted ventilation
Positive expiratory and pressure

References
Arms A A, Dines D E, Tinstman T C 1974 Aspiration
  pneumonia. Chest 65: 136-139
Mendelson C L 1946 The aspiration of stomach contents into
  the lungs during obstetric anaesthesia. American Journal of
  Obstetrics and Gynaecology 52: 191-205
Pradhan D J, Ikins P M 1976 Aspiration disease. American
  Surgeon 42: 186-191

Traumatic asphyxia

General features
Uncommon but striking clinical picture
Caused by compression of trunk
  In crowds
  In road accidents
  In crushing injuries (industrial or agricultural)

Clinical features
Petechiae in upper chest, arms, neck and head
May be almost confluent
Facial edema and cyanosis
Areas of pressure or markings of clothes outlined
  by paucity of petechiae
Subconjunctival hemorrhages
Mucosal petechiae present in mouth
Hemoptyses – small volumes
Clouding of consciousness of varying degree
Rib fractures often present
Retinal petechiae may dim vision

Radiological features
Patchy lung opacities
Rib fractures   } May be present
Ruptured diaphragm }

Pathological features
Due to sudden rise of venous pressure in upper
  part of body
Effects may be exacerbated if glottis is closed at
  moment of pressure
Petechiae occur in every organ
Rapid resolution of signs

Treatment
Unconsciousness:
  Head injury observation system
  Steroids
  Diuretics   } To diminish cerebral
  Intravenous mannitol) }   Edema

References
Leech P, Cuthert H 1972 Brachial plexus lesions associated
  with traumatic asphyxia. British Journal of Surgery 59:
  539-541
Sandiford J A, Sickler D 1974 Traumatic asphyxia with
  severe neurological sequelae. Journal of Trauma 14: 805-
  810

Oxygen toxicity

General features
Unrecognised until recent decades
Major mishap: Rentrolental fibroplasia in
  premature infants

Clinical features
Steady reduction in respiratory efficiency in a
  patient receiving excess oxygen
i.e. At 1 at. pressure
    by Mask
    or artificial ventilation
  At 1+ at. pressure:
    Rare circumstances of diving
      accidents and pressure chamber mishaps
Reduced lung compliance
High pO_2
Reduced pCO_2

Radiological features
Patchy opacification of lung fields
Later becoming confluent

Pathological features
Critical features of excess oxygen
  1. Duration   } not yet fully defined
  2. Partial pressure }
Possible ill effects in man
  6-36 hours at 100% oxygen at 1 at.
  6-12 hours at 100% oxygen at 2 at.
Much animal experimentation, little human
  information

Macroscopic changes
Heavy lungs
Interstitial edema

Microscopic changes
Alveolar thickening
Vascular congestion
Lymphatic dilatation
Disruption of endothelial cells from basement
  membrane

Unknown relationship between
Macrophage activity
Surfactant synthesis
Pulmonary mechanics
Oxygen tension

Treatment
Provide therapy that keeps arterial oxygen at
   80–100 mmHg. (10.6-13.3 KPa)
Careful bronchial toilet
Diuretics
Steroids
Antibiotics

References
Barber R E, Lee J, Hamilton W K 1970 Oxygen toxicity in
   man. A prospective study in patients with irreversible brain
   damage. New England Journal of Medicine 283: 1478-1484
Clark J M 1974 The toxicity of oxygen. American Review of
   Respiratory Diseases 110: 40-50
Singer M M et al 1970 Oxygen toxicity in man. A
   prospective study in patients after open heart surgery. New
   England Journal of Medicine 283: 1473-1477

11

ABDOMINAL INJURIES

With the assistance of A. I. Davidson,
W. H. H. Garvie

Gastro-intestinal injuries
Genito-urinary injuries

Management and assessment of abdominal injuries

Firstly
Secure airway
Control external hemorrhage
Splint fractures
Take blood for grouping and crossmatching
Put up an intravenous line

Secondly
Obtain history of injury
Examine abdomen –
  Wounds, swellings, guarding, rigidity, hernial
    orifices shifting dullness, abnormal
    resonance, auscultate abdomen
Examine Perineum:
  Scrotum or vulva
  Rectum

Thirdly
Begin to plot
  Pulse rate
  Blood pressure
  Respiratory rate
  State of consciousness
  Fluid balance
  Abdominal girth

Fourthly
Intubate
  Great veins for central venous pressure
  Bladder for hourly urinary output
  Stomach for aspirated contents

Fifthly
Investigations
Baseline:
  Hematological and Biochemical profile
Radiography:
  Abdomen   Erect and supine films if possible
  Chest
  Pelvis
  I.V.P Cystogram Urethrogram
Ultrasonic Scan }
Isotope Scan   } Unproven value at present

Peritoneal puncture
  Abdominal (4 quadrants)
  Upper vaginal
    Negative results do not exclude damage
Peritoneal lavage more certain

Sixthly
If serious doubt persists, consider laparotomy
  +/- thoracotomy

References

Clarke J W 1969 Culdocentesis in evaluation of blunt
  abdominal trauma surgery. Gynaecology and Obstetrics
  129: 809-810
Martin J D (ed) 1969 Trauma to the thorax and abdomen.
  Thomas, Springfield
Northfield T C, Smith T 1972 Physiologic significance of
  central venous pressure in patients with haemorrhage.
  Surgery, Gynaecology and Obstetrics 135: 267-270
Perry J F, Demeules J E, Root H D 1970 Diagnostic
  peritoneal lavage in blunt abdominal trauma surgery.
  Gynaecology and Obstetrics 131: 742-744

Injuries of stomach

General features
Stomach is protected from blunt trauma by its
  mobility and the lower ribs
More liable to corrosive chemical injury or
  foreign body injury than other parts of
  intestines
Other vital organs may be damaged in
  perforating injuries

Clinical features
Abdominal pain
Often hypovolemic shock
Lacerations contusions or perforations of
  abdominal wall or lower ribs may be present
Hematemesis likely in corrosive injuries or in
  perforations from foreign bodies
Peritoneal soiling results in:
  Tenderness, guarding
  Absent bowel sounds,
  Distension, Pyrexia, later

Radiological features
Gas under diaphragm if stomach is perforated
Stomach initially dilated in corrosive injuries
Peritoneal extravasation of contrast medium
Fractures of the lower ribs +/- lumbar spine may
  be present
Rupture of diaphragm

Pathological features

Mechanisms of Injury:

Gunshot wounds { may penetrate chest
or abdominal walls

Stab wounds { Profound blood loss
may occur

Foreign bodies:
Swallowed by children or mentally disturbed
adults
i.e. razor blades, pins etc.

Blunt injuries:
May contuse gastric walls or avulse part of
omentum

Corrosives:
Swallowed accidentally or intentionally
Alkalis damage esophagus worst
Acids damage stomach worst
Cause coagulative necrosis of gastric walls

Surgical damage:
From endoscopy etc.

Bursting injuries:
Compressed air accidents
Water-ski-ing accidents

Treatment

Restoration of blood volume
Full diagnosis
Nasogastric intubation

Gastroscopy } Rarely indicated in fit
Contrast studies } patients where doubt exists

Laparotomy:
Resection of devitalised parts
Repair of lacerations
Peritoneal toilet

Corrosives
Immediate gastric lavage with appropriate
antidote
Monitor vital signs
Esophagogastrectomy may be required in worst
cases

References

Chung R S K, Denbesten L 1975 Fibreoptic endoscopy in
treatment of corrosive injury of the stomach. Archives of
Surgery 11: 725-728
Marsh B R 1975 The problem of the open safety pin. Annals
of Otology, Rhinology and Laryngology 84: 624-626
Nicosia J F et al 1974 Surgical management of corrosive
gastric injuries. Annals of Surgery 180: 139-143
Ritter F N et al 1971 The rationale of emergency
esophagogastrectomy in the treatment of liquid caustic
burns of the esophagus and stomach. Annals of Otology,
Rhinology and Laryngology 80: 513-520 et seq.

Welch T P, Prathnadi P, Narco S 1971 Complete transection
of the stomach and pancreas as a result of blunt trauma.
British Journal of Surgery 58: 874-876
Yee K F, Schild J A, Holinger P H 1975 Extra luminal
foreign bodies (coins) in the food and air passages. Annals
of Otology, Rhinology and Laryngology 84: 619-623

Injuries of duodenum

General features

Uncommon, but increasing in frequency
Caused by
1. Blunt injury to abdomen or loin
2. Penetrating wounds, stabbing, gunshot
wounds
Often associated with other abdominal injuries,
particularly in warfare
Diagnosis may be delayed if injury is
retroperitoneal

Clinical features

External wound or bruising
Hypovolemic shock may be present
Intraperitoneal damage:
Pain
Guarding, rigidity
Distension, Ileus
Retroperitoneal damage:
Pain particularly on movement
Swelling in loin
Abscess development
Renal damage: Hematuria
Pancreatic damage:
Riased serum amylase
Blood on peritoneal lavage

Radiological features

Gas under diaphragm
Rarely in retroperitoneal tissues
Obscured psoas shadow
Contrast studies may show:
Duodenal leakage
Renal damage
Peritonitis:
Distended loops of bowel
Fluid levels

Pathological features

Intraperitoneal damage:
Moderate peritoneal contamination
Sterile at first

Damage to pancreas and other organs is
immediately serious and rapidly worsening

Retroperitoneal damage: (2nd part of duodenum)
Most often due to blunt trauma
Infected hematoma develops in loin
Eventually leads to a duodenal fistula

Duodenal fistula
Most serious outcome of injury
Loss of fluids
electrolytes
calories
Excoriation of skin
Rapid development of cachexia leading to death

Treatment
Exploration of external wound
Laparotomy: Mobilise duodenum when in doubt
Repair duodenal rent
Reinforce repair:
Omental graft for minor injury
Overlying jejunostomy for major injury
Decompress duodenum:
Nasogastric tube or
Gastrostomy
(Gastrojejunostomy may lead to stomal
ulceration)
Maintenance of nutrition:
Feeding jejunostomy
or Intravenous alimentation

References
Corley R D, Norcross W J, Shoemaker W C 1975 Traumatic
injuries to the duodenum. A report on 98 patients. Annals
of Surgery 181: 92-98
Heyse-Moore G H Blunt pancreatic and pancreatico-
duodenal trauma. British Journal of Surgery 63: 226-228

Injuries of small intestine

General features
Caused by blunt injuries
Road or industrial trauma
Penetrating injuries
Gun shot wounds
Stabbing incidents
Other abdominal injuries may be present

Clinical features
External wound may be obvious

Early
Abdominal pain
Guarding. Rigidity
Paracentesis may produce a little blood

Later
Distension. Peritonitis
Ileus
Severe injuries will produce hypovolemic shock

Radiological features

Early
Often no abnormality on 'scout' film
Rarely gas under diaphragm

Later
Fluid levels in distended loops of bowel

Contrast studies
I.V.P. to exclude renal injury
Aortography may show site of hemorrhage if
time allows

Pathological features

Deceleration or blunt injuries may cause
Mesenteric trears (devitalisation of bowel if large)
Rarely mucosal tears
Mural hematomata

Penetrating injuries
Single or multiple penetration of bowel and/or
mesentery
Peritoneal contamination not initially severely
infected

Treatment
Two schools of thought:
1. Explore every wound or injured abdomen
2. Observe carefully those abdomens without
obvious abnormal physical signs after full
non-surgical investigations

Laparotomy
Minor penetrations – Repair
Major penetrations }
Devitalised bowel   } Resect loop of bowel
Mesenteric tears – Close holes

References
Chappell J S 1974 Perforation of bowel associated with blunt
abdominal trauma in children. South African Medical
Journal 48: 2396

Mathewson C 1969 Routine exploration of stab wounds of abdomen. Journal of Trauma 9: 1028

Nance F C, Cohn I (Jnr) 1969 Surgical judgement in the management of stab wounds of abdomen. A retrospective and prospective analysis based on a study of 600 stabbed patients. Annals of Surgery, 170 560 580

Injuries of colon

General features
Causes
- Gunshot wounds
- Stabbing, etc.
- Blunt abdominal trauma
- Compressed air lines, etc.

Penetrating wounds often associated with injuries of other organs

Clinical features
External wound may be present
Abdominal pain
Guarding, rigidity, ileus
Severe injuries cause hypovolemic shock

Delayed diagnosis
Pyrexia
Peritonitis
Extraperitoneal sepsis in loin or pelvis

Radiological features

Initially
None due to colonic damage
Gas under diaphragm ⎫
Fractures ⎭ from other injuries

Later
Gas under diaphragm
Bowel distension with fluid levels
Space occupying shadows on right or left side of abdomen

Contrast studies
Dangerous for large bowel
I.V.P. may show associated renal or ureteric damage or shift

Pathological features
Sepsis is chief problem

Minor wounds
May self-seal by protruding mucosa or omental adhesions

Gunshot wounds
Complicated by
blood loss
damage to other abdominal organs
damage to thoracic contents
Major mesenteric injuries may cause colonic infarction

Treatment

Considerations:
Number of injuries
Delay before treatment
Degree of shock
Amount of fecal contamination

Minor wounds
Primary repair +/- cecostomy if right colon is injured

Major wounds with contamination
1. Primary repair with defunctioning colostomy
   Peritoneal toilet and drainage

Major wounds without contamination
1. Hemicolectomy if wound is suitably placed
2. Primary anastomosis after resection
   (Exteriorisation of anastomosis still unproven)

Complications
Wound infection
Abdominal or pelvic abscesses
Disruption of suture line
Stenosis of colon

References
Bartizal J K, Boyd D R, Rolk F A 1974 A critical review of management of 392 colonic and rectal injuries diseases of colon and rectum 17: 313-318

Beall A C (Jnr) et al 1971 Surgical considerations in the management of civilian colon injuries. Annals of Surgery 173: 971-978

Bowell H S, Bartizal J F, Freeark R J 1976 Blunt trauma involving the colon and rectum. Journal of Trauma 16: 624-632

Shrock T R, Christensen N 1972 The management of perforating injuries of the colon. Surgery, Gynaecology and Obstetrics 135: 64-68

Injuries of rectum

General features
Causes:
Falling on spiked objects
Gun shot wounds
Iatrogenic:
Enemas
Signoidoscopy
Associated with damage to bladder and other abdominal organs

Clinical features
Pain
Rectal hemorrhage
If severe:
Hypovolemic shock
Fractured pelvis ⎫
Perineal wounds ⎭ May be present
Peritoneal Damage:
Abdominal distension
Guarding. Rigidity. Ileus
Delayed diagnosis:
Pelvic or Peritoneal Sepsis

Radiological features
Variable features may be visible
i.e. Fractured pelvis
Gas in tissues
Gas under diaphragm
Cystogram may show bladder damage

Pathological features
Wounds of warfare more severe than those of civilian life
Sepsis is the major problem
Rupture – below peritoneum—pelvic tissues involved
Rupture above peritoneum—Abdominal cavity involved
Anterior wall of rectum most often damaged with involvement of bladder
Fractures of sacrum rarely cause rectal damage

Treatment
Catheterise bladder. Cystogram if indicated
Inspect rectum by proctoscope

1. Damage below peritoneal reflexion
Debride perineal wound
Repair rectal mucosa
Drain retro-rectal fossa
Antibiotics
Low residue diet

2. Damage above peritoneal reflexion
Left lower laparotomy
Colostomy
Repair rectal wound
Close peritoneum
Drain pre-sacral space and peritoneum
Antibiotics

References
Bartizal J K, Boyd D R, Folk F A 1974 A critical review of management of 392 colonic and rectal injuries. Diseases of Colon and Rectum 17: 313-318
Trunkey D, Hays R J, Shires G T 1973 Management of rectal trauma. Journal of Trauma 13: 411-415

Injuries of pancreas

General features
Uncommon
Due to
Massive blunt abdominal trauma
Seat belt injuries
Penetrating wounds:
Stabbing
Gun shot
Associated frequently with other major thoracic and/or abdominal injuries

Clinical features
Acute
Hypovolemic shock
Abdominal pain and guarding
Damage to other abdominal organs obscures the clinical picture
Delayed
Pancreatitis
Abscess
Fistula
Hypogastric swelling of pseudopancreatic cyst

Radiological features
Rarely seen
Fractures of ribs and/or spine
Hemopneumothorax
Subphrenic gas
Limited value
Ultrasonic scan
Hepatic scan

Pancreatic scan
Aortic angiography

Pathological features
Types of injury
  Contusion
  Laceration
  Transection
  Crushing
Sites of Injury
  Tail – often with splenic injury
  Body – often with gastric injury
  Head – often with duodenal injury
Effects of Injury
  Abrupt rise in serum amylase
  Release of enzymes into retroperitoneal tissues
  Massive local edema and hemorrhage

Diagnosis
High index of suspicion
Serum amylase levels
Abdominal paracentesis (Amylase level of
  peritoneal fluid)

Treatment
Rapid massive resuscitation
Explore penetrating wounds of trunk
Closed injury: Continued good
    condition – observe
              Poor condition – laparotomy

Findings

1. Superficial contusion—drain abdomen

2. Tail and body
Contusion—Drain
Perforation – Resect
Transection – Resect

3. Head alone
Perforation (Duct intact)
  Debride and drain
Perforation (Duct destroyed):
  Child procedure
  Drain body
  Roux-en-Y
Destroyed
  Whipple procedure
  Roux-en-Y

4. Head and duodenum
Perforation (duct intact)
  Duodenostomy
Duodenum damage (duct intact):
  Whipple procedure

Duodenum and pancreas destroyed:
  Whipple procedure

Complications
Delayed pancreatitis
Fistulae
Pancreatic insufficiency
Pseudopancreatic cyst

References
Anane-Sefah J, Norton L W, Eiseman B 1975 Operative
  choice and technique following pancreatic injury. Archives
  of Surgery 110: 761-766
Balasegaram M 1976 Surgical management of pancreatic
  trauma. American Journal of Surgery 131: 536-540

Injuries of spleen

General features
Varied causes and effects, i.e.,
  Diffuse major violence:
    Rupture with injuries to other systems and
    organs
  Discrete major violence:
    Rupture of spleen alone
    Perhaps fractures of lower left ribs
  Discrete minor violence:
    No injury unless spleen is already diseased
    (i.e. Malarious)
Spontaneous rupture very rarely ocurs

Clinical features
3 Types:
  1. Immediate, leading to collapse (and perhaps
     death)
  2. Latent, appearing during or after
     resuscitation
  3. Delayed – appear after 1-14 days
A. Pain in left hypochondrium
     Worse on respiration or movement
     Often felt in tip of left shoulder
     Local brusing and tenderness
B. Hypovolemic shock:
     Rising pulse
     Falling blood pressure, etc.
C. Guarding and rigidity of abdomen most
     noticeable in left hypochondrium
     Shifting dullness to percussion
     Abdominal distension after a few hours

Radiological features

Some or all may be present

i.e. Fractures of left lower ribs

Absence of bowel shadows in hypochondrium

Indentation of gastric gas shadow

Elevation of left diaphragm

Psoas outline obscured

Pathological features

Trivial split

Subcapsular hematoma

Minor split

Capsular defect

Some intraperitoneal blood

Major split

Large capsular defect

Fragments of spleen detatched (splenosis very rare)

Left Kidney, Tail of pancreas, diphragm, etc. may be damaged

Delayed onset of signs and symptoms may be due to

1. Subcapsular hematoma giving way
2. Damaged pancreas digesting splenic hematoma
3. Greater omentum, surrounding the initial injury giving way

Pre traumatic splenic disease

Malaria

Leukemia

Glandular fever

Portal hypertension, etc.

Treatment

Resuscitation and replacement of blood

Immediate splenectomy

Autotransfusion of intraperitoneal blood if necessary

Watch for hemostatic defects

Complications

Left basal pulmonary atelectasis

Ileus

Hiccup (diaphragmatic irritation)

Hematemesis (gastric veins tied off)

Pancreatitis (damage to pancreas)

Increased incidence of infection in children for years afterwards

Splenosis

References

Cerise E J, Pierce W A, Diamond D L 1970 Abdominal drains, their role as a source of infection following splenectomy. Annals of Surgery 171: 764-769

Lorimer W S (Jnr) 1964 Occult rupture of the spleen. Archives of Surgery 89: 434-440

Naylor R, Coln D, Shires G T 1974 Morbidity and mortality from injuries to the spleen. Journal of Trauma 14: 773-778

Symbas P N, Levin J M, Ferrier F L 1969 A study of autotransfusions from hemothorax. Southern Medical Journal 62: 671

Injuries of liver

General features

Causes:

1. Major blunt trauma to right hypochondrium
2. Penetrating injuries often thoraco-abdominal from stabbing or gun shot wounds

Spontaneous rupture of normal or diseased liver is rare

Clinical features

Hypovolemic shock

Right hypochondral pain

Guarding and rigidity

Later abdominal distension and ileus

Blunt trauma

Often pain and crepitus from fractured ribs

Additional respiratory distress if right diaphragm is ruptured

Penetrating injuries

Other vital structures damaged

Hemo-pneumothorax

Radiological features

Elevated right diaphragm

Blunt trauma

Displacement of bowel shadows from right abdomen

Fractured ribs

Penetrating injuries

Hemopneumothorax

Gas under diaphragm } Possible

Widened mediastinum } Findings

Other methods

Isotope scintigraphy

Ultrasonic scan } Time Consuming,

Selective angiography } Variable Value

Cholangiography

Pathological features

Liver may be bruised (subcapsular hematoma, rarely intrahepatic hematoma)
  lacerated
  ruptured
  pulped
Massive hemorrhage likely
Biliary tree may be damaged
Life possible after loss of 75% liver substance

Treatment

Surgical exploration mandatory
Massive transfusion facilities may be required
Right thoracolaparotomy gives best exposure
Control hemorrhage –
  free edge of lesser omentum
  Hepatic veins
Remove pulped tissue
Suture rents
Major resection if required
Repair other damaged structures
  (Hilar damage may require operative cholangiography or partial venography)
Biliary decompression with T tube
Adequate drainage to pleura and peritoneum

Complications

Shock:
  Hypovolemic
  Bacteremic
Repeated hemorrhage
Hepatorenal failure
Wound disruption
Infection:
  Subphrenic
  Peritonitis
Biliary peritonitis
Hematobilia:
  (Recurrent pain
    Biliary obstruction initially
    Observe gastro-intestinal hemorrhage)

References:

Evans G W et al 1972 Scintigraphy in traumatic lesion of liver and spleen. Journal of American Medical Association 222: 665-667
Foster J H et al 1968 Recent experience with major hepatic resection. Annals of Surgery 167: 651-666
Hanna W A, Wisheart J D 1969 Management of hilar injury of the liver. Annals of the Royal College of Surgeons of Edinburgh 14: 328-331
Lucas C, Walt A J 1970 Critical decisions in liver trauma. Archives of Surgery 101: 277-283
Madding F G, Kennedy P A 1971 Trauma to liver, 2nd ed. W B Saunders Co, Philadelphia
Wright P W, Orloff M J 1964 Traumatic haemobilia. Annals of Surgery 160: 42-53

Injuries of kidney

General features

Mechanism
Diffuse major violence (Road accidents, etc.)
Discrete moderate violence
  Punch or blow in loin
Minor violence if kidney is abnormal (polycystic or hydronephrotic)
Penetrating wounds – stabbing or gun shot injuries

Clinical features

Pain, tenderness, bruising in loin
Guarding and rigidity of abdomen in some cases if peritoneum is involved.
Hematuria
Hypovolemic shock in very severe injuries
Distension and meteorism after 24-48 hours

Radiological features

Scoliosis is usually present
Blurred psoas shadow
Local fractures may be present
  (lower ribs, transverse processes)
Contrast studies:
  1. I.V.P. or high dosage nephrotomogram may show calcyceal irregularities or extrarenal contrast medium
  2. Selective renal angiography may show damaged renal vessels
Ultrasonic scan shows swelling or irregular renal outline

Pathological features

Kidney may be avulsed from pedicle
  (1 hour of warm ischemia will destroy function)
Incomplete split of renal cortex
  Intracapsular hematoma
  Damage to calces – hematuria
Complete split of renal substance
  Blood and urine in perinephric fat
    (rarely intra-peritoneal)
  Clots may obstruct ureter with severe pain and delayed hematuria
Kidneys have big capacity for repair
Partial renal ischemia may lead to post-traumatic hypertension
Intra-peritoneal rupture more common in children

Treatment:
Replacement of blood volume
I.V.P. to confirm presence of opposite kidney
        to define extent of damage
Other radiological investigations as indicated
Minor damage:
    Watchful waiting. No surgery at first
    Urinary catheterisation. Comparison of hourly
        samples
    85% avoid surgery
Major damage:
    Open peritoneum to exclude other injury
    Cystoscopy to exclude damage to lower renal
        tract
    Exploration. Conserve renal tissue
        Renal tear – Repair
        Severe local damage: Partial nephrectomy
        Avulsion
        Severe general } Total nephrectomy
            damage

Complications
Retroperitoneal extravasation of urine
Perinephric abscess
Urinary fistula
Renal necrosis
Hypertension

References
Cockett A T K et al 1973 Recent advances in the diagnosis
    and management of blunt renal trauma. Journal of
    Urology 113: 750-754
Greene L F, Fraser R A, Hartman G W 1976 Bolus
    nephrotomography in diagnosis of lesions of kidney
    urology 7: 221-227
Holcroft J W, Trunkey D D, Minagi H 1975 Renal trauma
    and retroperitoneal haematomas. Indications for
    exploration, Journal of Trauma 15: 1045-1052
Lang E K 1975 Arteriography in the assessment of renal
    trauma. The impact of arteriographic diagnosis on
    preservation of renal function and parenchyma. Journal of
    Trauma 15: 553-566
Radwin H M, Fitch W P, Ribison J R 1976 A unified
    concept of renal trauma. Journal of Urology 116: 20-22

Injuries of ureter

General features
Uncommon. Caused by blunt or penetrating
    injuries
Often delayed diagnosis
Associated with intra-abdominal lesions
Lesion in lower ureter often due to surgery

Clinical features
Pain in loin. Later swelling
Diminished urinary output
Hematuria-very variable
Shifting dullness
Ureteric fistula with "incontinence" in lower
    lesions

Radiological features
Features of other injuries if present
Blurring of psoas shadow
I.V.P. may show:
    Non functioning kidney on injured side or
        extravasation of dye into tissues from ureter
        with dilation of ureter above fistula

Pathological features
Ureter fairly mobile with posterior peritoneum
Upper: Associated with renal, duodenal and
    splenic injuries
Middle: Gun shot wounds or penetrating injuries
Lower: Damaged by pelvic surgery particularly in
    women or by obstetrical surgery

Treatment
Drainage –
    affected ureter, or damaged kidney at
    site of injury
Repair – mid – upper regions
Re-implantation – lower regions: avoid reflux

Surgical injury
Immediately recognised –
    ureteric catheterisation
    immediate repair

Delayed recognition A. Unilateral
1. No symptoms – renal atrophy. No action
2. Lumbar pain } Nephrostomy
   Hydronephrosis } Secondary ureteric repair
   Pyonephrosis
3. Urinary fistula } Nephrostomy
                   } Secondary ureteric repair

Delayed recognition B. Bilateral
Anuria
Explore surgical wound
Remove ligatures
Repair ureter over catheter
    or re-implant ureter into bladder

References
Eikenberg H U, Amin M 1976 Gunshot wounds of ureter.
    Journal of Trauma 16: 562-572
Evans R A, Smith M J 1976 Violent injuries to the upper
    ureter. Journal of Trauma 16: 558-561

Intraperitoneal injuries of bladder

General features
M : F = 70.1
Usually due to blunt abdominal trauma
Less often due to penetrating injuries
   i.e. gun shot wounds
      stabbing, etc.
Virtually always occurs when bladder is full
Diagnosis may be delayed for several days

Clinical features
Abdominal pain—may pass off temporarily if
   patient is drunk or drugged
External wound may be present
A few drops of blood stained urine
Inability to urinate thereafter
Impalpable bladder

Later
Abdominal distension
Paralytic ileus
Shifting dullness
Paracentesis may produce urine

Radiological features
Abdominal films usually normal at first
(Unless penetrating wounds produce
   foreign bodies or
   gas under diaphragm)

Contrast studies
I.V.P.
Cystogram } Extra vesical leakage of contrast
False negatives are possible

Pathological features
Other organs may be damaged by penetrating
   wounds
Dome of bladder usual site of rupture
Urine in peritoneum remains sterile for long
   periods, unless bladder is infected at time of
   injury

Treatment
Laparotomy. Peritoneal toilet
Suture of bladder
Drainage of bladder and peritoneum

References
Brosman S A, Paul J G 1976 Trauma of the Bladder.
   Surgery, Gynaecology and Obstetrics 143: 605-608
Carswell J W 1974 Intraperitoneal rupture of the bladder.
   British Journal of Urology 46: 425-429
Cass A S 1976 Bladder trauma in the multiple injured
   patient. Journal of Urology 115: 667-669

Extra peritoneal injuries of bladder

General features
Usually due to fractures of pelvis
Less commonly due to penetrating wounds
   i.e. rectal trauma
      gun shot wounds, etc.
Extra-peritoneal rupture : Intra-peritoneal
   = 6 : 1

Clinical features
Pain
External wound may be present
A little blood stained urine may be passed
Thereafter inability to micturate: There may be
   an intense desire to do so
Bladder is impalpable
Prostate in normal position – distinguishes
   rupture of membranous urethra
Extravasation of urine into pelvis and lower
   abdominal wall may be mistaken for a full
   bladder
Catheterisation produces a small volume of
   blood stained urine

Note
30% of fractured pelves suffer retention of urine
   without bladder damage
30% of hematuria is due to bladder contusion
   without rupture

Radiological features
Fracture of pelvis usually present – usually pubic
   rami
Penetrating wounds may lead to gas above
   diaphragm
Contrast studies:
   I.V.P.
   Cystogram } Extra vesical leakage of contrast
False negatives are possible
'Tear drop' bladder shape is characteristic

Pathological features

Other pelvic injuries may be present (particularly rectum)

Rupture occurs around base of bladder

Urine leaks into tissues of pelvis and lower abdominal wall

Infection and abscess formation possible if neglected

Iatrogenic injuries to bladder

Surgical:

  Herniorrhaphy

  Hysterectomy

  Excision of rectum

  Endoscopy of bladder

Sexual perversions

Treatment

1. Operative

Suprapubic extra peritoneal approach

Repair of rupture

Drainage of bladder and prevesical space

2. Conservative:

Indications:

  1. Long delayed treatment

    Distance

    Delayed diagnosis

    Multiple trauma

  2. Urine is sterile

Procedure

Urinary catheter

Antibiotics

References:

Carswell J W 1974 Intraperitoneal rupture of the bladder. British Journal of Urology 46: 425-429

Cass A S 1976 Bladder trauma in the multiple injured patient. Journal of Urology 115: 667-669

Robarts V L et al 1976 Treatment of rupture of the bladder. Journal of Urology 116: 178-179

Injuries of membranous urethra.

General features

Usually due to pelvic fractures

Less often due to

  gunshot wounds

  rectal injuries

  urethral instrumentation

Clinical features

Pain swelling

Tenderness Bruising } in perineum

Urethral bleeding

Inability to micturate } Cardinal signs

Palpable bladder

Prostate will be high or impalpable on rectal examination

Subcutaneous extravasation of urine may occur if patient attempts to micturate

Radiological features

Abnormal urethrogram with contrast in retropubic and perineal tissues

Fractures of pubic rami or pubic symphysis usually present with displacement of fragments

Pathological features

Prostate and bladder become widely displaced from distal urethra in complete ruptures

Stricture formation in 60-80% of repairs

Sexual impotence in 60%

Treatment

Direct suture is technically impossible

2 schools of thought

(1) Suprapubic exploration and bladder drainage

  Attempted urethral repair

  Bladder traction through urethral catheter

(2) Suprapubic cystostomy immediately

  Much later, urethral exploration if necessary

References

Blandy J 1975 Injuries of the urethra in the male. Injury 7: 77-83

Comisarow R H 1978 Posterior urethral injuries in the fractured pelvis. Annals of Royal College of Surgeons of Canada 11: 319-320

Jackson D H, Williams J L 1974 Urethral injury: a retrospective study. British Journal of Urology 46: 665-676

Mitchell J P 1975 Trauma to the urethra. Injury 7: 84-88

Injuries of bulbous urethra

General features
Common. M : F = 10 : 1
Caused by falling astride sharp objects
  Fractures of pelvis
  Gunshot wounds
Bulbous urethra more often injured than
  membranous urethra

Clinical features
Pain, tenderness ⎫
Swelling, Bruising ⎭ in perineum
Inability to micturate when injury is severe
Urethral bleeding
Bladder becomes palpable
Prostate in normal relationship on rectal
  examination
If patient attempts to urinate, subcutaneous
  extravasation of urine occurs in lower
  abdominal wall and perineum

Radiological features
Abnormal urethrogram with extravasation of
  contrast into perineum
Fracture of pubic rami or symphysis may be
  present

Pathological features
Variable damage:
  Mucosal tear
  Incomplete rupture
  Complete rupture
  Urethral fistula
Due to crushing or tearing
Tissues heal well but with fibrosis and stricture
  formation
Fistulae persist without formal repair

Treatment
Catheterise in operating room
Explore perineum
Repair urethra around catheter: suprapubic
  drainage
Prolonged search for divided ends may be
  necessary.
  Complete suture may be impossible but as
    much as the circumference is possible should
    be anastomosed around catheter.

References
Blandy J 1975 Injuries of the urethra in the male. Injury 7: 77-83
Kiracofe H L, Pfister R R, Peterson N E 1975 Management of non-penetrating distal urethral trauma. Journal of Urology 114: 57-62
Macleod D A D 1976 Anterior urethral injuries. Injury 8: 25-30

Injuries of uterus

General features
Rare from external trauma
Commoner from surgical or obstetrical mishaps
Usually occurs in the gravid uterus

Clinical features
Pain
Hypovolemic shock
Abdominal guarding and tenderness
Fetus may be unusually palpable
  Inactive
  Absent heart sounds

Radiological features
Gas under diaphragm in penetrating wounds
Fractured pelvis ⎫
Fetal fractures ⎬ may be present
Foreign bodies ⎭

Pathological features

Gravid uterus: mechanisms
Rupture from abdominal blow
  seat belt injury
  fracture of pelvis
Lacerations from stab wounds
  gun shot wounds
  abortion attempts
  fetal monitoring procedures
Death of fetus may follow injury

Non gravid uterus: mechanisms
Avulsion from severe pelvic fractures
Puncture from uterine sound or curette
  endometrial biopsy
  contraceptive device
Lacerations from stab wounds
  gunshot wounds

Treatment

Gravid uterus:
Blood volume replacement
Laparotomy
Removal of products of conception
Repair of uterus
Hysterectomy for
    large tear
    massive hemorrhage

Non-gravid uterus
Repair uterus
Hysterectomy considered in old women

Puncture of uterus
Observe vital signs
Aspirate stomach
Maintain fluid balance
Laparotomy for hemorrhage or infection

References

Allen J R et al 1972 Removal of intra-uterine contraceptive
    devices after uterine perforation. Obstetrics and
    Gynaecology 40: 225-230
Haver Kamp A, Bowes W A 1971 Uterine perforation, a
    complication of continuous fetal monitoring. American
    Journal of Obstetrics and Gynaecology 110: 667-669
Knapp R C, Drucker D H 1972 Self inflicted stab wounds to
    pregnant uterus and fetus at term. New York State Journal
    of Medicine 72: 391-392
McNabney W K 1972 Penetrating wounds of the gravid
    uterus. Journal of Trauma 12: 1024-1028
Rubvits F E 1964 Traumatic rupture of the pregnant uterus
    from seat belt injury. American Journal of Obstetrics and
    Gynaecology 90: 828-829
Sprague A D, Jenkins V R 1973 Perforation of the uterus
    with a shield intra-uterine device. Obstetrics and
    Gynaecology 41: 80-82
Williams J J 1974 Uterine injuries complicating hypertonic
    saline abortion. Canadian Medical Association Journal
    111: 1223-1224

Injuries of vagina

General features
Rare
Usually present to a Casualty Department or a
    Gynaecologist
May occur in isolation or in association with
    abdominal and pelvic injuries

Clinical features
Pain. Vaginal bleeding.
Perineal lacerations may be visible

Rarely:
    Intestinal prolapse
    Urinary incontinence
    Pelvic fracture(s)
Neglected cases
    Pyrexia and malaise: Pelvic abscess
    Abdominal distension and vomiting: Paralytic
        Ileus

Radiographic features
Usually none
Pelvic fracture ⎫
Foreign bodies ⎬ may be visible
Gas under diaphragm if peritoneum has been
    perforated

Pathological features

Mechanisms of injury
Increased pressure:
    Compressed air
    Syringing
    Water ski-ing accidents
Coitus
Pelvic fractures
Childbirth
Surgery
Self inflicted in abortion attempts

Pre-disposing factors
Previous pelvic surgery or radio therapy
Postmenopausal involution

Situations of lesion
Vault:
    Tears ⎫
    Perforations ⎬ Intestines may prolapse
Walls:
    Lacerations ⎫
    Tears ⎬ Profuse bleeding may occur
    Vesico-vaginal fistula after childbirth produces
    urinary incontinence

Treatment
Accurate diagnosis
Urinary catheterisation for all but minor injuries
Suture of lacerations
Repair of vault ruptures with replacement of
    viscera
Repair of a vesico-vaginal fistula is a specialist
    gynaecological procedure

References
Ikempe J O, Morison C R 1970 Vaginal avulsion
    complicating pelvic fracture. British Journal of Surgery 57:
    317-318

Rolf B B 1970 Vaginal evisceration. American Journal of Obstetrics and Gynaecology 107: 369-375

Tweedale P G 1973 Gynaecological hazards of water ski-ing. Canadian Medical Association Journal 108: 20-22

Wilson T, Swartz 1972 Coital injuries of the vagina. Obstetrics and Gynaecology 39: 182-184

Injuries of vulva

General features
Uncommon
Usually associated with other injuries.

Clinical features
Pain
Hemorrhage

Pathological features
Types of Injury:
Lacerations ⎫
Avulsion   ⎬ Profuse bleeding may occur
Mutilation ⎭
Female circumcision (in Africans)
Burns – Clothing
Chemical Injury: Abortion with Potassium Permanganate

Treatment
Debridement
Lacerations: Suture
Burns: Exposure
Skin grafting for total skin loss
Chemicals: Irrigation to remove remaining chemicals
Exposure and later skin grafting for areas of total skin loss

Injuries of testis

General features
Uncommon because of position and mobility
Bilateral injuries very uncommon

Clinical features
Severity of injury often overlooked
Pain
Swelling and bruising of scrotum
Avulsion of testes produces shock
Lacerations produce severe bleeding

Radiological features
Nil per se.
Pelvic fracture(s) may be present

Pathological features
Hematoma:
Usually associated with a hematocele
Rupture:
Testis is mobile and has a firm covering
Must be trapped against symphysis pubis for rupture
Dislocation:
Usually displaced into lower abdominal wall
There appears to be no record of subsequent post traumatic testicular viability, or biopsy.
Torsion:
May occur spontaneously or after minor injury in adolescence
Testicular atrophy may follow
Avulsion:
Usually occurs in machinery accidents ('Power take-off' tractor injuries)
Penis and Scrotum also avulsed

Differential diagnosis:
Hematoma, Rupture, Torsion, may mimic Epididymo-orchitis or hydrocele

Treatment
Explore scrotum if in doubt about diagnosis:
Hematoma:
Scrotal support, Cold compress, Analgesics Drain hematocele

Rupture   ⎧ Explore scortum
Dislocation ⎪ Relocate testis
Torsion   ⎨ Repair rupture (Orchidectomy if devitalised)
            ⎩ Drain scrotum
Avulsion:
Tie off cord structures
Skin graft symphyseal region if required
Re-establish urethral orifice
Gunshot Wounds
& Lacerations:
Wound toilet
Repair structures
Drain scrotum

References
Goulding F J 1976 Traumatic dislocation of testis. Addition of 2 cases with a changing etiology. Journal of Trauma 16: 1000-1002

Schulman C C 1974 Traumatic rupture of the testicle. An underestimated pathology. Urology International 29: 31-33

McGinnis T B, Redman J F, Bissada N K 1974 High bilateral funiculo-orchiectomy. Secondary to avulsion injury. Urology 4: 596-597

Injuries of scrotum

General features:
Uncommon because of situation and mobility of scrotum and contents
Machinery accidents and gun shot wounds main causative agents
Testes, penis and urethra may also be damaged.

Clinical features
Pain
Hemorrhage
Shock is variable
Minimal:
  in skin avulsion
Maximal:
  if testes are avulsed
  if pelvic fracture is present
Hematocele:
  Tense, painful discoloured swelling

Radiographic features
None per se
Pelvic fracture(s) may be present
Urethrography may show associated urethral damage

Pathological features
Avulsions:
  Minor: Trouser zipper injury
  Major:
    Moving machinery may tear clothing and scrotal skin (Power take off drive in tractors)
  Testes usually intact
Lacerations:
  Gun shot wounds – usually warfare
  (Self) Mutilation
  Genitalia and pelvis may have other injuries
Contusions:
  Caused by
    falling astride
    blow from football
    kick in perineum
  Large hematocele possible as scrotal skin is so distensible
Burns:
  Arise from clothing burning or scalding from hot liquids or steam
  Corrugated scrotal skin usually partly survives in the depressions
  Full thickness burns are uncommon

Treatment
Hematocele: Drainage
Avulsion of scrotal skin:
  Partial loss: suture
  Total loss:
    Bury testes in thigh skin pouches
    Graft penis as required
Lacerations:
  Check penis, urethra, perineum, rectum and abdomen
  Explore scrotum and contents
  Suture and drain
  Treat other injuries as required
Burns:
  Exposure treatment
  Urethral catheter may be necessary
  Graft rarely required
Full thickness loss:
  Excise
  Suture remaining skin if possible
  Otherwise bury viable testis in thigh skin pouch

References
Culp D A 1977 Genital injuries. Etiology and initial management. Urologic Clinics of North America 4:, 143-156

Glover W L et al 1974 Massive scrotal subcutaneous and retroperitoneal emphysema following scortal laceration. A case report. Journal of Urology 112: 498-500

Malherbe W D 1975 Injuries to the skin of the male external genitalia in Southern Africa. Southern African Medical Journal 49: 147-152

Redman J F, Rountree G A, Bissada N K 1976 Injuries to the scrotal contents by blunt trauma. Urology 7: 190-191, et seq.

Sangmit S 1975 Reconstruction of the penoscrotal skin after avulsion. International Surgery 60: 563-565

Injuries of penis

General features
Uncommon because of position and mobility
Gunshot wounds most mutilating
Often associated with other genital and pelvic injuries

Clinical features
Pain
Hemorrhage
Retention of Urine or Dysuria
Avulsion injuries lead to shock
Fracture produces deformity

Radiological features
Nil per se.
Fracture(s) of pelvis may be present
Urethrography may show leakage of contrast

Pathological features
1. Degloving of skin: Machinery accidents
2. Avulsion: Machinery accidents
3. Amputation:
    Gunshot wounds
    Mutilation/Stabbing
    Accidental at circumcision
4. Preputial lacerations: Zipper accidents
5. Fracture:
    Violence during erection
    May later lead to chordee
6. Gangrene: Constricting bands (often from sexual perversions)

Treatment
1. Degloving: Grafting – split skin grafts or avulsed skin
2. Avulsion:
    Wound toilet
    Refashion urethral orifice
    Graft degloved perineum
3. Amputation:
    Surgical wound toilet and repair of urethra
    (Microsurgical replantation may be possible)
4. Preputial lacerations:
    Remove zipper if trapped
    Repair laceration or circumcise
5. Fracture: Suture of corpora cavernosa
6. Gangrene:
    Amputation
    Repair of urethral orifice
7. Burns:
    Preserve as much as possible
    Graft areas of total skin loss

References
Culp D A 1977 Genital injuries etiology and initial management. Urologic Clinics of North America 4: 143-156
Flowerdew R, Fishman I J, Churchill B M 1977 Management of penile zipper injury. Journal of Urology 117: 671
Gross M, Arnold T L, Peters P 1977 Fracture of the penis with associated lacerations of the urethra. Journal of Urology 117: 725-727
Sharma L K, Koshal A, Prakash A 1973) Degloving injury of the penis. International Surgery 58: 648
Tamai S, Nakamura Y, Motomiya Y 1977 Microsurgical replantation of a completely amputated penis and scrotum. Plastic and Reconstructive surgery, 60: 287-291
Taguchi H, Saito K, Yamada T 1977 A simple method of total reconstruction of the penis. Plastic and Reconstructive Surgery 60: 454-456

SPINAL INJURIES

Anatomy of odontoid

Ossification
A. 1 centre for body of axis
    Appears at 4th intrauterine mouth
B. 2 lateral centres for odontoid base
    Appear at 5th intrauterine mouth
C. 1 centre for apex of odontoid
    Appears between 2 and 5 years
2 centres of B fuse in 2nd year
A and B fuse at 3 or 4 years
B and C fuse between 10 and 13 years

Radiographic appearance
Os odontoideum:
    Smooth rounded appearance
    Lies above level of lateral processes of atlas
Fracture of base of odontoid:
    Irregular transverse line
    Lies below level of lateral processes of atlas
Odontoid may be absent

Blood supply
Paired ascending posterior and anterior vessels
    from vertebral arteries
Anastomosis around apex of odontoid
Additional vessels in accessory ligaments

Injury
Odontoid – Anterior atlantal arch measurements
    1-3 mm. Normal in children
    4-5 mm. Normal in adults
    5-6 mm. Disruption of transverse ligament
    6-10 mm. Additional ligamentous damage
    10 + mm. All ligaments damaged
Ondine's curse: sleep induced apnoea

References
Schiff D C M, Parke W W 1973 The arterial supply of the odontoid process. Journal of Bone and Joint Surgery 55A: 1450-1456
Wollin D G 1963 The os odontoideum. Journal of Bone and Joint Surgery 45A: 1459-1471

Fractures of atlas

General features
Rare
Caused by:
    blow on vertex
    falling on feet with body extended
May cause instant death by medullary damage
50% survive

Clinical features
Occipital pain worsened by movement
Patient holds his head in his hands
Local tenderness
Rarely:
    Occipital neurological deficit
    Retropharyngeal swelling

Radiological features
Interpretation often difficult because
1. Congenital anomalies may be present
2. 4 mm. asymmetry is within normal variation in A.P. views
3. Mandible and teeth may obscure A.P. views
Open mouth views – lateral masses may be splayed apart
Oblique lateral views centred on C3 will show whole of atlantal ring.
Tomography may resolve difficulties

Pathological features
Anterior and/or posterior part of ring may fracture – Usually posterior
Transverse ligament may rupture
Delayed or mal union may cause atlanto-axial instability
Vertebral artery may rupture causing medullary compression and death

Treatment
Displaced: Skull traction 4-6 weeks
Undisplaced: Cranio-thoracic orthosis
Persistent pain
Instability }Later atlanto-axial-occipital fusion

References
Childers J C, Wilson F C 1971 Bipartite atlas. Journal of Bone and Joint Surgery 53A: 578-582
Fielding J W et al 1974 Tears of the transverse ligament of the atlas. Journal of Bone and Joint Surgery 56A: 1683-1691
Sherk H H, Nicholson J T 1970 Fractures of the atlas. Journal of Bone and Joint Surgery 52A: 1017-1024

Fractures of odontoid

General features
Occur from flexion or extension forces
Usually in road accidents
Often associated with other atlanto-axial fractures
Differentiation from congenital non-fusion of odontoid may be difficult
Rare in children

Clinical features:
Pain in occipital region
Local tenderness
Limited movement
Diagnosis often delayed, particularly in the elderly

Radiological features
Usual fracture line lies transversely through base of odontoid
Open-mouth AP views essential
Lateral views to show relationship of odontoid and anterior arch of atlas
Tomography valuable
Congenital non-fusion usually shows as a transverse gap above odontoid base

Pathological features
Displacement may cause instant death
Survivors usually have a moderately stable fracture
Displacement can be gently corrected
Osseous union occurs in only 50%
Late myelopathy may arise from instability

Treatment
Displacement:
    Reduction by skull or halter traction
    Flexion or extension as indicated by radiographs
Splintage:
    Youngsters:
        Minerva cast
        Halo pelvic fixation
Oldsters:
    Moulded occipito-cervical collar
Non Union:
    Youngsters:
        Occipito-cervical fusion or atlanto axial fusion

Oldsters:
    No treatment, little significant morbidity

References
Anderson L D, D'Alonzo R T 1974 Fractures of the odontoid process of the atlas. Journal of Bone and Joint Surgery 56A: 1663-1674
Schiff D C M, Parke W W 1973 The arterial supply of the odontoid process. Journal of Bone and Joint Surgery 55A: 1450-1456
Simon L P 1977 Fracture of the odontoid in young children. Journal of Bone and Joint Surgery 59A: 943-948
Wollin D G 1963 The os odontoideum. Journal of Bone and Joint Surgery 45A: 1459-1471

Posterior axial fractures

Synonym
Hangman's fracture

General features
Rare
Usually from road traffic accidents
(Also occurs from hanging)
Diagnosis may be delayed

Clinical features
Pain, limited movement
Local tenderness
Pharyngeal edema
Occipital neuritis
Transient quadriplegia
Skin markings in hanging accidents

Radiological features
Fracture through lateral masses or pedicles of axis
Odontoid not fractured
Fragments distracted in hanging accidents
Spondylolisthesis of anterior axis may occur

Pathological features
Instant death may occur
Survival with no notable neurological deficit is the alternative
C2-3 inter-body ankylosis often occurs during healing phase

Treatment
Skull traction for reduction (but not, in hanging or distraction injuries)

Splintage:
    Custom made plastic collar
    Minerva plaster
    Occipito-cervical fusion not often required

References
Brashear H R, Venters G C, Preston E T 1975 Fractures of
    the neural arch of the axis. Journal of Bone and Joint
    Surgery 57A: 879-887
Williams T G 1975 Hangman's fracture. Journal of Bone and
    Joint Surgery 57B: 82-88

Atlanto-axial fracture dislocation

General features
Uncommon
Due to violent forces acting on the head in
    flexion or extension

Clinical features
Pain, limited movement
Local tenderness
No deformity visible
sometimes present:
Pharyngeal swelling
Occipital neuritis

Radiological features
Fracture through base of odontoid
Atlas and odontoid move –
    Forward in flexion injuries
    Backwards in extension injuries

Pathological features
Less damage to cord than in dislocation of atlas
    alone (rupture of transverse ligament)
Flexion injuries commoner in youngsters
Extension injuries commoner in oldsters

Treatment

Reduction
Skull or halter traction
Radiographs indicate flexion or extension
    movements to restore normal alignment

Splintage
Oldsters:
    Moulded cervical collar

Youngsters:
    Minerva cast
    Halo pelvic fixation
    Occipito-cervical fusion

Late instability
Occipito-cervical fusion or atlanto-axial fusion

Reference
Fried L C 1973 Atlanto-axial fracture dislocations. Journal of
    Bone and Joint Surgery 55B: 490-496

Traumatic atlanto-axial dislocation

General features
Very rare without a local fracture
Caused by major violence to head
Odontoid slips out of atlantal ring

Clinical features
Transient quadriplegia
Pain and stiffness of neck
Laryngeal and pharyngeal paralysis
Occipital neuritis
Other injuries often present

Radiological features
Odontoid lies anterior to atlas

Pathological features
Retro-pharyngeal hematoma
Gross instability of atlanto-axial joint
Sudden movement may provoke fatal cervical
    cord damage

Treatment

Skull traction
Increasing traction in extension
Reduced weight in flexion after reduction

Splintage
Youngsters:
    Minerva plaster
    Occipito-cervical fusions or atlanto-axial fusion
Oldsters:
    Custom made collar

References

Patzakis M et al 1974 Posterior dislocation of the atlas on the axis. Journal of Bone and Joint Surgery 56A: 1260-1262

Sassard W R, Heinig C F, Pitts W R 1974 Posterior atlanto-axial dislocation without fracture. Journal of Bone and Joint Surgery 56A: 625-628

Wigren A, Amici F 1973 Traumatic atlanto-axial dislocation without neurological disorder. Journal of Bone and Joint Surgery 55A: 642-644

Non-traumatic atlanto-axial subluxation

General features

Uncommon

Associations:

Youngsters:

Sepsis in nasopharynx or cervical spine

Mongolism

Mucopolysaccharoidoses

Oldsters:

Rheumatoid Arthritis

Symptoms arise and diagnosis made after a minor injury in some cases

Clinical features

Insidious onset usually

Stiff painful neck

Tilting and rotation of head (See Pathology section)

Occipital neuritis

Transient quadriplegia on movement

Radiological features

Normal measurements

Anterior Atlas Arch to Odontoid

2-3 mm. in children

4-5 mm. in adults

Increased in subluxation

Cineradiography shows abnormal atlanto-axial movement

Pathological features

Caused by laxity or softening of transverse atlantal ligament

Sullivan's classification

Anterior Unilateral:

Head rotated away but tilted towards affected side

Posterior Unilateral:

Head rotated towards affected side

Anterior arch of atlas impalpable in pharynx

Anterior Bilateral:

Head tilted forwards

No rotation

Treatment

Youngsters

Correct infective focus if causative

Skull traction for reduction

Atlanto-axial fusion for stability

Oldsters

Cervical collar

Occipito cervical fusion rarely required or tolerated

References

Fielding J W, Hawkins R J, Ratzan S A 1976 Spine fusion for atlanto-axial instability. Journal of Bone and Joint Surgery 58A: 400-407

Hunter G A 1968 Non-traumatic displacement of the atlanto-axial joint. Journal of Bone and Joint Surgery 50B: 44-51

Sullivan A W 1949 Subluxation of the atlanto-axial joint sequel to inflammatory processes of neck. Journal of Pediatrics 35: 451-464

Atlanto-axial rotatory fixation

General features

Usually transient with spontaneous recovery ("Wry neck")

Rarely persistent – diagnosis often long delayed

Clinical features

Torticollis. Head in 'listening' position

Deformity can be increased but not reversed

Painful neck movements

Local infection may be present

Radiological features

Atlanto-axial asymmetry visible on conventional films

Often difficult to interpret because of persistent angulation of neck and head

Tomography ⎱ confirm fixed rotatory subluxation

Cineradiography ⎰ of atlanto-axial joint

Pathological features

Causes
Local infection
Trauma (Minor or major)
Precise nature of rotatory fixation is uncertain

Treatment

Transient fixation:
Intermittent manual or halter traction
Analgesics and muscle relaxants
Persistent fixation:
Skull traction for reduction and
immobilisation
Occipito-cervical arthrodesis

Reference

Fielding J W 1977 Atlanto-axial rotatory fixation. Journal of Bone and Joint Surgery 59A: 37-44

Flexion injuries of cervical spine

General features

Caused by unrestricted flexion of head often with
element of rotation
i.e. Blow on back of head
Deceleration accidents
Frequently associated with
Neurological deficit
Head injuries

Clinical features

Pain. Worse on movement
Local tenderness
Skin injuries to front or back of head
Occasionally associated with 'stove-in chest'

Neurological changes

Spinal Cord: Complete or incomplete section
Cervical Roots: Radicular pain or deficit

Radiological features

Injury usually occurs between C4 and C7

Lateral films

Forward shift of one vertebral body on one
below
Variable fractures:
Front of vertebral bodies
Facets and pedicles
Posterior elements

Widened gap between spinous processes
Essential to visualise spine down to C7

A-P films

Difficult to interpret
Lateral displacement of spinous process may
indicate unilateral facetal dislocation

Oblique films

Show facetal displacement or dislocation
Identification of side is difficult (Beatson, 1963)
i.e. Right side down nearest plate
¾ face down: Right facets seen
¾ back-down: Left facets seen
Twinings manoeuvre may show lower cervical
facets in thickset individuals (lateral view with
one arm and shoulder pulled cranially and the
other depressed caudally)

Pathological features

No correlation between displacement and
neurological damage
i.e. Gross displacement but no neurological
change or No displacement and quadriplegia
Forward displacement can occur from:
Fracture of vertebral body(s) and posterior
elements
Overlapping of one or both facets
Reduction may occur if patient lies flat and still
Irreducible ¼ diameter displacement may indicate
dislocation of one facetal joint.
Irreducible ½ diameter displacement may
indicate dislocation of both facetal joints

Treatment

Reduction

1. Skull traction. Increasing weights ½ hourly
Frequent radiographs
Bilateral facetal dislocations:
Slight flexion
Extension when reduced
Unilateral facetal dislocations:
Flexion and lateral flexion
2. Manipulation under anesthesia
Swift but hazardous
3. Open reduction: indications:
Irreducible fractures
Advancing neurological deficit

Immobilisation

Skull traction : Quadriplegics
Halo-pelvic traction: Youngsters
Minerva plaster cast: Doubtful value
Plastic collar: Oldsters with stable fractures
Internal fixation: Unstable fractures

Posterior fusion with open reduction
Anterior fusion of doubtful value

Neurological deficit
Skilled nursing
Bladder and bowel drainage
Physiotherapy
(See section on paraplegia)

References

Beatson T R 1963 Fractures and dislocations of the cervical spine. Journal of Bone and Joint Surgery 45B: 21-35
Braakman R, Vinken P J 1968 Old luxations of the lower cervical spine. Journal of Bone and Joint Surgery 50B: 52-60
Burke D C, Berryman D, 1971 The place of closed manipulation in the management of flexion rotation dislocations of the cervical spine. Journal of Bone and Joint Surgery 53B: 165-182
Callahan R A et al 1977 Cervical facet fusion for control of instability following laminectomy. Journal of Bone and Joint Surgery 59A: 991-1001
Evans D K 1976 Anterior cervical subluxation. Journal of Bone and Joint Surgery 58B: 318-321
Stauffer E S, Kelly E G 1977 Fracture-dislocations of cervical spine. Instability and recurrent deformity after anterior interbody fusion. Journal of Bone and Joint Surgery 59A: 45-48
Torg J S et al 1977 Spinal injury at the level of the third and fourth cervical vertebrae from football. Journal of Bone and Joint Surgery 59A: 1015-1019

Bursting injuries of cervical spine

General features
Uncommon
Caused by
1. Blow on top of head
2. Falling on feet with spine extended
Usually an element of flexion or lateral flexion at site of injury

Clinical features
Pain, limited movement
Local tenderness
Usually a severe neurological deficit
1. Complete motor paralysis
   Incomplete sensory paralysis
   Preservation of some proprioception and touch
   Order of recovery: legs, bladder, arms
2. Complete quadriplegia
   No recovery

Radiological features
Vertical height of vertebral body (bodies) is reduced
Body fragments bulge backwards into spinal canal
Fractures of facets or posterior elements are unusual
Cervical spine may be abnormally flexed at point of injury
Myelogram shows blockage but may be contra-indicated in complete lesions

Pathological features
Disc and bone fragments may impinge on front of spinal cord
Posterior columns may be unchanged
Denticulate ligaments may prevent spinal cord riding backwards
Tear drop fragments of bone produce flexion instability of cervical spine

Treatment

Reduction
Skull traction
Consider laminectomy with division of denticulate ligaments to decompress spinal cord

Immobilisation
Skull traction 6 weeks
Occipito-thoracic splintage 6-12 weeks
Consider anterior fusion if no previous laminectomy

References

Petrie J G 1964 Flexion injuries of the cervical spine. Journal of Bone and Joint Surgery 46A: 1800-1806 et seq.
Schneider R C 1955 The syndrome of acute anterior spinal cord injury. Journal of Neurosurgery 12: 95-122
Schneider R C, Kahn E A 1956 Chronic neurological sequelae of acute trauma to the spine and spineal cord. Journal of Bone and Joint Surgery 38A: 985-997

Whiplash injuries of cervical spine

General features
Usually occur in road traffic accidents
Acute acceleration or deceleration forces on unprotected and unsuspecting neck
Rare before motor vehicles

Clinical features
Pain, local tenderness
Restricted neck movement, spasm of trapezius
Brachial neuritis. Usually subjective
Neurological deficit is rare
Persistent symptoms ½-3 years
Worse in the elderly with pre-existing cervical
    spondylosis
Worse when compensation claims are unsettled

Radiological features
Usually none

Early
Rarely tiny avulsion fractures of anterior margins
    of vertebral bodies
Post-oesophageal soft tissue swelling
Restricted movement at one or more cervical
    joints on screening

Later
Kinking of normal cervical lordosis may be
    present

Very late
Local osteophyte formation

Pathological features
Ill defined
Surgical or postmortem examination rarely
    possible
Probably muscular and ligamentous damage to 1,
    2 or 3 intervertebral joints

Treatment
Collar
Analgesics (No addictive drugs)
Reassurance
Physiotherapy:
    Heat
    Traction
    Exercises
Anterior cervical fusion for
    Persistent symptoms
    Localised demonstrable lesions
    Young patient

Reference
Hohl M 1974 Soft tissue injuries of the neck in automobile
    accidents. Journal of Bone and Joint Surgery 56A: 1675-
    1682

Hyperextension injuries of cervical spine

General features
More commonly recognised
30% of all cervical injuries
Mechanism:
    Blow on front of head
    Acceleration of body (as in rear end collisions)

Clinical features
Pain, worse on movement
Local tenderness
No deformity visible

Cord lesion varients
1. Sensation and proprioception lost below level
    of injury
    Pain and temperature lost with some motor
    loss
2. Acute central cord injury
    Paralysed hands, weak arms
    Paralysed sphincters, weak legs
3. Complete quadriplegia

Cervical root lesions
Brachial neuritis. Pain and paresthesia
Radicular motor and sensory loss

Radiological features
Alone or in combination (sometimes none seen)
Anterior soft tissue swelling posterior to
    esophagus
Fragment(s) avulsed from anterior margins of
    vertebral bodies
Fractures of posterior elements
No correlation of radiographic and clinical
    findings

Pathological features
The more rigid the spine, the more severe the
    skeletal and/or neurological damage
    (ankylosing spondylitis and cervical
    spondylosis)
Rupture of anterior longitudinal ligament
Buckling of ligamentum flavum may damage
    posterior tracts of cord

Fracture of articular masses
Recoil of head may lead to a final position of flexion dislocation

Treatment

No cord lesion
Youngsters
   No fracture: Collar
   Fracture   Collar (cranio-thoracic)
                 Minerva cast of doubtful value
   Late Instability: Anterior cervical fusion
Oldsters
   No fracture: Collar
   Fracture: Collar
   Late Instability: Collar
                 Consider fusion

Cord Lesion
Youngsters
   Skull traction
   Posterior cervical decompression
Oldsters
   Collar
   Physiotherapy
   Late Instability: Consider anterior
                    cervical fusion

References

Burke D C 1971 Hyperextension injuries of the spine. Journal of Bone and Joint Surgery 53B: 3-12
Guttman L 1966 Traumatic paraplegia and quadriplegia in ankylosing spondylitis. Paraplegia 4: 188-203
Lewin W 1965 Cerebral effects of injury to the vertebral artery. British Journal of Surgery 52: 223-225
Marar B C 1974 The pattern of neurological damage as an aid to the diagnosis of the mechanism in cervical spine injuries. Journal of Bone and Joint Surgery 56A: 1648-1654

Fractures of cervico-dorsal spines

Synonym
Shovellers' fracture

General features
Less common nowadays with less laborious work
Due to muscular pull

Clinical features
Sudden pain and tenderness during hard physical activity
Relieved by rest, worsened by activity

Radiological features
Fracture of spine of T1, less often C7 or C6
Difficult to obtain clear views of this region due to skeletal overlap

Pathological features
Fibrous union common
Does not impede function

Treatment
Rest until pain subsides
Extension or internal fixation never required

References

Hall R D McK 1940 Clay shoveller's fracture. Journal of Bone and Joint Surgery 22: 63-75
Zollinger F 1937 Isolierte dormfortsatzbruche mit besondere berucksichtigung der muskelzugfrakturen (schipper krankheit). Schweizishe Medizinische Wochenschrift 18: 485-505

Fractures of thoracic spine

General features
Normal bone: Injured by major violence
Abnormal bone: Injured by trivial violence
Usually flexion-compression effects
Fractures are splinted by rib cage
Overlapped fracture of sternum may be present

Clinical features
Pain, worse on movement
Tenderness over local kyphus
Minimal swelling and bruising visible

Neurological changes
5% of all thoracic spinal injuries
Paraplegia below level of injury
Local radiculitis is unusual

Radiological features

Normal bone
1 or 2 vertebral bodies variably compressed
Displacement only in very violent injuries

Abnormal bone
1 or several bodies compressed
Bone destruction –
   neoplasm
   infection
Rarefaction:
   Osteoporosis
   Osteomalacia
   Osteogenesis imperfecta
Paravertebral shadows: infection
Hemothorax may be visible on erect films

Paraplegia
Local blockage to CSF flow on myelogram

Pathological features
Spinal canal narrows in thoracic region
Even minimal further narrowing may result in
   paraplegia

Normal bone
Fractures usually stable
Rapidly become pain free

Abnormal bone
Very wide range of conditions may lead to
   compression fractures
Single vertebra or whole skeleton may be
   involved
Condition may be progressive

Treatment

1. No neurological change
Normal bone:
   Bed rest until pain free
   Extension exercises
   Thoracolumbar brace for 6-12 weeks for more
      severe injuries (doubtful value)
Abnormal bone:
   Make accurate diagnosis
   Vertebral biopsy if necessary
   Give appropriate treatment, i.e. Antibiotics,
      Vit. D., Radiotherapy, etc.
   Thoraco-lumbar brace until fracture has healed
      (doubtful value)

2. Neurological change
Normal bone:
   Consider decompression of cord
   Bed rest for 6 weeks
   Special nursing care
   Paraplegic rehabilitation
Abnormal bone:
   Decompression – accurate diagnosis

   Bed rest
   Special nursing care
Youngsters:
   Paraplegic rehabilitation
Oldsters:
   Consider brace or corset
   Rehabilitation within limits of physique and
      life expectancy

Fractures of thoraco-lumbar spine

General features
Common injury
Normal bone: Major violence
Abnormal bone: Minor violence

Clinical features
Tender localised kyphus
Pain – worsened on attempted movement
Later:
   paralytic ileus } often occurs after
   bruising in loin } major violence

Neurological changes
Unlikely in minor injuries with normal bone
If present may be (progressively)
1. Local radiculitis – pain and hyperesthesia in
   lower abdomen, groin and legs
2. Perineal anesthesia and absent perineal reflexes
3. Paraplegia

Radiological features
Indications of instability
Compression of one or more vertebral bodies
Displacement
Fractures of neural arches
(Reduction may have occurred by laying patient
   supine)
Hematoma may obscure psoas shadows

Pathological features
Varieties of neurological damage

Cord and roots
Complete paraplegia below level of injury
Roots may recover

Cord only
Perineal anesthesia

Paralysis of bladder and bowel
Recovery unlikely

Roots only
Paralysis of legs
Variable recovery likely
Retroperitoneal hematoma may cause
hypovolemic shock. Paralytic ileus for 1-3 days

Later
Spinal deformity may persist
Local osteo-arthrosis
30% symptomless
50% some symptoms
20% incapacitated – mostly in patients treated
conservatively

Treatment
Abnormal bone: Make accurate diagnosis

No neurological change
Stable fracture:
Bed rest 6 weeks
Early extension exercises
Spinal brace 6-12 weeks
Unstable:
Internal fixation
Bed rest 6-12 weeks: Turning beds useful
Later protection with brace

Neurological changes
Stable fracture:
Bed rest with skilled nursing
If not available:
Internal fixation rarely indicated
Unstable fracture:
Open reduction
Internal fixation
Paraplegic nursing regime
Open reduction
Particularly indicated for
Irreducible dislocation
Advancing neurological deficit
Internal fixation is temporary and will cut out
unless supplemented by local fusion as a
primary or secondary procedure

References
Burke D C, Murray D D 1976 The management of thoracic and thoraco-lumbar injuries of the spine with neurological involvement. Journal of Bone and Joint Surgery 58B: 72-78
Cullen J C 1975 Spinal lesions in battered babies. Journal of Bone and Joint Surgery 57B: 364-366
De Oliveira J C 1978 A new type of fracture dislocation of the thoraco-lumbar spine. Journal of Bone and Joint Surgery 60B: 481-488

Flesch J R et al 1977 Harrington instrumentation and spine fusion for unstable fractures and fracture dislocations of the thoracic and lumbar spine. Journal of Bone and Joint Surgery 59A: 143-153
Holdsworth F W 1963 Fractures, dislocations and fracture dislocations of the spine. Journal of Bone and Joint Surgery 45B: 6-20
Laaveg S J, Sprague B L 1978 Traumatic chylothorax, a complication of fracture – dislocation of the spine. Journal of Bone and Joint Surgery 60A: 708-709
Lewis J, McKibbin B 1974 The treatment of unstable fracture-dislocations of the thoraco-lumbar spine accompanied by paraplegia. Journal of Bone and Joint Surgery 56B: 603-612

Fractures of lumbar vertebral bodies

General features
Commonly seen in osteoporotic spines
Trivial violence
Less often seen in normal spines
Major violence
Usually due to flexion or flexion-rotation
mechanism

Clinical features
Pain, worse on movement
Local tenderness, local bruising in loin
Patient may be able to stand
Gap in interspinous ligament may be palpable
Neurological changes <50%
Perineum spared in fractures below L1
Motor and sensory changes in legs and feet

Radiological features
Indications of instability
Compression of one or more vertebral bodies
Displacement
Fractures of neural arches
Associated fractures of transverse processes
Psoas shadows may be obscured by hematoma

Pathological features
Lumbar spinal canal relatively capacious
Occupied by only canda equina below L1
Nerve roots protected by nerve sheaths
Relatively good prognosis for neurological deficit
Flexion-distraction forces cause horizontal
fracture of posterior elements extending into
body
Flexion-lateral flexion forces cause fracture of
transverse processes

Flexion-rotation forces cause unstable fracture dislocations

Flexion forces alone cause vertebral compression

Treatment

Stable fractures
Bed rest 1-4 weeks
Extension exercises
Spinal brace or corset up to 12 weeks

Unstable fractures
Reduction in hyperextension abandoned
1. Bed rest 6-12 weeks
   Skilled nursing
   Spinal brace or corset 12-20 weeks
2. Internal fixation (Harrington rods and fusion)

Neurological deficit
Maintain joint mobility
Develop remaining muscles
Splint weak joints i.e. Calipers
                      Ankle arthroses
                      Knee arthroses

References

Jacobs R R 1977 Bilateral fracture of the pedicles through the fourth and fifth lumbar vertebrae with anterior displacement of the vertebral bodies. Journal of Bone and Joint Surgery 59A: 409-410
Kaufer H, Hayes J T 1966 Lumbar fracture dislocation. Journal of Bone and Joint Surgery 48A: 712-730
Smith W S, Kaufer H 1969 Patterns and mechanisms of lumbar injuries associated with lap seat belts. Journal of Bone and Joint Surgery 51A: 239-254

Fractures of lumbar transverse processes

General features
Caused by major violence
Resisted lateral flexion of spine
Often associated with other fractures of lumbar spine or pelvis

Clinical features
Severe pain, worse on movement
Local tenderness and later bruising in loin
Hypovolemic shock ⎫ if fractures are
Paralytic ileus   ⎭ widely separated
Neurological changes are rare

Radiological features
Avulsion fractures of one or more transverse processes on one side
Renal and ureteric displacement on I.V.P. if retroperitoneal hematoma is large

Pathological features
Widespread tearing of lumbodorsal fascia
Retroperitoneal hematoma often large
Occasional inter-transverse fusion

Treatment
Bed rest
Blood volume replacement
Progressive physiotherapy
Lumbar belt sometimes required

Reference:
Jackson D W 1975 Unilateral osseous bridging of lumbar transverse processes following trauma. Journal of Bone and Joint Surgery 57A: 125-126

Fractures of sacrum

General features
Isolated fractures are rare
Fractures involving part of pelvic ring are more common
See sections on pelvic fractures
Caused by falling in sitting position

Clinical features
Severe pain. Local tenderness
Little local swelling or bruising visible in fat people
Inability to stand normally
Occasionally:
    Fresh blood per rectum
    Saddle anesthesia
    Bladder and bowel paresthesia

Radiological features
Pars articularis fractures easily visible
Transverse fractures more obscure
Tomography and/or oblique views may give clarification

Pathological features
Displaced fractures may tear rectal walls
– Dangerous – Pelvic sepsis – death possible

Sacral canal may be blocked –
Lower sacral nerve roots compressed
– Good prognosis if decompressed

Treatment

1. No visceral or neurological complications
Bed rest 3-4 weeks until comfortable

2. Rectal Damage
Colostomy and abdominal drainage
Rectal drainage
Antibiotics

3. Saddle paralysis
Sacral laminectomy
Internal fixation by wires or pins rarely required

References

Bucknill T M, Blackburn J S 1976 Fracture dislocations of
   the sacrum. Journal of Bone and Joint Surgery 58B: 467-
   470
Fountain S S, Hamilton R D, Jameson R M 1977 Transverse
   fractures of the sacrum. Journal of Bone and Joint Surgery
   59A: 486-489
Heckman J D, Keats P K 1978 Fracture of the sacrum in a
   child. A case report. Journal of Bone and Joint Surgery
   60A: 405-406

13

SPINAL CORD INJURIES

Treatment of traumatic spinal paralysis

Initial
Resuscitation
Determination of level of paralysis
Diagnosis of other injuries
Diagnosis of nature of spinal injury

Urgent
Reduction of dislocation and/or fracture by
 manipulation or distraction
Stop blood loss, i.e. laparotomy or thoracotomy
Removal of compression forces on spinal cord (if
 any can be identified) usually by laminectomy
 to divide denticulate ligaments (in cervical
 region) and to remove fragments of bone and
 cartilage

Less urgent
Drainage of bladder
Adjustable bed and/or mattress

Non-surgical measures
Turning 2-4 hourly to relieve pressure points
Large regular fluid intake (to avoid urinary stone
 formation)
Regular physiotherapy
 Passive movement of paralysed limbs
 Active exercise for normal muscles
 Breathing exercises
 Avoidance of contractures
Bowel management by Aperients, suppositories
 or manual evacuation
Drugs: Antibiotics for respiratory or urinary
 infections
  Anticoagulants for phlebothrombosis

Gunshot injuries of cord

Other injuries
from bullet or shrapnel passing through chest or
 abdomen
from the fall induced by cord section

from violent muscle spasm induced by cord
 section

Types
Division of cord
Fragment lies intramedullary
 or intradurally
 or extradurally
Ricochet injury of cord – cavitation from high
 velocity bullets
Blast injuries

Treatment
Complete debridement
Laminectomy or opening of dura if required
Antibiotics

References
Haynes W G 1946 Acute war wounds of the spinal cord.
 American Journal of Surgery 72: 424-433
Matson D M 1948 The treatment of acute compound injuries
 of the spinal cord due to missiles. Thomas, Springfield.
Yashon D, Jane J A, White R J 1970 Prognosis and
 management of spinal cord and cauda equina. Bullet
 injuries in sixty five civilians. Journal of Neurosurgery 32:
 63-170

Stab wounds of spinal cord

Clinical features
Rare except in colored South Africans

Often
1. Deliberate attempts to maim by sharp thin
 instruments
2. Thoracic region
3. Other intra-thoracic lesions
4. Incomplete cord lesions (i.e. Brown-Sequard
 syndromes)

Rarely
C.S.F. leakage
Persistent infection
Damage to vertebral column

Treatment
Careful debridement
Antibiotics
Paraplegic nursing care

References

Editorial 1978 British Medical Journal 1: 1093
Lipschitz R 1967 Associated injuries and complications of stab wounds of the spinal cord. Paraplegia 5: 75-81

Spinal cord damage from trauma

General features

Highest level with survival
    Immediate resuscitation and
        permanent respiratory assistance C 1/2
    Permanent respiratory assistance C 3/4
    Without respiratory assistance C4/5
Absence of recovery within 12 hours means
    permanent neurological deficit

Clinical effects of spinal cord section

Immediately
Sensory paralysis
Flaccid motor paralysis
Paralysis of bladder and bowel
Peripheral vasodilation and priapism in levels
    above T9
i.e. A state of 'spinal shock'

Later
Recovery of vasomotor tone 2-3 weeks
Spasticity of paralysed muscles 3-6 weeks
Bladder regains automatic emptying in response
    to peripheral and endogenous stimuli

General
Loss of paralysed muscle mass
Demineralisation of unused part of skeleton
Trophic changes in desensitised skin

Patterns of neurological damage in cervical cord injuries

General features

Often no correspondence to degree of skeletal
    damage
Arms held in statue of liberty position (complete
    C5/6 lesion)
Arms held crossed on chest. No finger flexion.
    (complete C6/7 lesion)
Perineal paralysis and anaesthesia (complete
    S2/3 lesion)
Ipselateral motor paralysis } Brown-Sequard
Contralateral pain and } lesion
    temperature loss
Late onset of paralysis indicates
    1. Mechanical instability at site of injury
or 2. Ischemia of spinal cord

Clinical features

Total transection of cord corresponding to skeletal level
Due to:
    Bursting fractures
    Bilateral dislocation of facets

Total motor loss and patchy sensory loss
Recovery of power in legs, bladder, arms
(Schneider's "acute central spinal cord" injury)
Due to:
    Hyperextension injuries
    Unilateral dislocation of facets

Total motor loss: complete sensory retention
Only arms recover
Due to:
    Compression fractures
    Tear drop fractures

Partial motor loss, no sensory loss
Due to:
    Unilateral fracture dislocations
    Fractures of arch of atlas

Brown Sequard Syndrome
Almost complete motor and sensory recovery
    may be possible

Due to:
Unilateral fracture dislocations
Bursting fractures

Reference

Marar, B. C., (1974) The Pattern of Neurological Damage as an Aid to the Diagnosis of the Mechanism in Cervical Spine Injuries. Journal of Bone and Joint Surgery 56a: 1648-1654

Spinal shock

General features
The results of section of the spinal cord
Duration related to degree of encephalisation
   i.e. 5 minutes in frog
      2+ weeks in man. Prolonged in infection or malnutrition
All spinal reflexes profoundly depressed
Cause is uncertain: Perhaps loss of impulses from above
Cause of recovery is uncertain: Perhaps sprouting of collaterals from injured neurones to give more excitatory endings

Clinical features
Loss of all reflexes
Hypotonia
Hypotension

Recovery
Leg flexors usually first
Other reflexes gradually – threshold steadily falls
Withdrawal reflexes
Positive supporting reflexes
Negative supporting reflexes
Mass reflex to varying noxious stimuli
   i.e. Evacuation of bladder and rectum
      Sweating, pallor
      Hypertension
      Withdrawal response
Labile blood pressure
Fragmented sexual responses

Metabolic changes
Negative nitrogen balance
Catabolism of body protein
Negative calcium balance
(Hypercalciuria, Renal calculi)

Local structural changes from spinal cord section

Recent

Macroscopic
Swollen
Blue/red. Minor hemorrhages
Anterior spinal artery interrupted

Microscopic
Hemorrhages, particularly in grey matter
Edema
Chromatolysis of cells
Fragmented, banded axon cylinders

Later

Macroscopic
Flatter thinner cord
Pial and arachnoid adhesions

Microscopic
Lymphocytic invasions
Absorption of axon cylinders
Microglial proliferation

Remote

Macroscopic
Local vacuolation of cord at or *above* site of injury

Microscopic
Fibroblastic proliferation in cord at and below site of injury

Post-traumatic symptomatic changes
Ascending neural deficit after traumatic cord section probably due to local vascular changes
Axonal regeneration at site of cord section does occur but is functionally ineffective except in very rare cases

References
Wolman L 1963 The neuropathology of traumatic paraplegia. Paraplegia 1: 233-247
Wolman L 1966 Axon regeneration after spinal cord injury. Paraplegia 4: 175-183

Vasomotor changes in spinal paralysis

Lesions above T5:
Normal vasomotor responses lost
Hypotension
Postural fainting
Vasodilation

Hypotension:
Effects worsened by head up position
        lessened by exercise and practice
                Deep breathing

Hypertension:
(often with bradycardia)
Due to:
    distended bladder
    distended intestines
    labour

References
Johnson R H, Park D M, Frankel H L 1971 Orthostatic hypotension and the renin-angiotensin system in paraplegia. Paraplegia 9: 146-152
Nanda R N et al 1974 Cerebral blood flow in paraplegia. Paraplegia 12: 212-217
Silver J R 1970 Vascular reflexes in spinal shock. Paraplegia 8: 231-242

Sweating disturbances in spinal paralysis

Sweating occurs from
1) External environmental changes:
    Lesions above T2 lead to no sweating in any part of body
Incomplete lesions above T2 lead to
    unilateral or segmental sweating
    Lesions below L2 leave normal sweating
    In thoracic cord lesions down to T10 sweating occurs in anesthetic skin several segments below lesion
Quadriplegics tend to be poikilothermic

2) Visceral changes:
    Usually bladder distension
    Lesions above T6: Reflex sweating involves whole body except legs
    Lesions below T6: Irregular onset of sweating
    Vasodilation occurs with sweating
3) Sensory stimulation:
    Catheterisation
    Enemata
    Change of posture
    Induction of spasms

Reference
Guttman L, Silver J, Wyndham C H 1958 Thermoregulation in spinal man. Journal of Physiology (London) 142: 406-419

Skin pressure problems in spinal paralysis

Average tolerable pressure in normals
$1\frac{1}{2}$ lb./in^2 or 80 mm. Hg.
Average permissible pressure in paraplegics
1 lb./in^2 or 50 mm. Hg.

Factors leading to ulceration
Age
Thinness
Malnutrition
Restlessness
Inertia

Sites at risk
Buttocks
Sacrum
Trochanters
Heels
Elbows

Prophylaxis
Skilled nursing care with regular turning night and day

Special beds
Pillows
Water bed
Rotating frames
    Circular
    Horizontal

Rolling frame
Sand bed

Local measures
Pads
Sheepskins
Rubbing with alcohol and powder

General measures
Avoidance of incontinence
Avoidance of anemia
Give vitamin C (ascorbic acid)
Zinc Sulphate (unproven)

Treatment
Buttocks and sacrum:
   Excision of slough
   Removal of sequestra
   Rotation of large dorsal flaps
Trochanters:
   Excision of slough and sequestra
   Small ulcers: Heal by contracture
   Large ulcers: Rotation Flap
Heels:
   Excision of slough
   When cleanly granulating whole thickness skin
    graft
Minor surgery only if patient is very fit

References
Carpendale M, 1974 A comparison of 4 beds in the prevention of tissue ischaemia in paraplegic patients. Paraplegia 12: 121-130
Editorial 1978 Treating pressure sores. British Medical Journal 1: 1232
Guttman L 1955 The problem of treatment of pressure sores in spinal paraplegics. British Journal of Plastic Surgery 7: 196-213
Scales J T et al 1974 The prevention and treatment of pressure sores using air support systems. Paraplegia 12: 118-131

The bladder in spinal paralysis

Normal neurological control

Filling
Contraction of internal sphincter
Relaxation of bladder wall
Relaxation of abdominal wall

Emptying
Relaxation of internal sphincter
   Sympathetic inhibition (T10-12)

Contraction of bladder wall
   Parasympathetic activity (S3-4)
Contraction of perineal musculature
   Pudendal nerve (S1-2)
Contraction of diaphragm and abdominal wall

Effects of neurological lesions

1. Upper motor neurone injury
(i.e. Damage to spinal cord above sacral segments)
Initially:
   Flaccid paralysis
   Overfilling
   Trickling overflow incontinence
Later:
   Gradual return of tone in bladder wall
   Intermittent partial emptying (in response to stimuli)

2. Lower motor neurone injury
(i.e. Damage to sacral segments of spinal cord or to sacral roots)
   Flaccid paralysis – persists
   Large volume, low pressure

Aims of bladder management
Prevention of
   infection
   over-distension
   damage to urethra or bladder
Maintenance of
   normal capacity
   freedom from catheter

Vasomotor changes from bladder distension
Sweating
Headache
Bradycardia
Hypotension

Patterns of bladder emptying in chronic spinal lesions
1. Co-ordinated vesical reflex
   Single contraction. 200-400 ml. voided 2-4 hourly
   Most often seen in incomplete transverse lesions
2. Unco-ordinated vesical reflex
   Irregular incomplete emptying
   Variations with state of heath, infection, spasms
   Worst effects with an uninhibited hypertonic bladder voiding small amounts of urine frequently

Reference
Yeates W K 1974 Neurophysiology of the bladder. Paraplegia
12: 73-82

Treatment of paralysed bladder

Early stages: three current methods

1. Continuous catheterisation
Always leads to eventual infection

2. Intermittent catheterisation
Requires devoted expert staff
Regular attention

3. Intermittent suprapubic cystostomy
Very thin tubing
Dangers of infection of pelvis or hematoma
    formation

Three older methods abandoned
1. Suprapubic cystostomy
2. Tidal drainage
3. Urethrostomy

Later stages
From 2-3-4 weeks
Remove catheter
Allow bladder to fill
Attempt to stimulate contraction
    1. Sensory stimulation in groin area
    2. Manual compression of bladder

Results
Failure:
    Replace catheter. Repeat in one week
Success:
    Regular emptying procedure
    Drink large volumes day and night

Maintenance
Check residual urine volume 3 monthly
Should be 5-10% of bladder capacity
I.V.P. yearly
Culture urine when unwell

Complications of bladder management

Investigation of bladder problems
Culture Urine
Radiograph of Pelvis to exclude calculi
Intravenous Pyelogram with pre and post
    emptying films of bladder
Cystoscopy
Pressure measurements of bladder and sphincters

1. Infection

Prophylaxis
Aseptic catheterisation
Large volume throughput
Long term urinary antiseptic
Avoidance of residual urine
Circumcision if phimotic

Treatment
Culture
Appropriate antibiotic
Increase urine volume
Acidification

2. Stone formation

Prophylaxis
Large urine volume
Regular movement of patient
Avoidance of
    infection
    residual urine

Treatment
Removal
    Litholapaxy
    Ultrasonic fragmentation
    Cystostomy

3. Persistent incontinence

Consider
Overflow distension
Stone or infection
Damage to perineum

Treatment
Order of desirability:
  Correction of above
  Parasympathetic stimulators
    Probanthine, Atropine
  Intrathecal alcohol
  Electrical stimulation of sphincters
  Urinals

4. Incomplete emptying (High residual urine)

Causes
Inefficient bladder contraction
Contracted sphincters
Prostatic hypertrophy
If bladder contraction is inefficient:
Give Acetyl Choline Analogues
or Anti-Choline Esterases

Treatment
A. Transurethral resection of prostate (T.U.R.)
   if median bar of prostate and bladder
   contractions are present
B. Pudendal neurectomy
   if sphincteric spasm is present. Unilateral
   surgery may be sufficient. Bilateral section
   causes impotence in males
C. Electrical stimulation of bladder or conus
   medullaris (Experimental)

5. Vesico-ureteric reflux
Eventually present in 20% of paraplegics
Demonstrated by cystography

Causes
Bladder contractions in presence of unrelaxed
  sphincters

Treatment
Better drainage of bladder
Ileal loop conduit
No consistently successful method

6. Suprapubic fistulae
From previous cystostomy

Treatment
Free urethral bladder drainage until healed

7. Urethral fistulae and diverticulae

Causes
Repeated catheter trauma

Treatment
Temporary suprapubic bladder drainage
Plastic repair of urethra

8. Hydronephrosis or pyonephrosis

9. Renal failure
See separate section

References
Bors E, Comarr A E 1954 Effect of pudendal nerve
  operations on the neurogenic bladder. Journal of Urology
  72: 666-670
Boyarsky S et al 1966 Clinical evaluation of bladder pressure
  studies in urological patients by combined cystometry and
  uroflometry. Journal of Urology 95: 778-780
Gibbon N O K, Ross J C, Damanski M 1964 Bladder neck
  resection in the paraplegic report on over one hundred
  cases. Paraplegia, 2: 264-274
Gibbon N O K 1974 Later management of the paraplegic
  bladder. Paraplegia 12: 87-98
Gibbon N O K 1975 A further look at the rationale of
  external sphincterotomy. Paraplegia 13: 243-246
Kracht H, Buscher H K 1974 Formation of staghorn calculi
  and their surgical implications in paraplegics and
  tetraplegics. Paraplegia 12: 98-110
Melzak J 1967 The incidence of bladder cancer in paraplegia.
  Paraplegia, 4: 85-95
Nashold B S et al 1972 Electromicturition in paraplegia.
  Archives of Surgery 104: 195-202
O'Flynn J D 1974 Early management of the neuropathic
  bladder in spinal cord injuries. Paraplegia 12: 83-86
Smith P M, Cook J B, Rhind J R 1971 Manual expression of
  the bladder following spinal injury. Paraplegia 9: 213-218
Susset J G et al 1966 Implantable electrical vesical stimulator.
  Canadian Medical Association Journal 95: 1128-1131
Vivian J M, Bors E 1974 Experience with intermittent
  catheterisation in the south west regional system for
  treatment of spinal injury. Paraplegia 12: 158-166

Persistent muscle spasm in spinal paralysis

Clinical features
Present in some degree in all patients
Worst in complete transverse cord lesions
May:
  prevent walking or sexual activity
  interfere with sitting or lying
  produce pressure ulcers
Exacerbated by:
  Stretch reflexes
  Infection
  Heat or cold
Relieved by:
  Fatigue
  Passive movements

Treatment

Pharmacology
Diazepam the only drug of proven effect
Non-paralysed muscles also affected

Chemotherapy
Intrathecal alcohol
Intrathecal phenol

Surgery
Anterior rhizotomy. Major operation
Posterior rhizotomy. Major operation
  Only temporarily effective
Cordectomy: Major operation
Peripheral neurectomy
Tenotomy:
  Adductors of Hips ⎱
  Hamstrings ⎰ Temporarily
  Achilles tendon ⎰ Effective

References
Apolinario E et al 1966 et seq. Follow up of a series of phenol spinal blocks. Paraplegia4: 162-175
Kelly R E, Gautier-Smith P C 1959 Intrathecal phenol in the treatment of reflex spasms and spasticity. Lancet 2: 1102-1105
Kerr-Sutcliffe A 1966 Anterior rhizotomy for the relief of spasticity. Paraplegia 4: 154-162

Soft tissue calcification in spinal paralysis

Synonyms
Para-articular ossification
Para-osteo-arthropathia
Osteosis neurotica para-articularis
Neurogenic ossifying fibromyopathy
Myositis ossificans circumscripta traumatica

General features
Develops in 5%-20% of all paraplegics
Always develops below level of neurological lesion
Similar condition arises after some severe head injuries

Clinical features
Patient may not notice any abnormality

Induration and local heat around major joint within 2-6 months after injury
Increasing joint stiffness. Usually bilaterally

Common sites
Medial femoral condyle
Upper anterior third of femur
Gluteal muscles
Anterior and posterior to elbow
May prevent sitting or feeding

Pathological features

Theories of causation
Immobility
Excessive passive movements
Changes in local tissue pH
Unnoticed local injury to soft tissues

Stages
Swelling and induration
Calcification
Ossification
Raised alkaline phosphatase
Abnormal bone scans

Differential diagnosis
(Depends on site)
Deep venous thrombosis
Soft tissue tumour
Hematoma

Treatment
1. Excision of osseous mass, when mature
    i.e. 1-2 years after initial injury
      Recurrence is common
2. Osteotomy to improve function
3. Diphosphonates to inhibit calcification

References
Damanski M 1961 Heterotopic ossification in paraplegia. Journal of Bone and Joint Surgery 43B: 286-299
Dejerine M, Cellier A, Dejerine Y 1919 Para-osteo-arthropathies des paraplegiques par lesion medullaire. Revue de Neurologique 26: 399-402
Stover S L, Niemann K M W, Miller J M 1976 Disodium etidronate in the prevention of post operative recurrence of heterotopic ossification in spinal cord injury patients. Journal of Bone and Joint Surgery 58A: 683-688
Tibone J et al 1978 Heterotopic ossification around hip in spinal-cord injured patients. Journal of Bone and Joint Surgery 60A: 769-775
Wharton G W, Morgan T H 1970 Ankylosis in the paralysed patient. Journal of Bone and Joint Surgery 52A: 105-112

Persistent spinal pain in spinal paralysis

Attempt to localise origin
   History
   Examination
   Investigations
   Local anesthesia
to elucidate cause

Treatment
Paravertebral local anesthetics (long acting
   varieties)
Intrathecal alcohol or phenol
Localised posterior rhizotomy
Arthrodesis of unstable painful segment
   +/- internal fixation
Physiotherapy +/- Psychotherapy

Fractures of paralysed limbs in spinal injuries
Occur in osteoporotic bones
Trivial violence
Usually 2 years after paralysis
Painless

Treatment
Minimal immobilisation in pillows or soft splints
Casts: Bad results from skin ulcers
Surgery: Poor results

References
Botterell E H, Callaghan J C, Jousse A T 1954 Pain in
   paraplegia, clinical management and surgical treatment.
   Procedings of Royal Society of Medicine 47: 281-288
Freehafer A A, Mast W A 1965 Lower extremity fractures in
   patients with spinal cord injury. Journal of Bone and Joint
   Surgery 47A: 683-694

Respiratory problems in spinal paralysis

Pre-trauma factors:
Age
Chronic bronchitis and other respiratory
   deficiences
Obesity

Trauma factors:
Level of paralysis
   (Minimal below T10)
   (Maximal at C5)
Injury to rib cage
Inhalation of foreign bodies

Post-trauma factors:
Skill of nursing care
Vigor and skill of physiotherapy
Atelectasis
Infection

Paralytic mechanism of respiration
Variations in root supply of diaphragm
Diaphragmatic excursion is diminished by a lax
   abdominal wall
Paralysed intercostals may yet reflexly contract
   when stretched
Accessory muscles of respiration
   (i.e. M. Trapezius and M. Sterno-mastoid)
will hypertrophy over a period of months

Measurable parameters
Vital capacity   (VC) ⎫ all
Forced expiratory volume   (FEV) ⎬ diminished
Maximal breathing capacity (MBC) ⎭
Maximum loss in high quadriplegics
V.C. may be as low as 0.3 litre
Parameters improve:
   In head down position
   With practice in recovery phase

References
Guttman L, Silver J R 1965 Electromyographic studies on
   reflex activity of the intercostal and abdominal muscles in
   cervical cord lesions. Paraplegia 3: 1-21
Hemingway A, Bors E, Hobby R P 1958 An investigation of
   the pulmonary function of paraplegics. Journal of Clinical
   Investigation 37: 773-782

Venous thrombosis and pulmonary embolism in spinal paralysis

Higher incidence than in any other class of patient 10-15% venous thrombosis in legs within 14 days of injury

Venous thrombosis
Diagnosis:
Swelling of leg(s) unchanged by elevation
Engorgement of superficial veins
Rise of temperature
Ultrasound
Venography
(No pain if sensation is lost)

Pulmonary embolism
Diagnosis:
Sudden rise in respiratory rate
Pain on respiration (may be absent in high levels of paralysis)
Pleural rub. Diminished breath sounds
Hemoptysis
Chest radiography
Lung scan
Pulmonary angiography

Prevention
Frequent change of position
Elevation of foot of bed
No compression of calves
Breathing exercises
No blood transfusion through paralysed limb (s)
Anticoagulants for transport in acute post injury stages
Low dosage heparin under evaluation

References
Hachen H J 1974 Anticagulant therapy in patients with spinal cord injury. Paraplegia 12: 176-185 et seq
Walsh J J, Tribe C 1965 Phlebo-thrombosis and pulmonary embolism in paraplegia. Paraplegia 3: 209-213

Sexual problems of spinal paralysis

Females
Normal menstruation continues after injury
Diminished fertility if pelvic or urinary sepsis is present
Normal pregnancy and delivery is possible
No sexual sensation
Orgasm is possible in partial cord lesions but may be unperceived
Flexor and/or adductor spasm may prevent penetration

Males
Marked variability in potency and fertility
Erection more frequently present than ejaculation
Incomplete cord lesions will allow both
Artificial ejaculation:
1. Intrathecal prostigmine 0.3—0.5 mgm. causes repeated ejaculation after 1-3 hours
2. Electrical stimulation of seminal vesicles Artificial insemination therefore possible
Ejaculation) accompanied by
Labour) vasomotor changes

References
Jackson R W 1972 Sexual rehabilitation after cord injury. Paraplegia 10: 50-55
Rossier A, Ruffieux M, Ziegler W H 1969 Pregnancy and labour in high traumatic spinal cord lesions. Paraplegia 7: 210-216

Late reconstruction in quadriplegics

General features
Confined to arm, wrist and fingers
Every case must be studied individually
No reconstruction should be considered until
1. Full potential of neurological recovery has been achieved
2. 2 years have passed since injury·
Many with lesions below C7 manage daily life without further surgery
Mobility of wrist is vital to tendon transfers

Possibilities

C5/6 lesion: B.R. → E.C.R.B.
Additional tenodesis of digital flexors may be
  desirable

C6/7 lesion: ECRL → E.P.L. + E.D.I.
       ECRB → APL
       PT → FDP
       FCR → Thumb opposition

C7/T1 lesion:- F.C.R. → F.D.P.
       B.R. → F.P.L.
       F.C.U. → Thumb Opposition

References

Freehafer A A, Vonhaam E, Allen V 1974 Tendon transfers
  to improve grasp after injuries of the cervical cord. Journal
  of Bone and Joint Surgery 56A: 951-959
Lamb D W, Landry R M 1971 The hand in quadriplegia.
  Paraplegia 9: 204-212
Lipscomb P R, Elkins E C, Henderson E D 1958 Tendon
  transfers to restore function of hands in tetraplegia
  especially after fracture dislocations of the sixth cervical
  vertebra on the seventh. Journal of Bone and Joint Surgery
  40A: 1071-1080
Zrubecky G 1972 Orthoses for restoration of prehensile
  function in tetraplegics. The Hand 4: 72-78

Physiotherapy for spinal paralysis

Aims
1. Prevention of pneumonia
2. Prevention of contractures
3. Hypertrophy of arm and shoulder muscles
4. Teaching of functional activities
5. Improvement of morale

Methods
1. Teaching of deep breathing
   Hypertrophy of accessory respiratory muscles
   Assisted coughing
   Percussion and postural drainage
2. Passive movements
   Electrical stimulation of paralysed muscles
   Splintage
3. Resisted active exercises
   Springs
   Weights
   Parallel bars

4. Learning to balance
     sitting (quadriplegics)
     standing (paraplegics)
   Self dressing, Relief of pressure points
   Transfers
     Bed – chair
     Chair – vehicle
5. Competitive exercises
   Swimming
   Sports meetings

Quadriplegics
M. Latissium dorsi and M. Trapezius important
  for sitting, balance and pelvic hitching
Hamstrings must be kept long to allow sitting
Finger flexors can be allowed to shorten to allow
  grasping on wrist extension

Paraplegics
Abdominal and trunk musculature important for
  standing and walking with calipers and
  crutches
3 point walking possible in most cases but
  expensive in energy
Spinal standing without splints for 10-15 minutes
  possible in lesions over T7

Reference
Hobson E P G 1956 Physiotherapy in paraplegia. Churchill,
  London

Information for paraplegics

Handbook of Spinal Cord Medicine. D. C. Burke, D. D.
  Murray. Macmillan Press 1975. London
Understanding Paraplegia. J. J. Walsh, Dolphin Publishing
  1964 London.
Practical Management of Spinal Injuries. A. G. Hardy, R.
  Elson, Churchill Livingstone, Edinburgh, 1976.

SHOULDER AND UPPER ARM INJURIES

Avulsion of upper limb
Birth injuries of brachial plexus
Upper plexus lesions
Lower plexus lesions
Postnatal injuries to brachial plexus
Rupture of M. pectoralis major tendon
Dislocation of sterno-clavicular joint
Fractures of clavicle
Acromio-clavicular dislocations
Fracture of scapula
Anterior dislocation of shoulder
Anterior recurrent dislocation of shoulder
Habitual dislocation of shoulder
Posterior dislocation of shoulder
Fracture dislocation of shoulder
Chronic dislocation of shoulder
Rupture of rotator cuff
Fractures of humeral head
Juxta epiphyseal fractures of upper humerus
Fractures of surgical neck of humerus
Bicipital tendinitis and rupture
Fractures of shaft of humerus
Supracondylar fractures of humerus in children
Supracondylar fractures with neurovascular
    complications
Established ischemia of forearm
Fracture of medial epicondylar epiphysis
Fractures of capitellum
Intercondylar fractures of humerus
Side swipe fracture of elbow
Fracture of lateral condyle of humerus
Dislocation of elbow
Recurrent dislocation of elbow
Displacement of lower humeral epiphysis

Avulsion of upper limb

General features
Rare injury
Nearly always due to machinery accidents
R > L

Clinical features
Arm may be missing at elbow or shoulder
Tendons, bones and muscle may be protruding
Hemorrhagic shock
Major vessels may not bleed

Radiological features
Part of upper limb missing
Associated fractures of remaining part of arm
   may be present
Neck and chest fractures possible

Pathological features
Tissues at site of avulsion may be crushed and
   devitalised
Traction injuries to remaining nerves are
   common
Post traumatic vasoconstriction may avoid fatal
   hemorrhage

Treatment
Resuscitation
Immediate wound toilet
   Formal amputation
   Skin flaps if necessary

References
Mardin C A 1967 Hay baler injuries requiring forequarter
   amputation. Journal of Trauma 7: 164-168

Birth injuries of the brachial plexus

General features
Three main types:
   Upper plexus: Erb's palsy
   Lower plexus: Klumpke's palsy
   Whole plexus: Always very rare

Incidence is falling due to better obstetrics
Associated with obstetrical problems
   i.e. Primiparity
         Contracted pelvis
         Large babies
         Breech presentation
         Other mal-presentations
         Precipitate delivery
         Obstetrical maneouvres and use of forceps

Specific features
Swelling or bruising at root of neck
Arm held immobile, flaccid paralysis is present
Absence of Moro and grasp reflexes
Occasional transient spastic paralysis of other
   limbs from hematomyelia

Differential diagnosis

In infants:
Fracture of upper humeral epiphysis (Putti-
   Scagletti lesion)
Fracture of clavicle
Septic arthritis
Syphilitic periostitis

In children
Scurvy
Poliomyelitis
Spinal cord tumour

Prognosis
Upper and lower plexus lesions often show a
   large measure of recovery
Whole plexus lesions have a bad prognosis

Upper plexus lesions

Synonym
Erb's Palsy

Clinical features
Paralysis of C5 and C6 motor function
Minimal sensory loss
Lack of:
   shoulder abduction
   elbow flexion
   forearm supination
Arm held in "waiters tip" position
i.e. shoulder adducted, elbow extended
      forearm pronated, wrist flexed

Radiological features
Posterior subluxation of humeral head
Later:
 Small humeral head
 Beaked acromion and coracoid
 Posterior subluxation of radial head
No changes in cervical spine

Pathological features
C5 and C6 roots are stretched or bruised at time
 of birth
Complete loss of function is unusual
The developing brain compensates for sensory
 loss by utilising stimuli arising from
 overlapping dermatomes in the arm

Early treatment
Aimed to achieve "Statue of Liberty" position
1. Abduction splints:
 Difficult to maintain
 May cause an abduction contracture of
 shoulder
2. Wrist tied to top of cot:
 May cause skin friction at wrist or edema of
 hand
3. Physiotherapy:
 Frequent passive movement of all joints

Later deformities
Shoulder:
 Adduction, internal-rotation contracture
Elbow:
 Lack of full extension
 Dislocation of head of radius
Forearm:
 Medial drift of radius and ulna across lower
 end of humerus

Later complaints
Abnormal appearance
Inability to reach up with arm or to supinate the
 hand
No sensory problems

Later treatment
Surgery after age 4
No complete cure nor unanimity of opinion
 about best procedure

Soft tissue procedures – best in early years
 1. Section of pectoralis major, subscapularis
 and coraco-brachialis (Sever's operation)
or 2. Transfer of latissimus dorsi and teres major
 to act as external rotators (L'Episcopo's
 operation)

or 3. Section of forearm flexor origin (Scaglietti's
 muscle slide)
or 4. Triceps → Biceps transfer

Bone operations
 1. Rotation osteotomy of upper third of
 humerus
or 2. Rotation osteotomy of radius
or 3. Arthrodesis of shoulder and/or wrist
or 4. Wedge osteotomy of neck of scapula

References
Adler J B, Patterson R L 1967 Erb's palsy, long term results
 of treatment in 88 cases. Journal of Bone and Joint
 Surgery 49A: 1052-1064
Erb W 1874 Uber eine eigenthumliche localisation von
 lahmungen im plexus brachialis verhandl. Naturist medizin
 2: 130-139
Green W T, Tachdjian M O 1963 Correction of residual
 deformity of the shoulder from obstetrical palsy. Journal of
 Bone and Joint Surgery 45A: 1544
L'Episcopo J H 1934 Tendon transplantation in obstetrical
 paralysis. American Journal of Surgery 25: 122-125
Tachdjian M O 1972 Pediatric orthopedics. Volume 2:
 p. 1036. W B Saunders Co., Philadelphia
Wickstrom J 1960 Birth injuries of the brachial plexus.
 Journal of Bone and Joint Surgery 42A: 1448-1449
Zachary R B 1947 Transplantation of teres major and
 latissimus dorsi for loss of external rotation at the
 shoulder. Lancet 2: 757-758

Lower plexus lesions

Synonym
Klumpke's Palsy

General features
Birth injury to lower cords of brachial plexus.
Initially total brachial plexus palsy may be
 present but this often improves to leave only a
 lower cord deficit

Clinical features
Paralysis of finger and wrist movement
Sensory loss in hand and forearm

Radiological features
None

Pathological features
Caused by traction injury to lower cords and
 roots (C7, 8: T.1)
1. Prolapse of arm in labour

2. Traction on arm in delivery
3. Suspension of infant by arm after delivery

Treatment
Early:
Sling
Passive movements of all joints
Late:
Muscle transfers may be indicated depending
on the exact pattern of residual paralysis
Best deferred until after age 6

Reference
Klumpke A 1885 Contribution a l'etude des paralysies
radiculares du plexus brachial. Paralysies radiculaires
totales paralysies radiculaires inferieures Revue de
Medecine 5: 591-616

Post-natal injuries to brachial plexus

General features
Usually young adults affected
Major violence involved – often road accidents
M > F

Clinical features
Lesion at root of neck
Common: Bruising and/or swelling
Uncommon: Laceration, Incision, Stab wound
Variable loss of power and sensation in arm
Upper plexus: Shoulder and elbow
Lower plexus: Wrist and fingers
Whole plexus: Whole upper limb
Horner's syndrome is frequent
Often other injuries are present elsewhere

Radiological features
Variable fractures:
Clavicle
First rib
Cervical transverse processes
Cervical radicular meningoceles on myelogram
Occasional loss of diaphragm function when
screened

Pathological features
Neurological lesions may be:

1. Supraclavicular
Preganglionic: Poor prognosis
Postganglionic: Better prognosis

2. Infraclavicular
Postganglionic:
Good prognosis
Associated with fractures and dislocations of
shoulder region
(Axonotmesis and neuronotmesis are difficult to
distinguish and are not helpful for prognosis)
Nature of lesion:
Laceration or incision (rarest)
Contusion
Avulsion (commonest)

Diagnostic tests
1. Cervical myelogram:
Presence of radicular meningoceles indicates
avulsion of nerve roots from spinal cord
No recovery
2. Histamine flare:
Subcuticular injection of 1 mg. of histamine in
adjacent dermatomes
Presence of a flare indicates a post-ganglionic
lesion and a better prognosis
3. Electromyography of posterior primary rami
extensor musculature:
Fibrillation potentials at 20 days indicates
denervated muscle and a poor prognosis
4. Cold vasodilation tests:
Elaborate. Little used
5. Activity of serratus anterior, rhomboids,
levator scapulae and diaphragm:
Contraction indicates a distal plexus lesion and
a better prognosis

Treatment

A: Initial
1. Lacerations, Incisions, Stab wounds:
Surgical exploration
Repair of divided nerve trunks
2. Contusions and avulsions
Passive movements of all joints
Splintage to prevent deformity
Regular galvanism of doubtful value

B: Secondary
When no further recovery is likely (After 2 years)
1. Upper Plexus:
Select appropriate operation:
Arthrodesis of shoulder
or Internal rotator transfer
or M. Pectoralis major transfer
or M. Brachio-radialis transfer
or Extensor-Flexor transfer at wrist
2. Lower plexus:
Arthrodesis of wrist or
Flexor tenodesis

3. Whole plexus:
   Amputation at mid humerus
   Arthrodesis of shoulder
   Posterior bone block of elbow
   Flexor tenodesis

References

Bonney G L W 1954 The value of axon responses in determining the site of lesion in traction injuries of the brachial plexus. Brain 77: 588-609

Bufalini C, Pescatori G 1969 Posterior cervical electromyography in the diagnosis and prognosis of brachial plexus injuries. Journal of Bone and Joint Surgery 51B: 627-631

Lain T M 1969 The military brace syndrome. Journal of Bone and Joint Surgery 51A: 557-560

Leffert R D, Seddon H 1965 Infraclavicular brachial plexus lesion. Journal of Bone and Joint Surgery 55A: 1159-1176

Seddon H J 1972 Surgical disorders of peripheral nerves. P. 178. Churchill-Livingstone, Edinburgh, London.

Yeoman P M, Seddon H J 1961 Brachial plexus injuries: treatment of the flail arm. Journal of Bone and Joint Surgery 43B: 493-500

Yeoman P M 1968 Cervical myelography in traction injuries of the brachial plexus. Journal of Bone and Joint Surgery 50B: 253-260

Rupture of pectoralis major tendon

General features
Rare
Caused by forced resisted adduction of upper arm

Clinical features
Sudden pain and swelling in anterior axillary fold
Local hematoma – when resolved anterior axillary fold is missing
Weak active adduction of upper arm

Pathological features
Rupture occurs at
   musculotendinous junction
      or
   within muscle belly

Radiological features
None

Treatment
Conservative early active exercises for intramuscular ruptures
Surgical repair for musculotendinous ruptures

Reference

Mcentire J E, Hess W E, Coleman S S 1972 Rupture of the pectoralis major muscle. Journal of Bone and Joint Surgery 54A: 1040-1046

Dislocation of sterno-clavicular joint

General features
Is the only articulation of the shoulder girdle on the trunk
Dislocation occurs from fall on point of shoulder

Clinical features
Pain, swelling, loss of function of shoulder
Posterior dislocations may produce dyspnoea and dysphagia

Pathological features
Disruption of capsule and meniscus
Anterior dislocations unstable and painful
Posterior dislocations stable and dangerous compressing carotid vessels, trachea and esophagus
Epiphyseal separation of medial end of clavicle very rare. (Age 14-16)

Radiological features
Difficult to visualise
Tomography more effective

Treatment
Anterior
Manipulation and figure 8 bandage
Recurrence
   Fascial repair or
   Subclavius tenodesis or
   Resection of inner half of clavicle

Posterior
Urgent manipulation
If this fails – open reduction and internal fixation
Epiphyseal Separation: Open reduction

References

Bateman J E 1968 Neurovascular syndromes related to the clavicle. Clinical Orthopaedics 58: 75-82

Dennam R H, Dingley A F 1967 Epiphyseal separation of the medial end of the clavicle. Journal of Bone and Joint Surgery 49A: 1179-1183

Howard F M, Schafer S J 1965 Injuries to the clavicle with neurovascular complications. Journal of Bone and Joint Surgery 47A: 1335-1346

Fractures of clavicle

General features
Very common
Indirect violence –
   oblique and transverse fractures.
Direct violence –
   comminution
   Compound
   Neurovascular damage

Clinical features
Fractures lateral to coracoid confused with acromio-clavicular subluxations
Fractures medial to coracoid displace unless weight of arm is supported
Pain, swelling, tenderness, loss of function

Radiological features
Easily visible on anterior-posterior films
Oblique/Tangential views aid definition
Greenstick fractures only in children

Pathological features
Rarely compound
Fragments may penetrate subclavian vessels
Damage to brachial plexus or pleura is very rare
Non union uncommon

Treatment

Conservative
nearly always adequate
Figure 8 bandage and sling 3 weeks
or Bed rest supine for 3 weeks

Operative
Essential for compounding and/or neurovascular damage
Desirable for long delayed union
Superfluous otherwise
   Plate or intramedullary nail used

Painful or deforming established non-union:
   Excision of outer half of clavicle

References

Howard F M, Schafer S J 1965 Injuries to the clavicle with neurovascular complications. Journal of Bone and Joint Surgery 47A: 1335-1346

Neer C S II, 1968 Fractures of the distal third of the clavicle. Clinical Orthopaedics 58: 43-50

Rowe C R 1968 An atlas of anatomy and treatment of mid-clavicular fractures. Clinical Orthopaedics 58: 29-42

Acromio-clavicular dislocations

General features
Caused by a blow or a fall on the point of the shoulder depressing the scapula downwards

Clinical features
Pain, tenderness and bruising
Elevation of outer end of clavicle
Concealed by supporting elbow
Worsened by allowing arm to hang down
Inability to move shoulder

Pathological features
Minor: Subluxation of acromio-clavicular joint
Incomplete: Dislocation of acromio-clavicular joint
Complete: Dislocation of acromio-clavicular joint and coraco-clavicular joint

Radiological features
Both sides best compared if both are visible on same film
Compare clavicular-acromial and clavicular-coracoid intervals
Displacement increased if arm is dependant-necessary to check full extent of injury
Fragments of coracoid may be avulsed

Treatment
Consider nature of injury, age and occupation of patient
Functional and anatomical results do not correspond
Good function is possible despite persistent dislocation

(1) Subluxation
Loop strapping and sling

(2) Acromio-clavicular dislocation

Loop strapping and sling. Often ineffective unless
carefully supervised
Fascial and tendon repairs
Internal fixation: intramedullary pin or wires.
Must be removed later

(3) Clavicular coracoid dislocation

Coraco-clavicular screw
Coraco-clavicular transfer
Internal fixation must be removed after 3 months
before it works loose

(4) Persistent deformity/pain

Removal of outer third of clavicle

References

Dewar F T, Barrington T W 1965 The treatment of chronic
acromio-clavicular dislocation. Journal of Bone and Joint
Surgery 47B: 32-35
Meyerding H W 1937 The treatment of acromio-clavicular
dislocation. Surgical Clinics of North America 17: 1199-
1205
Patterson W R 1967 Inferior dislocation of the distal end of
the clavicle. Journal of Bone and Joint Surgery 49A: 1184-
1186
Simmons E H, Martin R F 1968 Acute dislocation of the
acromio-clavicular joint. Canadian Journal of Surgery 11:
473-479
Spigelman L 1969 A harness for acromio-clavicular
separation. Journal of Bone and Joint Surgery 51A: 585-
586
Weitzman G 1967 Treatment of acute acromio-clavicular joint
dislocation by a modified Bosworth method. Journal of
Bone and Joint Surgery 49A: 1167-1177

Fracture of scapula

General features

Usually arise from road traffic accidents or other
direct violence
Associated with fractures of ribs, clavicle,
humerus
Fractures of coracoid alone occur from
(1) athletic muscular avulsion
(2) Part of dislocation of clavicle
(3) Gun recoil

Clinical features

Pain, swelling, loss of arm function
Symptoms and signs often obscured by other
injuries to neck, chest and arm

Radiological features

Fractures of body of scapula may not be visible
on anterior-osterior views
Shown better by tangential views

Pathological features

Most fractures are well splinted by scapular
muscles
Features of glenoid and coracoid may be
displaced
Costo-scapular adhesions very unusual

Treatment

Fractures of neck or body of scapula –
Velpeau bandaging and early active movement.
Fractures of coracoid – Internal fixation
sometimes indicated

References

Froimson A I 1978 Fracture of the coracoid process of the
scapula. Journal of Bone and Joint Surgery 60A: 710-711
Zoravkovic D, Damholt V V 1974 Comminuted and severely
displaced fractures of the scapula. Acta Orthopedica
Scandinavica 45: 60-65

Anterior dislocation of shoulder

General features

Usually requires major violence by falling on
outstretched hand
Anterior: Posterior = 50 : 1
Associated with muscular athletic individuals and
syndromes of joint laxity

Clinical features

Pain, swelling, tenderness, loss of function
Elbow supported away from trunk
Flattening of shoulder contour
Increased axillary girth
Humeral head sometimes palpable below
coracoid
10% circumflex nerve damage –
Deltoid paralysis
Anesthesia over deltoid
Rarely:
Brachial artery damage
Brachial plexus injury
Intrathoracic dislocation

Pathological features

Youngsters
Damage to glenoid labrum at osseous-cartilaginous junction

Elderly
Rent in anterior joint capsule

Subluxation
Humeral head hitched on edge of glenoid

Subcoracoid
Commonest situation
Humeral head lies under subscapularis

Subclavicular
Humeral head penetrates subscapularis
Extensive soft tissue damage
Delayed reduction may be dangerous from neurovascular adhesions

Luxatio erecta
Humeral head lies below glenoid

Radiological features

Easily diagnosed on A-P view
Axillary views give additional information
25% have fracture of greater tuberosity
1% fracture of glenoid
Postero-lateral notch on humeral head may be present

Treatment

Manipulation: methods
Abduction with traction
or Kochers' method (Traction, External rotation, Adduction, Internal rotation)
or Hippocrates method – may provoke a fracture dislocation or neurovascular damage if too violent
or Prone lying with forequarter dependent

After treatment:
Youngsters:
    Velpeau strapping for 3 weeks
    Mobilise for further 3 weeks
Oldsters:
    Sling for 3 weeks
    Mobilse therafter

Reference

Hippocrates translated by Withington E T 1927. Heinneman London.

Anterior recurrent dislocation of shoulder

General features

Variable incidence after first dislocation (20% to 50%)
Can occur despite good initial treatment
Usually occurs within one year
$M : F = 6 : 1$
$R = L$
Associated with
    Joint laxity syndromes
    Athletic pursuits
    Epilepsy

Clinical features

Involuntary dislocation from trivial actions
Becomes painless with repetition
Reduction:
    Under anesthesia firstly
    Patient learns reduction manoeuvre
    Voluntary reduction possible later
Lastly dislocation can take place at will with abduction and external rotation

Radiological features

Postero-lateral notch on humeral head
Special projection required
Fracture of glenoid rim ⎫
Loose body formation ⎬ Rare
Degenerative changes after several years

Pathological features

Voluminous joint capsule
Youngsters: Defect in glenoid labrum at the osseous-cartilaginous junction (Bankart lesion)
Oldsters: Defect in anterior rotator cuff

Treatment

Large variety of procedures advocated
Many are now of historical interest only
Best to learn one procedure well and use it whenever possible

Some procedures currently advocated
Overlapping of subscapularis (Putti-Platt operation)
Suturing of defect in labrum (Bankart operation)

Transfer of subscapularis to greater tuberosity
(Magnuson operation)
Repair of labrum defect by a small plate
(Moseley's operation)
Transfer of lateral coracoid to anterior edge of
glenoid (Bristow's operation)
Transfer of subscapularis to notch in humeral
head (If this is large and deep)

Prognosis
High success rates claimed for these methods by
those expert in their use. Further dislocation is
possible, however, if the patient is
Young
Athletic
Hypermobile
Careless

References:

Bankart A S B 1938 The pathology and treatment of
recurrent dislocation of the shoulder joint. British Journal
of Surgery 26: 23-29
Hall R H, Isaac F, Booth C R 1959 Dislocations of the
shoulder with special reference to accompanying small
fractures. Journal of Bone and Joint Surgery 41A: 489-494
Joessel D 1880 Ueber die recidive der humerusluxationen.
Deutsche zeitshrift chirurgie 13: 167-184
Lombardo S J et al The modified Bristow procedure for
recurrent dislocation of the shoulder. Journal of Bone and
Joint Surgery 58A: 256-261
Magnuson P B, Stack J K 1943 Recurrent dislocation of the
shoulder. Journal of American Medical Association 123:
889-892
Morrey B F, Janes J M 1976 Recurrent anterior dislocation
of the shoulder. Long term follow up of the Putti-Platt and
Bankart procedures. Journal of Bone and Joint Surgery
58A: 252-256 et seq
Moseley F 1961 Recurrent dislocation of the shoulder. E & S
Livingstone, Edinburgh, London.
Osmond-Clark H 1948 Habitual dislocation of the shoulder.
The Putti-Platt operation. Journal of Bone and Joint
Surgery 30B: 19-25

Habitual dislocation of shoulder

Definition
Repetitive or voluntary dislocation with
spontaneous reduction

General features
May begin after trauma
May develop spontaneously
Some association with generalised joint laxity

Clinical features
Dislocation anteriorly or posteriorly by certain
positions of arm or voluntary trick movements
Painless
Immediate spontaneous reduction
No neurovascular complications
After some years pain and crepitus develops
High incidence of psychotics

Radiological features
Pathological features
Those of acute or recurrent dislocation without
grooving of humeral head

Treatment
Avoidance of dislocation
Physiotherapy to develop weak musculature
Psychotherapy
Surgery: Usually fails unless patient is strongly
motivated to recover
Each operation tailored to patient

Reference
Rowe C R, Pierce D S, Clark J G 1973 Voluntary dislocation
of the shoulder. Journal of Bone and Joint Surgery 55A:
445-460

Posterior dislocation of shoulder

General features
Uncommon but commonly overlooked

Clinical features
Shoulder pain
Follows trauma or muscle spasm
Swelling mostly posterior when viewed from
above
All movements limited initially
External rotation particularly painful and very
restricted
Rarely recurrent

Radiological features

Abnormal circular appearance of humeral head
  on A-P view (Compare opposite side)
Humeral head appears to 'stand off' from glenoid
Axillary view shows posterior subluxation

Pathological features

May be due to
  Eclampsia
  Electric shock
  Epilepsy
Humeral head subluxes to lodge on posterior
  edge of glenoid. Groove in head results in
  absence of external rotation
Humeral head lies subspinous in complete
  dislocations

Treatment

Manipulation under anesthesia
Easy and stable in first few days

If unstable

Shoulder spica with arm partly abducted and
  externally rotated

Surgery

Wire fixation (Temporary) of gleno-humeral joint
  after manipulation
Open reduction with repair of capsule and
  labrum

References

Bloom M H, Obata W G 1967 Diagnosis of posterior
  dislocation of the shoulder with use of velpeau axillary and
  angle-up roentgenographic views. Journal of Bone and
  Joint Surgery 49A: 943-949
Lindholm T S 1974 Recurrent posterior dislocations of the
  shoulder. Acta Chirurgica Scandinavica 140: 101-106
O'Connor S J, Jacknow A S 1956 Posterior dislocation of the
  shoulder. Archives of Surgery, 72: 479-491
Roberts A, Wickstrom J 1971 Prognosis of posterior
  dislocation of the shoulder. Acta Orthopedica Scandinavica
  42: 328-347

Fracture dislocations of shoulder

General features

Occur from infraglenoid dislocations – Full
  abduction and vertical compression
Humerus is angled against acromion and
  fractures at surgical neck. Head moves to
  subcoracoid position and neck lies in glenoid

Clinical features

Pain, swelling, tenderness
Elbow close to waist
Neurovascular complications possible
Humeral head palpable beneath coracoid

Radiological features

Humeral head usually subcoracoid in position
Humeral neck lies in glenoid

Pathological features

Humeral head may penetrate the
  subscapularis – difficult reduction
Wherever it lies soft tissue attachments prevent
  ischemic necrosis

Treatment

None

Old frail patients
Sling and active exercises

Manipulations

Younger active patients
Often ineffective. Can be dangerous in full
  abduction

Surgery

Open reduction
Internal fixation of humeral neck fracture
  i.e. Wire sutures
  or Oblique screw
  or Transacromion transfixation pin penetrating
    humeral head and shaft
Replacement arthroplasty if humeral head is
  devoid of soft tissue

Reference
Gold A M 1971 Fractured neck of humerus with separation and dislocation of the humeral head (fractured dislocation of the shoulder, severe type). Bulletin of the Hospital for Joint Diseases, New York, 32: 87-89

Chronic dislocation of shoulder

General features
Term applied to dislocation of more than 3-6 weeks' duration

Clinical features
Initial pain, swelling and tenderness subsides
Deformity of shoulder persists together with neurological deficits
Limited function returns – power less and inability to work with arm above horizontal

Radiological features
Those of acute dislocation
Local osteoporosis later

Pathological features
False capsule formed in soft tissues beneath coracoid
Glenoid filled by adherent remnants of rotator cuff

Treatment
Manipulation 3-8 weeks. Hippocratic method
Care required to avoid fracture of neck of humerus and neurological or vascular damage

Elderly
No further action. Active exercises

Youngsters
Open reduction. 4 weeks – 2 years
May be very difficult
Temporary internal fixation to retain reduction
Vigorous physiotherapy thereafter

References
Bennett G 1936 Old dislocations of the shoulder. Journal of Bone and Joint Surgery 18: 594-606
Mouterde P, Pere C, 1977 Old dislocation of the shoulder. Annales Chirurgie, 31: 119-124

Schultz T J, Jacob S B, Patterson R L 1969 Unrecognised dislocation of the shoulder. Journal of Trauma 9: 1009-1023

Rupture of rotator cuff

Clinical features
M >F
Arises after fall or minor injury
Usually a manual worker over 40 years
Sudden brief shoulder pain
Worsens in a few hours
Inability to elevate arm against gravity (This may recover)
No loss of elevation on stooping
Tenderness under acromion
'Drop arm' sign in complete ruptures
Wasting of supra and infra spinatus, visible in thin patients after a few months
Power and movement eventually improve
Shoulder never useful for work above horizontal level

Radiological features
Normal A-P film
Arthrography will show contrast diffusing into subacromial bursa
Later cystic changes and roughening of great tuberosity

Pathological features
Rupture may be partial or complete
25% of asymptomatic persons over 50 years have some rupture
Rupture occurs at critical vascular area
Association with diabetes, rheumatoid arthritis, and alcoholics

Treatment
1. Surgical repair as soon as possible
   3-6 weeks post-operative splinting in abduction
   Results are often disappointing
   Contra indicated for age, frailty, occupation.
2. Neglected cases: Acromionectomy
3. Conservative treatment: Local anesthetic and steroids.

Reference

Bakalim G, Pasila M 1975 Surgical treatment of rupture of the rotator cuff tendon. Acta Orthopaedica Scandinavica 46: 751-757

Codman E A 1934 The shoulder. Private Printing, Boston

Cotton R E, Rideout D F 1964 Tears of the humeral rotator cuff. Journal of Bone and Joint Surgery 46B: 314-328

Debeyre J, Patie D, Elemelike E 1965 Repair of ruptures of the rotator cuff of the shoulder. Journal of Bone and Joint Surgery 47B: 36-42

Neviaser J S, Neviaser R J, Neviaser T J 1978 The repair of chronic massive ruptures of the rotator cuff of the shoulder by use of a freeze-dried rotator cuff. Journal of Bone and Joint Surgery 60A: 681-684

Fractures of Humeral head

General features

Associated with dislocation
Greater tuberosity
Lesser tuberosity
Groove fracture

Without dislocation
Greater tuberosity
Lesser tuberosity
'4-fragment' fractures
Anatomical neck

Clinical features
Major trauma
Pain swelling loss of movement
Occasional neurovascular complications

Radiological features
'4-fragment' fracture occurs through planes of fusion of epiphyses
Downward displacement of fragments usually an artefact

Pathological features
Single fragments are vascularised by their muscle attachments
Articular surface fragment liable to avascular necrosis
Long tendon of biceps separates lesser and greater tuberosity fragments

Treatment
Reduction of dislocation
4 fragment fractures:
  Early mobilisation: Best for oldsters
  Wiring of fragment: Difficult procedure
  Prosthetic replacement: Disappointing results

References

Hall R W, Isaac F, Booth C R 1959 Dislocations of the shoulder with special reference to accompanying small fractures. Journal of Bone and Joint Surgery 41A: 489-494

Kraulis J, Hunter G 1976 Results of prosthetic replacement in fracture dislocations of the upper end of the humerus. Injury 8: 129-131

Neer S, 1963 Prosthetic replacement of the humeral head. Surgical Clinics of Northern America 43: 1581-1597

Juxta-epiphyseal fractures of upper humerus

General features
Caused by falling on outstretched hand in childhood and early adolescence

Clinical features
Pain, swelling, loss of function
Circumflex nerve never damaged

Radiological features
Juxta-epiphyseal fracture with a metaphyseal fragment attached to head
(Salter type 2)
Humeral head may move into abduction and lateral rotation if fracture becomes disimpacted

Pathological features
Non-union unknown
Malunion common but function is unimpaired
Remodelling restores normal anatomy in 1-2 years

Treatment
Minimal displacement:
  Velpeau bandaging and sling
Moderate displacement:
  Manipulation
  Velpeau and sling

Major displacement:
Manipulation
If this fails:
Open reduction
Screw fixation
Plaster spicas in abduction have led to abduction
contractures.
Bayonet opposition sufficient in children under 5

Reference
Dameron T B, Reibel D B 1969 Fractures involving the
proximal humeral epiphyseal plate. Journal of Bone and
Joint Surgery 51A: 289-297

Fractures of surgical neck of humerus

General features
Rare in middle life
Caused by fall on outstretched hand
Usually a rotatory element

Clinical features
Pain, swelling, loss of function
Circumflex nerve palsy is rare

Radiological features
Fracture may be undisplaced
Humeral shaft may be abducted on head or
adducted on head
Impaction is common
Comminution is unusual

Pathological features
Malunion is frequent
Non-union is rare
Impacted adduction fractures may limit
abduction
Impacted abduction fractures may lever humeral
head from glenoid

Treatment
Undisplaced:
Sling and exercises
Adduction:
Oldsters:
Sling and exercises

Youngsters:
Manipulation by traction
Velpeau bandage and sling
Abduction:
Oldsters:
Sling and exercises
Youngsters:
Manipulation by traction
Velpeau bandage and sling
Displaced irreducible fractures may require open
reduction and internal fixation

Reference
Neer C S II 1970 Displaced proximal humeral fractures.
Journal of Bone and Joint Surgery 52A: 1077-1089

Bicipital tendinitis and rupture

General features
Part of degenerative changes in rotator cuff
Occurs in second half of life
M > F

Clinical features

Tendinitis
Pain in front of shoulder
Worsened by elbow flexion
Tenderness in bicipital groove
Palm up sign positive
(Elbow flexion against resistance with palm
supinated)

Rupture
Sudden pain in front of shoulder on exertion
Local pain and swelling
Biceps belly moves distally
Weak painful elbow flexion
Eventual recovery of almost full power

Radiological features
Soft tissue swelling

Pathological features
Ischemic changes in tendon
Disruption of collagen
Inflammation of synovium

Treatment

Prerupture
Local anesthetic and steroid injections
(May predispose to rupture)

Rupture
No treatment of lesion if patient is unconcerned
   about appearance
Surgery is chiefly for cosmesis
1) Suture of tendon to bicipital groove
2) Reroute tendon anteriorly to coracoid process

References

Crenshaw A N, Kilgore W E 1966 Surgical treatment of
   bicipital tenosynovitis. Journal of Bone and Joint Surgery
   48A: 1496-1502
Heckman J D, Levine M I 1978 Traumatic closed transection
   of the biceps brachii in the military parachutist. Journal of
   Bone and Joint Surgery 60A: 369-372
Hitchcock H H, Bechtol C O 1948 Painful shoulder.
   Observations on the role of the tendon of the long head of
   biceps brachii in its causation. Journal of Bone and Joint
   Surgery 30A: 263-273

Fractures of shaft of humerus

General features
Common injury
Direct blow – transverse fracture
Fall on hand – oblique fracture

Clinical features
Pain, swelling, loss of function
Visible soft tissue damage from a direct blow
Sometimes compound
Radial nerve paralysis in fractures of lower third
   of shaft – wrist drop

Radiological features
Transverse fractures sometimes comminuted
Spiral oblique fractures usually not fragmented.

Pathological features
Radial nerve may be damaged in spiral groove –
   Contused or divided
   Trapped on fracture edges
   Covered in callus
Brachial artery and other nerves rarely injured
Pathological fractures can occur at any age from
   large variety of lesions

Treatment

Conservative
Elderly:
   Bind arm to chest 4-6 weeks
Youngsters:
   Plaster U slab and sling
   If ununited at 6 weeks consider a plaster spica

Operative indications
Other injuries in same or other limbs
Pathological fracture
Method
   Intramedullary nail
   On-lay plate

Complications
Delayed or non-union:
   Nail + grafts + plaster spica
Radial Nerve paralysis:
   Explore if no sign of recovery at 2 months

References

Klenerman L 1966 Fractures of the shaft of the humerus.
   Journal of Bone and Joint Surgery 48B: 105-111
Loomer R, Kokan P 1975 Non-union in fractures of the
   humeral shaft. Injury 7: 274-278
Sarmiento A et al 1977 Functional bracing of fractures of the
   shaft of the humerus. Journal of Bone and Joint Surgery
   59A: 596-601
Shaw J L, Sakellarides H 1967 Radial nerve paralysis
   associated with fractures of the humerus. Journal of Bone
   and Joint Surgery 49A: 899-902

Supracondylar fractures of the humerus in children

General features
Common injury M > F : R > L
More frequent in summer
98% extension variety due to fall on outstretched
   hand
2% flexion variety due to fall on point of elbow
Age 2-12. Rare before 2 years

Clinical features
Pain, swelling, deformity, loss of function
Sometimes compound anteriorly
Brachial artery occluded } in 20-30%
Median nerve interrupted }

Radiological features

Juxta-epiphyseal fracture (Salter type 2)

Very wide displacement can occur

Distal fragment displaces
  posteriorly (extension type)
  or anteriorly (flexion type)

Difficult to diagnose in infants if no eiphyseal
  ossification is present

Lateral and rotatory displacements can also
  occur

Pathological features

Usually severe damage to M. Brachialis

Spike of humeral shaft may impale brachial
  artery and/or median nerve

Ulnar and radial nerves very rarely damaged

Treatment

(for those without neurovascular damage)

1. Little swelling

Early reduction
  in flexion (extension type)
  or extension (flexion type)

Splintage in extension can be used for both types
  of fracture

2. Much swelling

Elevation of arm

or, Dunlop traction

or, Traction by ASIF screw } until manipulation is safe

3. Unstable fractures

Dunlop traction

or, Olecranon pin traction or ASIF screw

or, Percutaneous pin fixation

4. Irreducibility

Usually due to soft tissue interposition

Open reduction +/- internal fixation

After treatment:

Remove splintage (internal and external) at 3
  weeks

Mobilisation 3-6 weeks

Full mobility may take 6-12 months

Complications

Non Union:
  Very rare

Mal Union:
  Common, may be due to
    1. epiphyseal damage
    2. poor reduction
    3. inadequate fixation

1. Anteroposterior tilting may limit
     flexion/extension
   Surgery very rarely required
   Remodelling may take three years
2. Varus tilting 'Gun stock' deformity
     Unusual
     Does not recover spontaneously
     Osteotomy of lower humerus required

References

D'Ambrosia R D 1972 Supracondylar fractures of humerus. Prevention of cubitus varus. Journal of Bone and Joint Surgery 54A: 60-66

Dodge H S 1972 Displaced supracondylar fractures of the humerus in children – treatment by Dunlop's traction. Journal of Bone and Joint Surgery 54A: 1408-1418

Elstrom J A, Pankovich A M, Kassab M T 1975 Irreducible supracondylar fracture of the humerus in children. Journal of Bone and Joint Surgery 357A: 680-681

Flynn J C, Matthews J C, Benoit R L 1974 Blind pinning of the displaced supracondylar fractures of the humerus in children. Journal of Bone and Joint Surgery 56A: 263-372

Gartland J J 1959 Management of supracondylar fractures of the humerus in children. Surgery, Gynaecology and Obstetrics 109: 145-154

Soltanpur A 1978 Anterior supracondylar fracture of humerus (flexion type). Journal of Bone and Joint Surgery 60B: 383-386

Supracondylar fractures in children

With vascular and neurological complications

Ulnar and radial nerves rarely damaged

Clinical features

Those of fracture

Often excessive swelling and bruising

Absent radial pulse. Poor capillary filling

Loss of sensation in radial half of palm

Loss of index and thumb flexion

Loss of sweating in radial half of palm

Pain on passive extension of fingers

Pathological features

Brachial artery

May be occluded by
  Hematoma
  Pressure of displaced bone end
  Internal tear
  Local vasoconstriction
  Dislocation into fracture site
  or divided by

Bone fragment
Ends retract: No bleeding

Median nerve
Contused
Divided very rarely

Radiological features
Arteriography very rarely reported
Blockage of brachial artery present
Collaterals usually occluded also

Treatment
Elevate arm, reduce fracture, partly extend elbow
Exploration is safest policy
Inevitably decompresses collateral vessels

Brachial Artery:
Divided: Tie off each end
Constricted: Apply papaverine (doubtful value)
Loss of brachial artery does not lead to
    ischaemia if the collaterals are open.
Intimal repair impractical unless operating
    microscope is available.

Median nerve
Continuity: Decompress
Divided: Repair

Fracture
Stabilise with percutaneous epicondylar pins

References

Elstrom J A, Pankovich A M, Kassab M T 1975 Irreducible
    supracondylar fracture of the humerus in children. Journal
    of Bone and Joint Surgery 57A: 680-681
Spinner M, Schreiber S N 1969 Anterior interosseous nerve
    paralysis as a complication of supracondylar fractures in
    children. Journal of Bone and Joint Surgery 51A: 1584-
    1590
Staples O S 1965 Dislocation of the brachial artery. Journal
    of Bone and Joint Surgery 47A: 1525-1532
Symeonides P P, Pagalides T 1975 Radial nerve enclosed in
    the callus of a supracondylar fracture. Journal of Bone and
    Joint Surgery 57B: 523-524
Wiens E, Lav S C K 1978 The anterior interosseous nerve
    syndrome. Canadian Journal of Surgery 21: 354-357

Established ischemia of forearm

Synonym
Volkman's Contracture

General features
Increasingly uncommon in Western World
Causes:
    Usually supracondylar humeral fracture in
        children
    Other fractures of upper limb
    Crushing injuries of upper limb
    Crush syndrome of arm (+/- drug overdosage)
Variable disability depending on degree of
    ischemia
In hemophilia, may occur from minor injury

Clinical features

Initially
Unrelieved pain and swelling of forearm
Pallor of hand
Absent radial pulse
Variable paralysis of musculature

Later
Median and ulnar nerve paralysis
Fixed flexion of wrist
Clawed fingers
Wasting of forearm

Pathological features
Ellipsoid muscle infarct centred on anterior
    interosseous artery
Due to arterial occlusion
Debate about effects of venous occlusion
Fibrosis of F.D.P. and F.P.L. muscles including
    median nerve

Radiological features
Generalised osteoporosis
Evidence of previous fracture
Arteriography may show brachial artery blockage
    and poor distal "run-off"

Treatment

Prophylaxis
Observation and elevation of injured limb

Early decompression
Splinting to avoid contracture
Passive and active exercising

Surgery
Excision of infarct if no recovery in 3-6 months
Nerve grafting

References

Page C M 1923 An operation for the relief of flexion contracture in the forearm. Journal of Bone and Joint Surgery 5: 233-234

Parkes A 1951 The treatment of established Volkmann's contracture by tendon transplantations. Journal of Bone and Joint Surgery 33B: 359-362

Seddon M J 1956 Volkmann's contracture. Treatment by excision of the infarct. Journal of Bone and Joint Surgery 38B: 152-174

Seddon M J 1964 Volkmann's ischemia. British Medical Journal 1: 1587-1592

Tsuge K 1975 Treatment of established Volkmann's contracture. Journal of Bone and Joint Surgery 57A: 925-929

Volkman R Vonn 1881 Die ischaemischen mustellahmungen und krontrakturer. Zentralblatt Fur Chirurgie 8: 801-803

Fracture of medial epicondylar epiphysis

General
Caused by valgus strain to the elbow
Occurs between 7 and 17 years (appearance to fusion)

Clinical features
Pain, swelling on inner side of elbow
Inability to move elbow
Ulnar nerve dysfunction in severe injuries

Radiological features
1st degree : Slight separation
2nd degree :Epicondyle level with elbow joint
3rd degree : Epicondyle included in elbow joint
4th degree : Avulsion of epicondyle and lateral dislocation of elbow

Pathological feature
No metaphyseal fragment
(Salter type I injury)
Ulnar nerve contused but never divided
May be part of dislocation of elbow with spontaneous reduction of dislocation
Fibrous union still allows normal function

Treatment
1st degree:
    Sling and bandage
2nd degree:
    Plaster cast below right angle
3rd degree:
    Open reduction and internal fixation with transposition of ulnar nerve
4th degree:
    Open reduction and internal fixation with transposition of ulnar nerve
(Electrical stimulation of flexor muscles to withdraw epicondyle from the elbow joint has been abandoned)
Flexion is quick but extension is slow to recover

References

Bede W B, Lefebure A R, Rosman M A, 1975 Fractures of the medical humeral epicondyle in children. Canadian Journal of Surgery 18: 137-142

Wilson J N 1960 The treatment of fractures of the medial epicondyle of the humerus. Journal of Bone and Joint Surgery 42B: 778-781

Fractures of capitellum

Synonym
Mouchet's fracture

General features
Caused by falls on outstretched hand with valgus strain to elbow.
Not seen before 14-15 years

Clinical features
Pain, swelling, loss of function

Radiological features
Forward and upward displacement of capitellum
Fractures of radial head may be present
Capitellar fragment usually larger than it appears on radiographs.

Pathological features:
Corresponds to lateral condylar fractures in children
3 Grades:
    Bruising of capitellar cartilage
    Undisplaced fracture) Often half lower humeral
    Displaced fracture   ) articular surface

Treatment
Immediate excision usually gives best results
Closed reduction with elbow extended) Poor
Open reduction +/- internal fixation) results

References
Alvarez E et al 1975 Fracture of the capitulum humeri. Journal of Bone and Joint Surgery 57A: 1093-1096
Fowles J V, Kassab M T 1974 Fracture of the capitulum humeri. Treatment by excision. Journal of Bone and Joint Surgery 56A: 794-798
Mouchet A 1898 Fractures de l'extremite inferieure de l'humerus 290-295. Paris, G Steinheil

Intercondylar fractures of humerus

General features
Caused by heavy fall on outstretched hand or violent blow over lower humerus
May be part of 'side-swipe' fracture
Very rare in children

Clinical features
Pain, swelling, loss of function
Neurovascular complications unusual
Rarely compound

Radiological features
'T' shaped fracture of lower humerus separating trochlear and capitellum from each other and humeral shaft
Further comminution in the elderly

Pathological features
Type   I: No displacement
       II: Trochlear and Capitellum separated but not rotated
       III: Trochlear and capitellum separated and rotated
       IV: Severe comminution and wide separation

Treatment

Oldsters
Bandage and sling. Early movement

Youngsters
Type I: Plaster cast and sling
      II: Manipulation, splint in extension

Types III & IV: (i) Open reduction and internal fixation
           (Variety of methods)
or (ii) Olecranon traction
or (iii) No reduction early active movements in elderly or infirm

References
Brown R F, Morgan R G 1971 Intercondylar 'T' shaped fractures of the humerus. Journal of Bone and Joint Surgery 53B: 425-428
Dickson R A 1976 Reversed dynamic slings. A new concept in treatment of post-traumatic elbow flexion contractures. Injury 8: 35-38
Riseborough E J, Radin E L 1969 Inter-condylar 'T' fractures of the humerus in the adults. Journal of Bone and Joint Surgery 51A: 130-141

Side-swipe fracture of elbow

Synonym
Baby-car fracture

General features
Caused by violent blow on flexed elbow—usually protruding from a vehicle
Sometimes compound

Clinical features:
Pain, swelling, loss of function
Neurovascular deficit not uncommon

Radiological features
Fracture of lower shaft of humerus
Fracture of olecranon and forward dislocation of elbow
Fracture of shaft of ulna and/or radius

Pathological features
Malunion is common
Serious disability if elbow dislocation is not fully corrected

Treatment:
1. Internal fixation of olecranon and reduction of dislocation
2. Splintage in extension
   or Internal fixation of humerus and/or ulna and radius

References

Scharplatz D, Allgower M 1975 Fracture dislocations of the elbow. Injury 7: 143-159

Watson-Jones R 1976 Fractures and joint injuries. Wilson J N (ed) 5th Edition, Volume 2, p. 653. Churchill-Livingstone, Edinburgh

Fractures of lateral condyle of humerus

General features

Occurs in children

Falls on outstretched hand with elbow flexed

Element of rotation and varus force

Similar injury to medial condyle is extremely rare as is separation of lateral epicondylar epiphysis

Clinical features

Occurs between 5 and 15

Loss of elbow function

Early ulnar nerve dysfunction is rare

Pain, swelling, worst laterally

Radiological features

Separation of triangular fragment of capitellar epiphysis and adjoining metaphysis (Salter type IV)

Variable displacement and angulation

Compare films of opposite elbow

Pathological features

Extensor musculature may cause fragment to turn upside down

Non-union is frequent. May be due to fibrinolysis in hemoarthrosis

Lack of growth laterally may lead to cubitus valgus and ulnar neutitis in late adolescence

Treatment

Surgery:
Open reduction
Internal fixation

Late cases:

Open reduction, grafting, internal fixation

Neglected cases:

Anterior transposition of ulnar nerve

References

Flynn J C, Richards J F, Saltzman R I 1975 Prevention and treatment of non-union of slightly displaced fractures of the lateral humeral condyle in children. Journal of Bone and Joint Surgery 57A: 1087-1092

Jakob R et al 1975 Observations concerning fractures of the lateral humeral condyle in children. Journal of Bone and Joint Surgery 57B: 430-436

Dislocation of elbow

General features

Occurs at any age

Fall on hand, elbow flexed—posterior dislocation

Blow on back of extended elbow—anterior dislocation

Clinical features

Pain, swelling, deformity, loss of function

Marked instability if radial head or olecranon is fractured

Ulnar nerve damage very common

Dislocation and supracondylar fractures distinguished by relationship of olecranon to the epicondyles.

Radiological features

Posterior or postero-lateral displacement of olecranon is commonest

(Anterior dislocation of olecranon with fracture uncommon)

Fractures of medial epicondyle or coronoid process may be present

Pathological features

Rupture of capsule

Contusion of ulnar nerve

Arterial occlusion unusual

Extra-articular ossification may occur from too early mobilisation

Treatment

Manipulation

Easy with elbow flexed to 90°

Hyperextension is dangerous

Splint for 3 weeks

Fracture of coronoid may be ignored usually

Surgery

Internal fixation of displaced medial epicondyle and fractured olecranon

Remove comminuted radial head (if present) not earlier than 3 weeks

Neglected Dislocations

4 weeks : Manipulation

6 months : Open reduction
: Consider excision arthroplasty or prosthetic arthroplasty

Complications

1. Irreducibility

Causes:

Medial epicondyle trapped in elbow joint (Unossified before 6 or 7)

Ulnar nerve ⎫
Brachial artery ⎬ All reported
Median nerve ⎭

Treatment:

Open reduction

2. Extra articular ossification

Persistent limitation of movement

Visible on radiographs

Treatment:

Usually responds to rest

Wait 6 months before considering excision

3. Recurrent dislocation

Vide infra

References

Protzman R R 1978 Dislocation of the elbow joint. Journal of Bone and Joint Surgery 60A: 539-541

Scharplatz D, Allgower M 1975 Fracture dislocations of the elbow. Injury 7: 143-159

Silva J F 1958 Old dislocations of the elbow. Annals of the Royal College of Surgeons of England 22: 363-381

Recurrent dislocation of elbow

General

Rare

Due to congenitally shallow olecranon notch or unsound repair after first dislocation with marginal fractures

Clinical features

Minor falls dislocate elbow after first major incident

Pain, swelling, deformity

Patient may reduce dislocation himself

Radiological features

Fracture of coronoid process may be present and ununited

Degenerative changes eventually appear

Pathological features

Lax capsule

Laxity of posterolateral ligaments

Marginal joint fractures may be present

Treatment

Conservatism

Indicated for age, frailty or general disease:

Hinged elbow splint

Surgery

1. Strengthening of anterior structures
   Rerouting biceps tendon through coronoid
   Bone block on coronoid

or 2. Reconstruction of postero-lateral ligaments

or 3. Posterior bone block

or 4. Deepening of olecranon notch

or 5. Combination of some of these procedures

Best methods still uncertain

References

Dreyfuss U, Kessler I 1978 Snapping elbow due to dislocations of the medial head of the triceps. Journal of Bone and Joint Surgery 60B: 56-57

Jacobs R L 1971 Recurrent dislocation of the elbow joint. Clinical Orthopaedics 74: 151-154

Osborne G, Cotterill P 1966 Recurrent dislocations of the elbow. Journal of Bone and Joint Surgery 48B: 340-346

Displacement of lower humeral epiphysis

General features

Rare

Caused by fall on point of elbow.

Children 3-8

Clinical features
Pain, swelling, loss of function
Neurovascular deficit very rare

Radiological features
Forward displacement of lower humeral
    epiphysis
Lateral film of normal elbow for comparison

Pathological features
Is an intracapsular supracondylar fracture with
    little displacement. (Salter, Type I)

Treatment
Manipulation backwards of displaced epiphysis
Splint in extension for 3 weeks

Reference
Watson-Jones R 1976 Fractures and joint injuries Wilson J N
    (ed) 5th Edition, Volume 2, p. 634. Churchill Livingstone,
    Edinburgh.

FOREARM AND HAND INJURIES

Pulled elbow

General features
Occurs only in children, 2-6 years
Caused by forcible traction on extended arms,
    usually in a recalcitrant child

Clinical features
Painful elbow
Tenderness over radial head
Supination restricted by pain
Full flexion and extension

Radiological features
No abnormality visible

Pathological features
Uncertain
Thought to be due to stretching of annular
    ligament and partial subluxation of radial
    head

Treatment
Forcible supination of forearm
No anesthesia usually required
May spontaneously recover in sling after 48
    hours

References
Hutchison A J 1885 On certain obscure sprains of the elbow
    occurring in young children. Annals of surgery 2: 91-97
Illingworth C M 1975 Pulled elbow: A study of 100 patients.
    British Medical Journal 2: 672-674
Ryan J R 1969 The relationship of the radial head to the
    radial neck diameters in fetuses and adults with reference
    to radial head subluxation in children. Journal of Bone and
    Joint Surgery 51A: 781-783

Fracture of head of radius

General features
Caused by fall on outstretched hand with valgus
    strain to elbow
R > L
Commonest in young and middle adult life

Clinical features
Local tenderness over head of radius
Little swelling

Supination most restricted
Weak grip

Radiological features
Chisel fracture
Segmental fracture
Communited fracture—"Exploded"
    head } Variable features
Fracture of neck of radius
Irregularity of capitellum

Pathological features
Damage to capitellum and medial ligament of
    elbow sometimes present
Displaced fragments become avascular
May form loose body in elbow or block elbow
    movement by lying in soft tissues nearby
Occasional damage to inferior radioulnar joint

Treatment
Bandage and sling early movements for
Chisel fracture
Small segmental fracture $<1/3$ Diameter
Removal of radial head
+/- silastic replacement: for
Large segmental fracture $>1/3$ Diameter
Communited fracture
Plaster cast 2-3 weeks early movements for
Fracture of radial neck:
Undisplaced fractures
Manipulation and Percutaneous pin fixation for
Displaced fractures
The smaller the fracture the better the results.
Rehabilitation may take several months in worst
    fractures.

References
Bakalim G 1970 Fractures of the radial head and their
    treatment. Acta Orthopaedica Scandinavica 41: 320-331
Rabin E L, Riseborough E J 1966 Fractures of the radial
    head. Journal of Bone and Joint Surgery 48A: 1055-1064

Fractures of olecranon

General features
Occur from falls on point of elbow
May be part of a Monteggia injury particularly
    in children:
(Fracture of radial shaft or dislocating of radial
    head)

Clinical features
Pain, bruising
Fracture site easily palpable. Often compound
Loss of elbow extension
Ulnar nerve rarely damaged

Radiological features
Variable angulation of fracture surface
Comminution often present in the elderly
Patella cubiti present from 10 to 16 years
(Films of opposite elbow will confirm)

Pathological features
Fracture fragments separated by triceps elasticity
Good elbow function still possible with only 20%
   of distal olecranon notch remaining
Fracture gap untreated will eventually fill with
   fibrous tissue

Treatment

Oldsters
Powerful extension never required
Bandage and sling

Others
Comminuted undisplaced fractures: Sling
   Separated fragments:
1. Sherman's or Lane's screws obliquely inserted
      to engage opposite cortex
or 2. Knowles screw for intramedullary fixation
or 3. Hooked plate
or 4. Figure 8 wire loop
or 5. Tension wire suture (AO Technique)
or 6. Excision of fragments if very comminuted

References
Colton C L 1974 Fractures of the olecranon in adults.
   Classification and management. Injury 5: 121-129
McKeever F M, Buck R M 1947 Fracture of the olecranon
   process of the ulna. Treatment by excision of fragment and
   repair of triceps tendons. Journal of American Medical
   Association 135: 1-5
Newell R L M 1975 Olecranon fractures in children. Injury 7:
   33-36
Theodorou S A 1969 Dislocation of the head of the radius,
   associated with fracture of the upper end of the ulna in
   children. Journal of Bone and Joint Surgery 51B: 700-706

Juxta-epiphyseal fractures of upper radius in children

General features
Caused by valgus strain of elbow
Mostly occur before 4
Can occur up to 12

Clinical features
Pain, loss of function
Variable swelling

Radiological features
   Greenstick fracture of neck of radius
or Displacement of upper radial epiphysis
      Associated injuries: Fracture of medial
                           epicondyle
                  or Fracture of upper ulna

Pathological features
Removal of radial upper epiphysis leads to
   shortened radius and dislocation of inferior
   radio-ulnar joint
If upper epiphysis is retained extensive
   remodelling can occur

Treatment

Tilt < 30°:
No manipulation
Bandage and sling

Tilt 30° - 60°
Manipulation: Extended elbow, varus strain,
                  pressure over radial head

Tilt > 60°
Cautious surgery; levering epiphysis into place
Percutaneous pin fixation if very unstable
No treatment if fracture is over 3 weeks old

Complications of surgery
Heterotopic ossification
Turning epiphysis upside down
Avascular necrosis of epiphysis
Radio-ulnar synostosis

References

Henrikson B 1969 Isolated fractures of the proximal end of
  the radius in children. Epidermology, treatment and
  prognosis. Acta Orthopedica Scandinavica 40: 246-260
Jones E R L, Esah M 1971 Displaced fractures of the neck of
  the radius in children. Journal of Bone and Joint Surgery
  53B: 429-439

Fracture of ulna with dislocation of radial head

Synonym
Monteggia's fracture

General features
Caused by direct blow on mid forearm
Sometimes caused by forced pronation
Extensor type 85-90%
Flexor type 10-15%
Difficult to treat successfully
May be compound

Clinical features
Pain, swelling deformity
Loss of function of wrist and elbow

Radiological features
Minor changes in children. Easily missed
  i.e. Bowed ulna and lateral displacement of
    radial head

Flexor type
Ulna bowed posteriorly
Radial head displaced posteriorly

Extensor type
Ulna bowed anteriorly
Radial head displaced anteriorly
Isolated fracture of upper ulna requires repeated
  checking of position of radial head
Isolated dislocation of radial head is rare

Pathological features

Type I
Anterior dislocation of radial head
Fracture of ulnar diaphysis with anterior
  angulation

Type II
Posterior or posterolateral dislocation of radial
  head
Fracture of middle or proximal third of ulna

Type III
Lateral dislocation of radial head
Fracture of proximal ulnar metaphysis

Type IV
Anterior dislocation of radial head
Fracture of middle or proximal third of ulna
Fracture of middle third of radius
Posterior interosseous nerve often paralysed
Vascular deficit unusual

Treatment

Flexor type
Manipulation
Splintage with elbow extended in full pronation

Extension type
1. Internal fixation of ulna
   Intramedullary nail or compression plate
2. Open reduction of radial head if it fails to
   reduce manually

Complications
Late subluxation of radial head: Excision (only
  in adults)
Non union: Graft + internal fixation and
  external splintage
Mal union: Osteotomy and internal fixation
Cross union: (Usually with high ulnar fractures)
           Excision or osteotomy

References

Bado J L 1962 The Monteggia lesion. Blackwell, Oxford
Bruce H E, Harvey J P, Wilson J C 1974 Monteggia
  fractures. Journal of Bone and Joint Surgery 56A: 1563-
  1576
Mullick S 1977 The lateral Monteggia fracture. Journal of
  Bone and Joint Surgery 59A: 543-545
Peiro A et al 1977 Acute Monteggia lesions in children.
  Journal of Bone and Joint Surgery 59A: 92-97
Wiley J J, Horwich J P 1974 Traumatic dislocation of the
  radius at the elbow. Journal of Bone and Joint Surgery
  56B: 501-507

Fracture of radial head with disruption of inferior radio-ulnar joint

General features
Caused by a fall on the outstretched hand with
  axial compression of forearm
Wrist injury often overlooked

Clinical features
Pain, little swelling
Loss of function of elbow and wrist

Radiological features
Usually severe comminution of radial head.
Subluxation or dislocation of inferior radio-ulnar
  joint

Pathological features
Function of wrist and elbow affected

Treatment
Delay excision of head of radius
Closed reduction of inferior joint
Splint for three weeks
Vigorous physiotherapy thereafter
Remove radial head later if necessary

Reference
Essex-Lopresti P 1957 Fractures of the radial head with distal
  radio-ulnar dislocation. Journal of Bone and Joint Surgery
  33B: 244-247
McDougall A, White J 1957 Subluxation of the inferior
  radio-ulnar joint complicating fractures of the radial head.
  Journal of Bone and Joint Surgery 39B: 278-287
Taylor T K F, O'Connor B T 1964 The effect upon the
  inferior radioulnar joint of excision of the head of the
  radius in adults. Journal of Bone and Joint Surgery 46B:
  83-88

Fracture of radius with dislocation of ulnar head

Synonym
Galleazzi's fracture

General features
Caused by falling on outstretched hand
Corresponds to Monteggia fracture dislocation
Difficult to treat successfully
Not often compound

Clinical features
Pain, swelling, deformity
Loss of function of wrist

Radiological features
Fracture of lower third of radius
Dislocation or subluxation of inferior radio-ulnar
  joint

Pathological features
Triangular cartilage may be ruptured
Ulnar styloid may be avulsed
Neurovascular damage unusual
Subluxation of inferior joint may occur alone

Treatment
1. Manipulation and splintage in full supination
     Weekly x-rays required. Most success in
       children
2. Open reduction and internal fixation of radius
     Splintage in supination
       Radial plate and transverse wire across
         inferior radio-ulnar joint

Complications
Non union of radius: Graft, Plate, Splintage
Mal-union of radius: Excise lower end of ulna
                     +/- Osteotomy of radius

References
Mikic Z D 1975 Galeazzi fracture dislocations. Journal of
  Bone and Joint Surgery 57A: 1071-1080
Snook G A et al 1969 Subluxation of the distal radio ulnar
  joint by hyperpronation. Journal of Bone and Joint
  Surgery 51A: 1315-1323

Isolated fractures of ulnar shaft

General features
Unusual
Dislocation of superior radio-ulnar joint may be
  overlooked
Caused by direct blow

Clinical features
Pain and swelling
No deformity
Little loss of function

Radiological features
Greenstick fracture in children
Minor displacement +/- comminution in adults
Major displacement is unusual

Pathological features
Delayed union is frequent
Non-union not unusual

Treatment
Complete reduction difficult to obtain
Manipulation.
  Children: Splintage 3 weeks
  Adults   :   6-12 weeks
Delayed Union:
  Grafts and internal fixation
  Plate better than intramedullary rod
Functional Bracing may be most effective
  splintage

References
Hooper G 1974 Isolated fractures of the shaft of the ulna.
  Injury 6: 180-184
Sarmiento A et al 1976 Treatment of ulnar fractures by
  functional bracing. Journal of Bone and Joint Surgery
  58A: 1104-1107

Isolated fracture of radial shaft

General features
Caused by rotational forces
Dislocation of superior or inferior radio-ulnar
  joints may be overlooked

Clinical features
Pain, swelling, some deformity
Loss of function of elbow and wrist

Radiological features
Fracture may be present in any part of middle $\frac{3}{4}$
  of shaft

Pathological features
Relationship of M. Pron. Teres insertion to
  fracture site determines deformity and position
  of reduction
Interosseous membrane damaged.
Type   I: Fracture mid-upper third –
  Upper fragment supinated

    Lower fragment: pronated
Type II: Fracture in mid third: Fragments in
  mid position
Type III: Fracture in mid/lower third: Upper
  fragment pronated

Treatment: Manipulation +/- internal fixation of radius
Type   I: Forearm supinated
Type II: Forearm in mid position
Type III: Forearm pronated

References
Evans E M 1951 Fractures of the radius and ulna. Journal of
  Bone and Joint Surgery 33B: 548-561

Fractures of the radial and ulnar shafts

General features
Transverse and comminuted fractures caused by
  a direct blow
Spiral fractures caused by twisting, indirect
  violence, often at different levels in the radius
  and ulna
Crushing injuries cause major soft tissue damage

Clinical features
Pain, swelling, deformity
Loss of function
Neurovascular deficits commoner in crushing and
  compound injuries

Radiographic features

Greenstick fractures common in children

Whole of radius and ulna should be visualised

Difference in width of interosseous membrane above and below fracture means a rotational deformity at fracture site

Pathological features

Delayed or non-union is common

Cross union occurs only in the more severe injuries

Bowing of forearm without fracture may occur in children

Angular deformities of 10°-20° grow out in children under 7-8 years

Treatment

Some shortening is acceptable in children in bayonet-type fractures

Rotational and angular deformity must be corrected

Greenstick fractures

Manipulation. Long arm cast 3-4 weeks

Oblique spiral fractures

Manipulation. Long arm cast 6-8 weeks

Consider plating in adults if reduction is not perfect

Transverse and comminuted fractures

Conservative:

Traction, hitching and long arm cast 8-12 weeks

Surgical:

Plating. Compression plating if possible.

Initial delay of 2-3 weeks gives better long term results

Compound fractures

Wound debridement – Close if possible

Vascular repair if necessary

Otherwise:

Delayed primary closure

Delayed skin grafting

When skin is sound: Consider internal fixation

Nerve damage: Repair at internal fixation or at 3rd operation if necessary

Long arm cast for 8-12 weeks

Complications

Mal-Union: Osteotomy and plating

Non Union: Grafting compression platting

Loss of part of 1 shaft: Radio-ulnar fusion

Radio-Ulnar Synostosis: Excision

Neurovascular damage: Exploration and repair

References

Anderson L D et al 1975 Compression plate fixation in acute diaphyseal fractures of the radius and ulna. Journal of Bone and Joint Surgery 57A: 287-297

Borden S 1974 Traumatic bowing of the forearm in children. Journal of Bone and Joint Surgery 56A: 611-616

Castle M E 1974 One bone forearm. Journal of Bone and Joint Surgery 56A: 1223-1227

Elstrom J A, Pankovich A M, Egwele R 1978 Extra-articular low velocity gunshot fractures of the radius and ulna. Journal of Bone and Joint Surgery 60A: 335-341

Ghandi R K et al 1962 Spontaneous correction of deformity following fractures of the forearm in children. British Journal of Surgery 50: 5-10

Nicholl E A 1956 The treatment of gaps in long bones by cancellous insert grafts. Journal of Bone and Joint Surgery 38B: 70-82

Sarmiento A, Cooper J S, Sinclair W F 1975 Forearm fractures: early functional bracing: a preliminary report. Journal of Bone and Joint Surgery 57A: 297-304

Smith J E M 1959 Internal fixation in the treatment of fractures of the shafts of the radius and ulna in adults. The value of delayed operation in the prevention of non-union. Journal of Bone and Joint Surgery 41B: 122-131

Warren J D 1963 Anterior interosseous nerve palsy as a complication of forearm fractures. Journal of Bone and Joint Surgery 45B: 511-512

Fractures of lower forearm in children

General features

Falls on outstretched hand in forced pronation

Clinical features

Pain, swelling, loss of function, deformity

Rarely compound

Neurovascular damage very rare

Age 3-12

Radiological features

Type 1:

Greenstick fracture of lower quarter of radius

Type 2:

Fracture of lower quarter of radius

Greenstick fracture of lower ulna

Type 3:

Fractures of lower quarter of radius and ulna with displacement

Type 4:

Fracture of lower quarter of radius

Dislocation of inferior radio ulnar joint (Galleazzi fracture)

Pathological features
Interposition of tendons of A.P.L. and E.P.B.
muscles may prevent reduction of radius

Treatment

Manipulation
Worsen deformity to hitch displaced surfaces of
radius before attempting reduction

Open reduction
Required if manipulation fails from soft tissue
interposition percutaneous trans-carpal
intramedullary radial wire or nail gives
stability
Splintage 3-5 weeks

References
Rang M 1974 Children fractures. Chapter 13. J B Lippincolt
Co, Toronto

Displacement of lower radial epiphysis

Synonym
Children's Colles fracture

General features
Occurs from falls on outstretched hand
Age 3-12

Clinical features:
Those of any fracture
Dinner fork deformity may be present
No neurovascular impairment

Radiological features
Dorsal lateral angulation or displacement of
lower radial epiphysis
Triangular metaphyseal fragment present

Pathological features
Periosteal attachment always retained
Usually Salter Type 2
Avascular necrosis never occurs
Premature epiphyseal fusion is rare

Treatment
1. Manipulation
Difficult to over-reduce
Plaster cast 3-4 weeks
2. Open reduction and/or internal fixation never
required
3. Premature fusion of radial epiphysis:
Excise lower end of ulna at end of growth

References
Rang M 1974 Children's fractures, Chapter 13. J B
Lippencolt Co, Toronto

Dorsal fracture of lower radius

Synonym
Colles fracture

General features
Usually in old women
$M : F = 1 : 20$
Caused by a fall on the outstretched hand
In young people is caused by major violence
Rarely compound

Clinical features
Pain, swelling, tenderness
"Dinner fork" deformity
Dorsoradial displacement of lower radius with
tilting

Radiological features:
Fracture of lower radius, often comminuted
Fracture of ulnar styloid
Dorsal tilting of articular surface of radius with
impaction of fragments

Pathological features
Osteoporosis usually present
Avascular necrosis never occurs
Median nerve may be compressed
Friction attrition of M. Ext. Poll. Long. tendon
can occur at 4-8 weeks

Treatment
Not every fracture requires treatment
Decide on age, general condition, wrist deformity
and radiological appearance
Regional analgesia as good as general anesthesia

1. Elderly
Manipulation
Cast for 6 weeks (below elbow)

2. Youngsters
Manipulation. Aim for perfection
Above elbow cast
+/- Percutaneous pin fixation

Complications
Stiff forequarter:
    Particularly in elderly
    Physiotherapy often required for several
      months
Malunion:
    Excise lower end of ulna
Median Nerve Compression:
    Decompress
Rupture of E.P.L. tendon:
    Repair with E. I. tendon
Sudek's Osteodystrophy:
    Persistent active exercise
    Avoid drugs of addiction
Osteoarthrosis of wrist:
    Wrist strap
    Arthrodesis
Non Union (excessively rare):
    Bone graft

References
Colles A 1814 On the fracture of the carpal extremity of the radius. Edinburgh Medical and Surgical Journal 10: 182-186

Green D P 1975 Pins and plaster treatment of comminuted fractures of the distal end of the radius. Journal of Bone and Joint Surgery 57A: 304-310

Pool C 1973 Colles' fracture. A prospective study of treatment. Journal of Bone and Joint Surgery 55B: 540-544

Sarmiento A et al 1975 Colles fractures. Functional bracing and supination. Journal of Bone and Joint Surgery 57A: 311-317

Anterior fracture of lower radius

Synonym
Chauffeur's fracture. Smith's Fracture

General features
Occurs from:
    blow on back of wrist
    falls with hand palmar flexed
Usually in middle age or later

Clinical features
Pain, swelling, tenderness of wrist

Radiological features
Volar displacement of carpus and hand
Types   I Fractures of ulna and radius
          Articular surface of radius intact
      II Anterior marginal fracture of radius
         only.
         Damage to articular surface of radius
         (Barton's fracture)
     III Fracture of lower end of radius only
         No damage to articular surface of
         radius

Pathological features
Comminuted fractures involve the lower radial articular surface and may lead to osteoarthrosis

Treatment
Manipulation
    Forearm supinated
    Elbow flexed
    Full arm cast applied
Open reduction. Ellis plate. Best for Type II fractures
Mal-union

Complications
Median nerve compression
    Divide carpal ligament
Osteodystrophy
Osteoarthrosis of wrist
Late rupture of Flex. Poll. long tendon

References
De Oliveira J C 1973 Barton's fractures. Journal of Bone and Joint Surgery 55A: 586-594

Ellis J 1965 Smith's and Barton's fractures. A method of treatment. Journal of Bone and Joint Surgery 47B: 724-727

Smith R W 1847 A treatise in fractures in the vicinity of joints and on certain accidental and congenital dislocations, Hodges and Smith, Dublin, p 162-164

Thomas F B 1957 Reduction of Smith's fracture. Journal of Bone and Joint Surgery 39B: 463-470

Fractures of radial styloid

General features
Caused by a fall on outstretched hand
May be part of a complex of other injuries

Clinical features
Pain, very little swelling. No deformity
Local tenderness, loss of wrist function
Very rarely compound

Radiological features
Rarely displaced
Fracture line may pass through tip or base of styloid process

Pathological features
Attrition of E.P.L. tendon may occur
De Quervain's stenosing tendo-vaginitis a later possibility

Treatment
Splintage for 3-4 weeks in plaster
Internal fixation if initially displaced

Reference
De Palma A F 1970 The management of fractures and dislocations. 2nd Edition, Volume 2, p 927, W B Saunders Co, Philadelphia

Fracture dislocation of radio-carpal joint

General features
Major violence involved
Injuries in other systems frequent
Usually young adults

Clinical features
Pain, swelling, deformity
Loss of wrist and hand function
Neurovascular deficit is uncommon

Radiological features
Fractures of radial and ulnar styloids
Fractures of dorsal edge of radius
Varied intra-carpal injuries

Pathological features
Radiocarpal arthritis is a late sequel

Treatment
Swift manipulation to correct major deformity
Open reduction and internal fixation
Splintage for 6-8 weeks – pins and screws used according to individual lesions

References
Bilos Z J, Pankovich A M, Yelda S 1977 Dislocation of the radio carpal joint. Journal of Bone and Joint Surgery 59A: 198-203
Dunn A W 1972 Fractures and dislocation of the carpus. Surgical Clinics of North America 52: 1513-1538

Injuries of the distal radio-ulnar disc

General features
Uncommon
Probably caused by extreme pronation and extension of wrist
May be associated with local fractures (Diagnosis may be delayed until fractures have healed)

Clinical features
Pain on movement, particularly pronation and supination
Painful click often present
Local tenderness over distal radio-ulnar joint
Instability of joint

Radiological features:
Non per se
Apparent lateral shift of ulnar styloid
Arthrography of wrist delineates distal radio-ulnar joint in all cases but only 50% of normals.

Pathological features
Attachment at ulnar styloid may be torn off
No spontaneous healing
Occasionally disc may be calcified

Treatment
Excision from dorsal approach

References
Coleman H M 1960 Injuries of the articular disc at the wrist. Journal of Bone and Joint Surgery 42B: 522-529
Snook G A 1969 Subluxation of the distal radio-ulnar joint by hyperpronation. Journal of Bone and Joint Surgery 51A: 1315-1323
Spinner M 1971 Calcification of the triangular cartilage of the wrist. Bulletin of the Hospital for Joint Diseases, New York, 23: 21-26

Dislocation of carpal scaphoid

General features
Rare: Caused by fall on hand

Clinical features
Acute: Pain, swelling, loss of function.
Chronic: Pain and stiffness of wrist.
Recurrent: Intermittent pain and loss of function.

Radiological features
May be associated with
   Perilunar carpal dislocation
   Radiocarpal dislocation
   Fracture of radial styloid
   Loss of height of scaphoid seen in A.P. film
   Widening of lunate-scaphoid interval

Pathological features
Lunate-scaphoid ligament ruptured
May dislocate anteriorly or
Rotate on long axis
Radial styloid fracture may procede to malunion
   with recurrent dislocation

Treatment

Acute
Manipulation, splintage for 6 weeks
If unsuccessful: Open reduction
   or Excision and prosthetic replacement

Chronic
Open reduction
or Excision and prosthetic replacement

Recurrent
Open reduction
Repair of lunate-scaphoid ligament
or Lunate-Scaphoid fusion

References
Linscheid R L et al 1972 Traumatic instability of the wrist. Journal of Bone and Joint Surgery 54A: 1612-1632
Thompson T C, Campbell R D, Arnold W D 1964 Primary and secondary dislocation of the scaphoid bone. Journal of Bone and Joint Surgery 46B: 73-82

Fractures of scaphoid

General features
Caused by fall on outstretched hand
Most common fracture in young adults
Rare in children

Clinical features
Pain, slight swelling, no deformity
Tenderness distal to radial styloid
Some loss of wrist function

Radiographic features
Fractures may occur through
   distal/mid third
   Waist
   Proximal/mid third
Fracture line may not be visible for 10-14 days
Xerography or Tomography may aid definition
Early wide separation of fracture may mean a
   trans/scaphoid perilunar fracture dislocation
   has occurred
Sclerosis of adjacent surfaces and cyst formation
   may mean an old fracture is present
Radio-opacity of proximal pole indicates
   ischemia

Pathological features
Scaphoid is the link between proximal and distal
   rows of carpus and is most subject to
   mechanical stress
Blood supply enters dorsally and distally
Proximal pole may become ischemic in 20%
Scaphoid may be bipartite (os centrale)
(Bilateral condition, smooth sclerosed adjacent
   surfaces, no unusual density)

Treatment
No manipulation required
Distal pole:
   Scaphoid cast for 3 weeks
   Excellent prognosis
Other fractures:
   Scaphoid cast for 6 weeks
   If ununited – renew cast for further 6 weeks
Initial doubt:
   Treat as fracture in cast for 2 weeks
   New radiographs will clarify situation
Treatment of other scaphoid problems is
   debatable, i.e.

Factors involved
Age of patient,
Hand dominance
Presence of arthritis in wrist
Nature of Work,
Avascularity of proximal pole

Non-union at 12 weeks
Consider:
    Discarding cast – Non-manual workers
    Surgery – (Manual workers)
             Graft or screw fixation
    Retaining cast for further 12 weeks
             Doubtful value

Non-union at 12 weeks with avascular proximal
pole
Discard cast – Non manual workers
Removal avascular pole: Manual workers

Neglected fractures
No action:
    If painless and fully functional
Surgery:
    If painful and/or stiff, i.e.
1. Excision of avascular pole ⎫ Non manual
or Scaphoid plastic prosthesis ⎰ workers
2. Removable plastic orthosis ⎱ Manual workers
or Radial styloidectomy ⎭

Carpal arthritis with neglected fracture
    Consider: Removable plastic orthosis
or Radio-carpal arthrodesis
or Intra carpal arthrodesis
or Proximal row carpectomy

References
Barber H M 1974 Acrylic scaphoid prostheses: a long term follow up. Proceedings of Royal Society of Medicine 67: 1075-1078
Barnard L, Stubbins S G 1948 Styloidectomy of the radius. Journal of Bone and Joint Surgery 30A: 98: 102
Dwyer F C 1949 Excision of the carpal scaphoid for united fracture. Journal of Bone and Joint Surgery, 31B: 572-577
Fisk G R 1970 Carpal instability and the fractured scaphoid. Annals of the Royal College of Surgeons of England 46: 63-76
Graner O et al 1966 Arthrodesis of the carpal bones in the treatment of Keinboch's disease, painful united fractures of the navicular and lunate bones, with avascular necrosis and old fracture dislocations of the carpal bones. Journal of Bone and Joint Surgery 48A: 767-774
Jorgenson E C 1969 Proximal row carpectomy. Journal of Bone and Joint Surgery 51A: 1104-1111
Louis D S et al 1976 Congenital bipartite scaphoid. Fact or fiction? Journal of Bone and Joint Surgery 58A: 1108-1112
Maudsley R H, Chen S C 1972 Screw fixation in the management of the fractured carpal scaphoid. Journal of Bone and Joint Surgery, 54B: 432-441
Mulder J D 1968 The results of 100 cases of pseudarthrosis in the scaphoid bone, treated by the Matti-Russe operation. Journal of Bone and Joint Surgery 50B: 110-115
Southcott R, Rosman M A 1977 Non-union of carpal scaphoid fractures in children. Journal of Bone and Joint Surgery 59B: 20-23
Taleisnik J, Kelly P J 1966 The extra-osseous and intra-osseous blood supply of the scaphoid bone. Journal of Bone and Joint Surgery 48A: 1125-1137

Trans-scaphoid-perilunar fracture dislocations

General features
Uncommon
Usually caused by falling on outstretched hand
    with major violence
Other injuries often present

Clinical features
Pain, swelling, deformity
Loss of hand and finger function.
Neurovascular impairment common.

Radiological features
Fracture through waist of scaphoid
1. Lunate and proximal scaphoid may remain
    with radius and remainder of carpus
    dislocates
or 2. Lunate and proximal scaphoid dislocate and
    carpus remains aligned with radius.
Large variety of fractures and dislocations are
    possible

Pathological features
Median nerve frequently compressed
Ulnar nerve and arteries may be compressed in
    total carpal dislocations
Avascular necrosis of proximal scaphoid or
    radio- carpal arthritis give trouble later

Treatment
Traction and manipulation
Open reduction for persistent displacement and
    delayed diagnosis
Splintage required until scaphoid fracture heals

References

Campbell R D et al 1965 Indications for open reduction of lunate and perilunate dislocations of the carpal bones. Journal of Bone and Joint Surgery 47A: 915-932

Weiss C, Laskin R S, Spinner M 1970 Irreducible transscaphoid perilunate dislocation. Journal of Bone and Joint Surgery 52A: 565-568

Dislocation of carpal lunate

General features
Caused by falling with wrist dorsiflexed
Young adults mainly involved
M > F
Injury often overlooked

Clinical features
Pain, swelling, loss of function
Median nerve damage is very common

Radiological features
Lateral films of both wrist show anterior displacement more easily
AP films show triangular outline of dislocation and quadrilateral normal outline

Pathological features
Lunate usually stripped of soft tissue
Ischemica necrosis usually follows
Median nerve compression in carpal tunnel

Treatment
1. Gentle manipulation with wrist powerfully distracted in dorsiflexion
   Forceful maneouvres cause further damage to median nerve
2. Open reduction: Flexor approach
3. Removal of lunate: +/- Silastic replacement

References

Agerholm J C, Goodfellow J W 1963 Avascular necrosis of the lunate bone treated by excision and prosthetic replacement. Journal of Bone and Joint Surgery 45B: 110-116

Campbell R D, Lance E M, Yeoh C B 1964 Lunate and perilunar dislocations. Journal of Bone and Joint Surgery 46B: 55-72

Rarer carpal injuries

Naviculo-capitate fracture
Caused by forced dorsi-flexion of wrist
Proximal fragment of capitate rotates through 180°
Open reduction required (Meyers, 1971)

Transcaphoid, transcapitate, transtriquetral, perilunar fracture
More grossly displaced example of above (Wesley, 1972)

Disruption of proximal carpal arch
Caused by crush injuries (Primiano, 1974)

Others
Fractures of Trapezium   (McClain, 1955)
Fractures of Hamate   (Stark, 1977)
Fracture of Triquetrum   (Bartone, 1956)
Dislocation of Trapezium   (Siegel, 1969)
Dislocation of Hamate   (Mathison, 1975)
Dislocation of Trapezoid   (Stein, 1971)
Dislocation of Triquetrum ⎫
                          ⎬ Unrecorded as isolated injuries
Fracture of Trapezoid   ⎭

References

Bartone N F, Grieco R V 1956 Fractures of the triquetrum. Journal of Bone and Joint Surgery 38A: 353-356

McClain E J, Boyes J H 1966 Missed fractures of the greater multangular. Journal of Bone and Joint Surgery 48A: 1525-1528

Mathison G W, MacDonald R I 1975 Irreducible transcapitate fracture and dislocation of hamate. Journal of Bone and Joint Surgery 57A: 1166-1167

Meyers M M, Wells R, Hervey J P 1971 Naviculo-capitate fractures syndrome. Journal of Bone and Joint Surgery 53A: 1383-1386

Primiano G A, Reef T C 1974 Disruption of the proximal carpal arch of the hand. Journal of Bone and Joint Surgery 56A: 328-332

Siegel M W, Hertzberg H 1969 Complete dislocation of the greater multangulum (trapezium). Journal of Bone and Joint Surgery 51A: 769-772

Stark M M, Jobe F W, Boyes J H et al 1977 Fracture of the hook of the hamate in athletes. Journal of Bone and Joint Surgery 59A: 575-582

Stein A M 1971 Dorsal dislocation of the lesser multangular bone. Journal of Bone and Joint Surgery 53A: 377-379

Wesley M S, Barenfeld P A 1972 Transcaphoid, transcapitate, transtriquetral, perilunar fracture dislocation of the wrist. Journal of Bone and Joint Surgery 54A: 1073-1078

Infective tenosynovitis

General features
Much less common in the antibotic era
Can arise from trivial and/or major injuries
May progress rapidly

Clinical features
Severe pain and swelling
General malaise
Lymphangitis and lymphadenitis
Local loss of function
Increased tenderness over affected tendon sheath
Pain on active or passive movement of tendon

Radiological features
Usually none unless associated with a compound
    fracture and/or foreign body

Pathological features
Wide variety of pyogenic organisms may be
    responsible.
Intense inflammatory response in synovium
Fibrinous exudate which becomes purulent
Healing with fibrosis
Tendon becomes adherent and functionless

Tuberculosis
Low grade inflammatory changes
Fibrinous loose bodies form
Foci of tuberculosis elsewhere

Treatment
Wide decompression
Lavage with saline + antibiotics
Elevation of limb and analgesics
Systemic antibiotics
Early active exercises to prevent adhesions
See Figure 25

References
Bailey D A 1963 The infected hand. Chapter 13, Lewis,
    London
Pollen A G 1974 Acute infection of the tendon sheaths. The
    Hand 6: 21-25

Fig. 25 Incision for draining tendon sheaths.

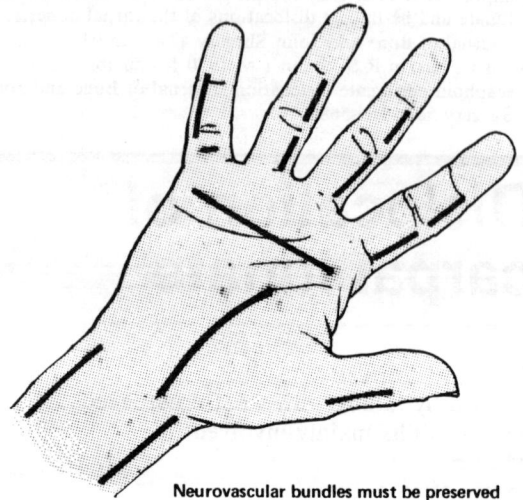

Neurovascular bundles must be preserved

Division of flexor tendons at wrist

General features
Common injury
Caused by
    Putting hand through glass
    Slashing injury
    Suicide attempt

Clinical features
Irregular varieties of wound on flexor surface of
    wrist
Variable loss of finger flexion depending on the
    tendon divided
Radial and/or ulnar arteries divided
Median nerve nearly always damaged
Ulnar nerve less commonly injured

Radiological features
Skeleton rarely injured
Lateral films usually show only a soft tissue gap
    or glass fragments

Pathological features
Proximal ends of tendons retract
Widespread fibrosis if untreated
Multiple tendon repairs become adherent unless
    wrapped in local synovium
Hand will survive ligation of ulnar and radial
    arteries

Treatment

Wide exposure and extension of wound under tourniquet

Certain identification of both ends of all tendons and nerves

Excise F.D.S. tendons if F.D.P. tendons also divided

Careful repair and splintage in flexion for 2-3 weeks

References

Boyes J H, Wilson J N, Smith J W 1960 Flexor tendon ruptures in the forearm and hand. Journal of Bone and Joint Surgery 42A: 637-646

London P S 1967 A practical guide to the care of the injured. Chapter 16, Livingstone, Edinburgh

Flexor tendon ruptures

General features

Usually occurs from powerful muscle action against resistance

(Extensor tendons rupture 3 times more often)

R > L

M > F

Usually young adults

Clinical features

Sudden pain

Local tenderness at site of rupture

Inability to flex digit(s) and/or wrist

Later minor bruising

Ring finger most often affected

Radiological features

Nil

Pathological features

Possible causes

Preceeding local trauma to tendon

Tenosynovitis

Mechanical attrition on sharp edge of bone

Early rheumatoid arthritis

Frequency

Usually:

digital profundus tendon alone

Less often:

profundus and sublimis tendons together

Least often:

sublimis tendons alone

Sites

Insertion	60%
Mid tendon	35%
Musculo-tendinous junction	5%

Treatment: F.D.P. tendon

at insertion:

Early case: Advancement and repair

Late case : No action

At mid palm:

Consider repair

Both tendons:

Repair or grafting

References

Boyes J H, Wilson J N, Smith J W 1960 Flexor tendon ruptures in the forearm and hand. Journal of Bone and Joint Surgery 42A: 637-646

Von Zander R 1891 Trommlerlammung. Inaugural Dissertation, Berlin

Injuries of extensor tendons over dorsum of hand

General features

Very common

Usually arise from lacerations

Dissolution or dislocation may occur from rheumatoid arthritis

Clinical features

Wound on dorsum

or Dislocation between meta carpal heads

Inability to extend one or more M-P joints

Radiological features

Usually none unless there is an associated fracture or signs of rheumatoid arthritis

Pathological features

Juncturae tendinum diminish loss of function

Wide anatomical variation

Lacerated tendons do not retract

Limited adhesion formation

Edematous paratenon with lymphocytic infiltrations in rheumatoid arthritis

Treatment
Surgical repair:
  Easy technique
  Figure 8 sutures sufficient
  MP joints splinted in extension for 1-2 weeks

References
Bunnell S 1948 Surgery of the hand (2nd edition) p. 448, D B
  Lippincott Co, Philadelphia
Kettelcamp D B, Flatt A E, Moulds R 1971 Traumatic
  dislocation of the long finger extensor tendon. Journal of
  Bone and Joint Surgery 53A: 229-240
Schenk R R 1964 Variations of the extensor tendons of the
  fingers. Journal of Bone and Joint Surgery 46A: 103-110
Vaughan-Jackson O J 1962 Rheumatoid hand deformities
  considered in the light of tendon imbalance. Journal of
  Bone and Joint Surgery 44B: 764-775
Wheeldon F T 1954 Recurrent dislocation of the extensor
  tendons of the hand. Journal of Bone and Joint Surgery
  36B: 612-617

1st carpo-metacarpal fracture dislocation

Synonym
Bennett's fracture

General features
$M : F = 9 : 1$
Caused by blow on knuckle of thumb

Clinical features
Pain and swelling at base of thumb
Minimal deformity
Loss of function of thumb

Radiological features
Intra-articular fracture of base of 1st metacarpal.
Proximal dislocation of shaft of metacarpal
Tension of thumb tendons dislocates shaft of
  metacarpal proximally

Pathological features
Malunion or non union leads to osteoarthrosis of
  1st carpo-metacarpal joint

Treatment
*Variety of methods available. Each has its
advocates*

Manipulation of thumb into full extension
Cast splintage for 4-6 weeks
or Percutaneous pin fixation +/- oblique
  traction
or Open reduction with screw fixation

Late osteoarthrosis
  Metacarpo-carpal fusion
or Excision of trapezium
or Replacement with silastic trapezium

References
Bennett E H 1882 Fractures of the metacarpal bones. Dublin
  Journal of Medical Science 73: 72-75
Griffiths J C 1964 Fracture at the base of the first metacarpal
  bone. Journal of Bone and Joint Surgery 46B: 712-719
Pollen A G 1968 The conservative treatment of Bennett's
  fracture subluxations of the thumb metacarpal. Journal of
  Bone and Joint Surgery 50B: 91-101
Spanzberg O, Thoren L 1964 Bennetts fracture, a method of
  treatment with oblique traction. Journal of Bone and Joint
  Surgery 45B: 732-736

2nd-5th carpo-metacarpal fracture dislocations

General features
Caused by blow on knuckles

Clinical features
Local pain and swelling
Some loss of function
Minimal deformity

Radiological features
Variable mixture of fractures and dislocations are
  possible
5th C-MC injury may simulate a Bennett's
  fracture of 1st metacarpal

Pathological features
2nd, 3rd, 4th MCs usually dislocate dorsally
2nd 5th MCs may develop exostoses over which
  E.D.C. tendons sublux
4th, 5th MCs may compress deep branch of
  ulnar nerve
5th MC may dislocate in front of base of 4th
  MC

Treatment
Manipulation by traction and pressure

Surgery:
Fixation by percutaneous pins
+/- open reduction

Cast
Splintage
3-4 weeks

References
Artz T D, Posch J L 1973 The carpo-metacarpal bones. Journal of Bone and Joint Surgery 55A: 747-752
Bora F W, Didizian N B 1974 The treatment of injuries to the carpo-metacarpal joint of the little finger. Journal of Bone and Joint Surgery 56A: 1459-1463
Harwin S F, Seolin E D 1975 Volar dislocation of the bases of the second and third metacarpals. Journal of Bone and Joint Surgery 57A: 849-851

Fracture of neck of 5th metacarpal

General features
Common
Usually male
Caused by blow on knuckle of 5th finger
Similar fractures can occur in other metacarpals

Clinical features
Local pain, swelling
Loss of movement of little finger
Minor deformity

Radiological features
Transverse fracture through neck of metacarpal
Head angled palmarwards

Pathological features
Persistent angulation may limit extension of little finger

Treatment
Minor angulation:
Strap adjacent fingers and carpus
Early active movement
Major angulation:
Manipulation using proximal phalanx as a lever.
Cast for 3 weeks

References
Hunter J M, Cowen N J 1970 Fifth metacarpal fractures in compensation clinic population. Journal of Bone and Joint Surgery 52A: 1159-1165
Jahss S A 1938 Fractures of the metacarpals. Journal of Bone and Joint Surgery 20: 178-186

Rupture of m.ext.poll. long tendon

Synonym
Drummer boy's palsy

General features
Uncommon
Often occurs during sleep

Clinical features
Drooping of thumb
Inability to extend interphalangeal joint

Radiological features
Evidence of fracture of lower end of radius or rheumatoid arthritis
Otherwise no changes

Pathological features

Causes
Rheumatoid arthritis
Fracture of lower end of radius
Closed injury
Ideopathic

Local cause:
Local ischemia
Attrition over spicule of bone
Lymphocytic infiltration

Treatment
Splintage ineffective as proximal end retracts
Surgery:
M. Ext. Ind. transfer best
M. Ext. Carp-Rad. Brev. transfer less effective
Arthrodesis of I-P joint undesirable
Free tendon graft possible

References
Duplay S 1876 Rupture sous-cutanee du tendon du long extensor du pouce de la main droite au niveau de la tabaticre anatomique. Paris 2: 788-791
Hamlin C, Littler J W 1977 Restoration of extensor pollicis longus tendon by an intercalated graft. Journal of Bone and Joint Surgery 59A: 412-414
Riddell D M 1963 Spontaneous rupture of the extensor pollicis longus. Journal of Bone and Joint Surgery 45B: 506-512

Repair of flexor tendons of hand

Primary repair:

Local excision of fibrous flexor sheath.
(Retain part as a local pulley)

Techniques:

Rectangular Bunnel stitch

Oblique interlacing stitch (+/- pull-out loop)

Epitendinous stitches + Transfixion needles

Advancement of profundus

Barbed wire sutures (Experimental)

Delayed primary repair:

Careful selection of cases – minimal
contamination

Expert technique required

Performed within 3-4 days

A. Wound toilet, close skin

B. Re-open wound
Discard F.D.S. tendon
Find and repair F.D.P. tendon

Fig. 24 Extension of wounds for primary flexor tendon
repair.

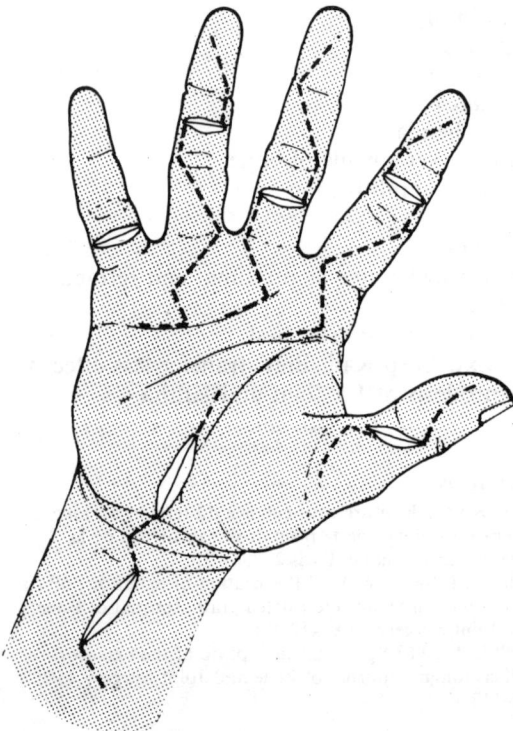

Secondary repair: methods

1. Attachment of tendons of different diameters
Interlacing tendons
Fish-mouth incision and closure
Wrap around technique

2. Tendon attachment to bone
Suture to periosteum and local fibrous tissue
Formation of tunnel in bone
Tendon looped on itself
Pulled through to opposite side
+/- Pull out loops for each method

Tenolysis conditions:

6-9 months after grafting surgery
Improvement ceased.
Passive range remains greater than active range
of movement
Followed by early vigorous active movements
See Figure 24

References

Brand P W 1961 Tendon grafting. Journal of Bone and Joint
Surgery 43B: 444-453

Fetrow K O 1967 Tenolysis in the hand and wrist. Journal of
Bone and Joint Surgery 49A: 667-685

Madsen E 1970 Delayed primary suture of flexor tendons cut
in the digital theath. Journal of Bone and Joint Surgery
52B: 264-267

Milford L 1971 Campbell's operative orthopaedics (editor: A
H Grenshaw). 5th Edition. Volume I. Chapter 4. C V
Mosley & Co, St. Louis

Shaw P C 1968 A method of flexor tendon suture. Journal of
Bone and Joint Surgery 50B: 578-587

Verdan C E 1972 Primary repair of flexor tendons. Journal
of Bone and Joint Surgery 42A: 647-657

Verdan C E 1972 Half a century of flexor tendon surgery.
Current status and changing philosophies. Journal of Bone
and Joint Surgery 54A: 472-491

Wagner C J 1958 Delayed advancement in the repair of
lacerated flexor profundus tendons. Journal of Bone and
Joint Surgery 40A: 1241-1244

Investigations into digital flexor tendon repair

Measurement of recovery

Fingers:

Distance from finger pulp to distal palmar
crease in full flexion

Thumb:
Range of movement of I-P joint (Pulvertaft, 1956)
Comparison of methods of measuring recovery (McKenzie, 1967)
Two-stage tenoplasty: F.D.S. reversal after F.D.S.-F.D.P. suture (Paneva-Holevich, 1969)
Gliding function recovery (Lane, 1976)
Factors in production of adhesions (Matthews, 1976)
Silastic rod to induce sheath formation (Hunter, 1971)
Prevention of adhesions: Paratenon and Silastic sheeting better than a multitude of other substances (Stark, 1977).

References

Hunter J M, Salisbury R E 1971 Flexor tendon reconstruction in severely damaged hands. Journal of Bone and Joint Surgery 53A: 829-858
Lane J M, Black J, Bora J W 1976 Gliding function following flexor tendon injury. Journal of Bone and Joint Surgery 58A: 985-990
McKenzie A R 1967 Function after reconstruction of severed long flexor tendons of the hand. Journal of Bone and Joint Surgery 49B: 424-439
Matthews P, Richards W 1976 Factors in the adherence of flexor tendons after repair. Journal of Bone and Joint Surgery 58B: 230-236
Paneva-Holevich E 1969 Two stage tenoplasty in injury of flexor tendons of hand. Journal of Bone and Joint Surgery 51A: 21-32
Pulvertaft R G 1956 Flexor tendon grafts for flexor tendon injuries in the fingers and thumb. Journal of Bone and Joint Surgery 38B: 175-194
Stark M M, Boyes J H, Johnston L, et al 1977 The use of paratenon polyethylene film or silastic sheeting to prevent restricting adhesions to the tendons in the hands. Journal of Bone and Joint Surgery 59A: 908-913

Flexor tendon grafting

Available tendons
Palmaris Longus (Absent in 25%)
Plantaris
Extensor Digitorum Longus to 3rd and 4th toes
Extensor Indices

Techniques

1. Free graft technique
Excision of avascular fibrous tissue and damaged tendons
Excision of fibrous flexor sheath except for local pulleys

Insertion of long graft
Tendon sutures inserted far from gliding planes.
Splintage for 2-3 weeks

2. Two stage silastic rod technique
(a) Excision of flexor tendons from insertion to mid palm
Insertion of silastic rod for 3-4 weeks
Active and passive exercises to preserve joint mobility
(b) Replacement of rod by tendon graft
Splintage for 2-3 weeks

References

Harrison S H 1958 Primary flexor tendon grafts. British Journal of Plastic Surgery 11: 106-110
Hunter J M, Salisbury R E 1971 Flexor tendon reconstruction in severely damaged hands. Journal of Bone and Joint Surgery 53A: 829-858
Pulvertaft R G 1960 The treatment of profundus division by free tendon graft. Journal of Bone and Joint Surgery 42A: 1363-1371

Division of thumb flexor tendon

At I-P joint:
Direct primary suture
Distal to mid phalanx:
Advancement
Distal to M-P joint:
Advancement with lengthening at wrist
Distal to M-C joint:
Free secondary tendon graft
At wrist:
Direct primary suture

References

Urbank J R, Goldner J L 1973 Laceration of the flexor pollicis longus tendon. Delayed repair by advancement free graft or direct suture. Journal of Bone and Joint Surgery 55A: 1123-1148

Ulnar artery thrombosis

Synonyms
Hypothenar Hammer Syndrome
Post-traumatic digital ischemia

General features
Rare
Often caused by repeated blows on ulnar side of hand

Clinical features
Painful tender mass in hypothenar region
Tingling and numbness in ulnar nerve territory of hand
Hand is cold, sensitive
Allen's test positive (Hand becomes ischemic on fist clenching with radial artery compressed)

Radiological features
Occluded ulnar artery on arteriography

Pathological features
Localised thrombosis of ulnar artery with surrounding fibrosis
Ischemic changes in ulnar nerve

Treatment
1) Total excision of thrombosed segment, may allow collateral vasodilation
2) Thrombectomy with microvascular surgery

References
Herndon W A, Hershey S L, Lambdin C S 1975 Thrombosis of the ulnar artery in the hand. Journal of Bone and Joint Surgery 57A: 994-995
Kleinert M E, Volianitis G J 1965 Thrombosis of the palmar arterial arch and its tributaries. Etiology and newer concepts of treatment. Journal of Trauma 5: 447-457

Disruption of metacarpo-phalangeal joint of thumb

Synonym
"Gamekeeper's thumb" (if caused by repetitive minor injury)

General features
Not uncommon despite normal mobility of MP joint
Sideways force disrupts lateral stability
(Hyperextension dislocations described separately)

Clinical features
Acute
Pain, swelling, loss of function

Chronic
Weakened pinch
Instability and discomfort

Radiological features
Avulsion of corner of base of proximal phalanx in 25%
Lateral stress films show instability

Pathological features
Ulnar collateral ligament damaged in 60%
Usually due to one episode of major trauma
Repetitive minor trauma may have some effect
Lengthened or torn collateral ligament
Partial tear of volar plate
Eventual osteo-arthrosis of MP joint

Treatment
Acute
Operative repair
+/- percutaneous pin to fix fracture
Plaster cast 4-5 weeks

Chronic
Conservative: Plastic or leather splint
Surgical:
    I ligamentous repair
or a) +/- M.Ext.Ind. transfer
or b) +/- M.Add. Poll. transfer
or c) +/- M.Ext.Poll. transfer
    II Arthrodesis of MP joint if osteo-arthrosis present

References
Bowers W H, Hurst L C 1977 Gamekeepers thumb, evaluation by arthrography and stress roentgenography. Journal of Bone and Joint Surgery 59A: 519-524
Campbell C S 1955 Gamekeepers thumb. Journal of Bone and Joint Surgery 37B: 148-149
Smith R J 1977 Post-traumatic instability of the metacarpo-phalangeal joint of the thumb. Journal of Bone and Joint Surgery 59A: 14-21

Fractures of metacarpal shafts

General features

Isolated fractures
Common
Transverse from direct blow
Spiral from blow on knuckles

Multiple fractures
Less common
Often crush injuries
Often compound

Clinical features
Pain, swelling, some loss of function
A mutilated hand may have many fractures
Recession of knuckle

Radiological features
1st Metacarpal:
   Juxta-epiphyseal in children
   Often comminuted in adults
Multiple fractures may show every variety of
   fissuring and displacement

Pathological features
Isolated fractures have no complications
Union occurs as rapidly as with ribs
Multiple fractures may be associated with a
   palmar hematoma and ischemia of fingers

Treatment
1st Metacarpal:
   Scaphoid type cast after manipulation
5th Metacarpal:
   Colles type cast
2nd, 3rd, 4th Metacarpals:
   Usually no manipulation required
   Strapping for support.
Multiple fractures   ⎱ Percutaneous pins
Single displaced fractures⎰ +/- open reduction

References
Lamb D W, Abernethy P A, Raine P A M 1973 Unstable
   fractures of the metacarpals. The Hand 5: 43-48
Rockwood C A, Green D F (eds) 1975 Fractures Vol. I
   Chapt. 6. Lippincott, Philadelphia.

Amputation of thumb

General features
Uncommon
Crippling injury. Worse in Dominant hand
Usually arise from machinery accident

Clinical features
Division can occur at any level
Usually an irregular laceration
Avulsion leaves wisps of protruding tendon
   and/or neurovascular bundles
Little blood loss
Other hand injuries may be present

Radiological features
Infinite variety of skeletal loss
Other fractures may be present

Pathological features
Avulsion damage may extend to wrist
Crush injuries jeopardise blood flow to
   remaining tissue

Treatment

Primary surgery
Retain as much of first ray as possible
Wound toilet, skin closure if possible.

Secondary surgery:
Various Possibilities
Factors in Choice of Procedure:
   Age
   Hand Dominance
   Occupation
   Sex
   Other hand injuries
   Wishes of Patient
1. Advancement pedicle flap
2. Elongation of remaining thumb by
   (a) Ribgraft or
       1st M-C distraction lengthening
   (b) Iliac peg graft and skin pedicle graft
   (c) Composite bone and skin groin flap
3. Pollicisation of digit
   Long neurovascular bundle essential for
      success
   2 or 3 stage procedure
   Pollicisation of Index for congenital absence of
      thumb

4. Free digital transfer
   Digit from other hand or great toe
   Microvascular technique
5. Restoration of thumb sensation
   Radial nerve skin transfer

References

Bralliar F, Horner R L 1969 Sensory cross finger pedicle
  graft. Journal of Bone and Joint Surgery 51A: 1264-1268
Buck-Gramcko D 1971 Pollicisation of the index finger.
  Journal of Bone and Joint Surgery 53A: 1605-1617
Butler B 1964 Ring finger pollicisation. Journal of Bone and
  Joint Surgery 46A: 1069-1076
Cobbett J R 1969 Free digital transfer. Journal of Bone and
  Joint Surgery 51B: 677-679
Finseth F, May J W, Smith R J 1976 Composite groin flap
  with iliac bone flap for primary thumb reconstruction.
  Journal of Bone and Joint Surgery 58A: 130-132
Matec I B 1970 Thumb reconstruction after amputation at
  the metacarpo-phalangeal joint by bone lengthening.
  Journal of Bone and Joint Surgery 52A: 957-965
Miura T 1973 Thumb reconstruction using radial innervated
  cross-finger pedicle graft. Journal of Bone and Joint
  Surgery 55A: 563-569
O'Brien B M et al Hallux to hand transfer. The Hand 7: 128-
  133 et seq
Posner M A, Smith R J 1971 The advancement pedicle flap
  for thumb injuries. Journal of Bone and Joint Surgery
  53A: 1618-1621

Dorsal dislocation of metacarpo-phalangeal joint of thumb

General features
Not uncommon: children > adults
Usually under 50
M > F. Usually from a hyperextension force

Clinical features
Pain and deformity
Loss of thumb function
Dorsal displacement of proximal phalanx
More rarely flexorwards

Radiological features
Dorsal dislocation of phalanx on metacarpal
Sesamoids may lie within joint

Pathological features
Head of metacarpal often buttonholed through
  flexor aspect of capsule

Treatment

Manipulation
Traction, followed by flexion
Splintage for 2-3 weeks

Surgery
Open reduction from flexor aspect
Splintage for 2-3 weeks

Reference
Coonrad R W, Goldner J L 1968 A study of the pathological
  findings and treatment in soft tissue injury of the thumb
  metacarpophalangeal joint. Journal of Bone and Joint
  Surgery 50A: 439-451

Dislocation of metacarpo-phalangeal joint of index

General features
Rare
Caused by falling on outstretched finger
Other hyperextension forces

Clinical features
Pain and deformity
Loss of index function
Index displaced dorsally
Palmar skin dimple

Radiological features
Dorsal or ulnar dislocation of phalanx on
  metacarpal
Widened joint space
Index sesamoid within joint
  (Not ossified before 13 years)

Pathological features
Rupture of metacarpal attachment of volar plate
Inversion of plate and sesamoids into M-P joint

Treatment
Surgery:
  Open reduction from palmar incision
  Brief splintage in flexion
  Early active movements

References

Becton J L et al 1975 A simplified technique for treating the complex dislocation of the index metacarpophalangeal joint. Journal of Bone and Joint Surgery 57A: 698-700

Green D P, Terry G C, 1973 Complex dislocation of the metacarpo-phalangeal joint. Journal of Bone and Joint Surgery 55A: 1480-1486

Mcelfresh E C, Dobyns J H, O'Brien E T 1972 Management of fracture dislocation of the proximal interphalangeal. joints by extension block splinting. Journal of Bone and Joint Surgery 54A: 1705-1711

Potenza A D 1973 A technique for arthodesis of finger joints. Journal of Bone and Joint Surgery 55A: 1534-1536

Salamon P B, Gelberman R H 1978 Irreducible dislocation of interphalangeal joint of thumb. Journal of Bone and Joint Surgery 60A: 400-401

Dislocations of interphalangeal joints of the hand

General features
Common
Caused by hyperextension forces
or falling with finger(s) outstretched

Clinical features
Pain, swelling, deformity
Loss of function of finger
Tendon insertions may be avulsed
Neurovascular bundles rarely injured

Radiological features
D.I.P. joints usually dislocate backwards
Marginal fractures often represent avulsion of tendons

Pathological features
Sprains of finger joints are often momentary subluxations or dislocations
Fractures of base of middle phalanx often end in persistent dorsal subluxation of middle phalanx
Anterior dislocation of P.I.P. joint is associated with rupture of central slip of extensor tendon

Treatment
No fracture:
Manipulation and splintage
Fracture:
Open reduction
Internal fixation by pin or screw
Persistent pain and deformity:
Arthrodesis

References

McCue F C et al 1970 Athletic injuries of the proximal interphalangeal joint requiring surgical treatment. Journal of Bone and Joint Surgery 52A: 937-955

Fractures of phalanges

General features
Very common
Often compound and/or multiple

Clinical features
Pain, swelling
Deformity, loss of function

Radiological features
Wide variety of fractures possible
Condylar fractures always unstable
Juxta-epiphyseal fractures occur in children with impaction and angulation

Pathological features
Extensor and flexor tendons frequently damaged.
Division of neurovascular bundles further imperils functional recovery

Treatment

Closed fractures of shaft
Middle and terminal phalanges:
Strap injured finger(s) to adjacent uninjured fingers.
Proximal phalanx:
Splint in flexion

Displaced and condylar fractures
Percutaneous pin fixation, open or closed

References

Coonrad R W, Pohlman M H 1969 Impacted fractures in the proximal portions of the proximal phalanx of the finger. Journal of Bone and Joint Surgery 51A: 1291-1296

Joshi B B, Chaudhari S S 1973 Dorsal relaxation incisions in burst fingers. The Hand 5: 135-139

Lee M L H 1963 Intra-articular and peri-articular fractures of the phalanges. Journal of Bone and Joint Surgery 45B: 103-109

Finger tip amputations

General features
Occur in all age groups
Crush injuries more frequent than lacerations

Clinical features
Painful wound of finger tip
Terminal phalanx often exposed
Nail and nail bed often damaged

Radiological features
Comminuted fracture of terminal phalanx is
frequent

Pathological features
Nail bed damage may give permanent deformity.
Soft tissue loss in young children often
regenerated
Adherent pulp scars often persistenly painful

Treatment

Children
Wound toilet
Minimal resection
Free skin graft

Adults
Wound toilet
Grafting procedure: various techniques available:

(a) Palmar flap
(b) Advancement flap
(c) Kutler flap
(d) Toe pulp free graft
(e) Nail bed graft

Thereafter, early active movements

References
Atasoy E et al Reconstruction of the amputated finger tip
with a triangular volar flap. Journal of Bone and Joint
Surgery 52A: 921-926
Barton N J 1975 A modified thenar flap. The Hand 7: 150-
151
Beasley R W 1969 Reconstruction of amputated finger tips.
Plastic and reconstructive surgery 4: 349-352
Fisher R H 1967 The Kutler method of repair of finger tip
amputations. Journal of Bone and Joint Surgery 49A: 317-
321
Flatt A E 1957 The thenar flap. Journal of Bone and Joint
Surgery 39B: 80-85

Posner M A, Smith R J 1971 The advancement pedicle flap
for thumb injuries. Journal of Bone and Joint Surgery
53A: 1618-1621

Ring injuries

General features
Uncommon
Caused by catching ring under a moving
obstruction

Clinical features
"Degloving" injury of finger involves at least
middle and distal phalanx
Considerable pain
Little blood loss

Radiological features
Usually no phalangeal fracture

Pathological features
Neurovascular bundles often avulsed
If skin grafts are successful finger remains stiff
and insensitive

Treatment
Consider each case individually
Amputations at site of election
Variety of grafting procedures possible

References
Bevin A G, Chase R A 1963 The management of ring
avulsion injuries and associated conditions in the hand.
Plastic and Reconstructive Surgery 32: 391-400

Boutonniere deformity

General features
Uncommon
Caused by
   1. forced flexion of an actively extended P.I.P.
   joint
   2. Laceration of dorsum of P.I.P. joint

Clinical features
Pain and swelling of P.I.P. joint
Fixed flexion of P.I.P. joint
Hyperextension of D.I.P. joint

Radiological features
Usually none
Rarely damage to base of middle phalanx on extensor surface

Pathological features
Essential feature is division of central slip of extensor tendon
Lateral bands of extensor tendon slip towards flexor surface of joint causing lack of full extension of P.I.P. joint but hyperextension of D.I.P. joint

Treatment
Splintage uninterruptedly in extension 6-8 weeks
    Deformity usually recurs
Surgical repair:
    Difficult
    Variety of techniques
    Results fair

References
Littler J W, Easton R G 1967 Redistribution of forces in the correction of Boutonniere deformity. Journal of Bone and Joint Surgery 49A: 1267-1274
Matev I 1964 Transposition of the lateral slips of the aponeurosis in treatment of long standing Boutonniere deformity of the fingers. British Journal of Plastic Surgery 17: 281-286
Souter W A 1967 The Boutonniere deformity. Journal of Bone and Joint Surgery 49B: 710-721

Division of finger flexor tendons in the hand

General features
Very common. Local adhesions cause bad results particularly within fibrous flexor sheath

Clinical features
Painful wound
Loss of flexion of associated finger
Loss of sensation if neurovascular bundle is damaged

Radiological features
None

Pathological features:
Laceration }
Incision   } Most common
Crushing }
Fractures } Worsen prognosis
Proximal cut ends of tendons retract.
Cut ends and suture lines adhere to flexor sheath and other structures.
Adhesions worsened by
    Infection
    Crushing
    Fractures
    Immobility

Requirements for Successful Grafting
Mobile finger
Good sensation
Co-operative patient
Careful technique

Treatment

Division at D.I.P. joint:
F.D.P. only is divided.
Acute   : Re-attachment to base of terminal phalanx
Chronic: D.I.P. arthrodesis

Division over middle phalanx:
F.D.P. only is divided.
Acute: Advancement of F.D.P. and re-attachment
Chronic: D.I.P. arthrodesis

Division at P.I.P. joint:
If 1) F.D.S. only is divided:
        Local excision of flexor sheath
        Reattachment to base of middle phalanx
If 2) F.D.S. and F.D.P. are divided:
    Acute: Local excision of flexor sheath
            Excision of F.D.S. remnants
            Repair of F.D.P. tendon
    Chronic: Secondary F.D.P. tendon graft

Division over proximal phalanx:
If 1) F.D.S. only divided
        Close skin. No further action.
If 2) F.D.S. and F.D.P. are divided
    Acute: Local excision of flexor sheath
            Excision of F.D.S. tendon
            Repair of F.D.P. tendon
    Acute/Chronic: Secondary F.D.P. tendon graft

Division at M-P joint
If 1) F.D.S. only divided
      a) Close skin. No further action.
  or b) Excise proximal tendon sheath.
          Repair F.D.S. tendon.
If 2) F.D.S. and F.D.P. are both divided
    Acute: Excise proximal tendon sheath.
          Excise F.D.S. tendon
          Repair F.D.P. tendon.
    Chronic: Secondary F.D.P. tendon graft.

Division in palm
F.D.S. and/or F.D.P. division
  Repair FDP tendon +/- FDS tendon
  Wrap suture lines in lumbrical muscle or in
    paratenon

References

Holms W 1974 Primary suture of flexor tendons in the
danger zone. The Hand 6: 17-20
Pulvertaft R G 1956 Tendon grafts for flexor tendon injuries
in the fingers and thumb. Journal of Bone and Joint
Surgery 38B: 175-194
Pulvertaft R G 1960 The treatment of profundus division by
free tendon graft. Journal of Bone and Joint Surgery 42A:
1363-1372
Pulvertaft R G 1965 Problems of flexor tendon surgery of the
hand. Journal of Bone and Joint Surgery 47A: 123-132
Shrewbsury M M, Kuczynski K 1974 Flexor digitorum
superficialis tendon in the fingers of the human hand. The
Hand 6: 121-133
Wilson W F, Hueston J T 1973 Intratendinous architecture.
The Hand 5: 33-38

Mallet finger

Synonym
Drop finger

General features
Very common
Index, Ring, Long and little finger affected in
  that order
Caused by forced flexion of an actively extended
  finger rupturing extensor insertion

Clinical features
Inability to extend terminal joint
Painful swelling over dorsum of middle or
  terminal phalanx

Radiological features
60% no abnormality
30% show marginal fracture of base of terminal
  phalanx

Pathological features
No fracture
Extensor tendon retracts to dorsum of middle
  phalanx

Fracture
Minimal retraction
Frequent spontaneous bony or fibrous union

Children
Separation of epiphysis of terminal phalanx
  Often compound

Treatment
Splintage of D.I.P. joint in hyperextension for
3-4 weeks
  Must be continous. Plaster plastic metal splints
    in use. 50% good results

Surgery
1. Percutaneous pin through D.I.P. joint in
   hyperextension for fresh injuries
2. Repair of extensor insertion by wire suture
3. Arthrodesis of D.I.P. joint for neglected cases

References

Lee M L H 1963 Intra articular and peri-articular fractures of
the phalanges. Journal of Bone and Joint Surgery 45B:
103-109
Mikic Z, Helal B 1974 The treatment of the mallet finger by
the Oakley spint. The Hand 6: 76-81

Skin cover for finger injuries

General considerations:
Rapid skin cover essential to minimise scarring
  and stiffness
Loss of skin sensation makes the hand "blind".
Split skin or whole thickness free grafts adequate
  only for small areas

Available methods

1. Cross over finger flap

Gives good quality skin for flexor surface with
  normal sensation
Covers exposed tendon or bone
Will replace a hyperesthetic scar or inadequate
  skin graft.
Contra-indications:
  Arthritis
  Vasospastic syndromes
  > 45 years

2. Neuro-vascular island pedicle graft

Graft of skin and subcutaneous tissue based on
  its neurovascular pedicle
Donor areas: Ulnar side of long and ring fingers
Recipient areas:
  Both sides of thumb
  Radial side of index and long fingers
  Ulnar side of little finger
Results:
  Slight loss of top quality sensation
  Sensation usually referred to donor site

3. Abdominal pedicle graft

Useful for dorsum of hand and thumb
Accurate planning and patient co-operation
  essential
Procedure requires at least three weeks

4. Cross arm bridge flap

Useful for flexor surfaces of fingers and palm
Immobilises both arms for 3-4 weeks

5. Full thickness skin grafts

Most easily taken from forearm
But, not thick enough for palm
  Leaves a colour difference in pigmented races
Sole of foot a possible donor site of palmar skin
Hypothenar skin donor site easily available
Assessment of Quality of Recovery variable
Delayed Primary Closure
Useful for war wounds of hand, or crushed,
  infected wounds
Need for skin grafting may be avoided

References

Burkhalter W E et al 1968 Experiences with delayed primary
  closure of war wounds of the hand in Vietnam. Journal of
  Bone and Joint Surgery 50A: 945-954
Johnson R K, Iverson R E 1971 Cross finger pedicle flaps in
  the hand. Journal of Bone and Joint Surgery 53A: 913-919
Kelleher J C et al 1970 Use of a tailored abdominal pedicle
  flap for surgical reconstruction of the hand. Journal of
  Bone and Joint Surgery 52A: 1552-1562
Krag C, Rasmussen K B 1975 The neurovascular island flap
  for defective sensibility of the thumb. Journal of Bone and
  Joint Surgery 57B: 495-499
Lie K K, Magargle R K, Posch J L 1970 Free full thickness
  skin grafts from the palm to cover defects of the fingers.
  Journal of Bone and Joint Surgery 52A: 1559-1561
McCash C R 1956 Cross arm bridge flaps in the repair of
  flexion contractures of the fingers. British Journal of
  Plastic Surgery 9: 25-33
Micks J E, Wilson J N 1967 Full thickness sole-skin grafts
  for resurfacing the hand. Journal of Bone and Joint
  Surgery 49A: 1128-1134
Murray J F, Ord J V R, Gaveling G E 1967 The
  neurovascular island pedicle flap. Journal of Bone and
  Joint Surgery 49A: 1285-1297
Mutz S B 1972 Thumb web contracture. The Hand 4: 236-
  246
Omer G E et al 1970 Neurovascular cutaneous island pedicles
  for deficient median nerve sensibility. Journal of Bone and
  Joint Surgery 52A: 1181-1192
Porter R W 1968 Functional assessment of transplanted skin
  in volar defects of the digits. Journal of Bone and Joint
  Surgery 50A: 955-963

Reconstruction of the mutilated hand

General features

Minimal requirements:
Pincer grip
Sensation in pincer
Some cosmetic acceptability
Best results by a specialist hand surgeon
Patient co-operation required
Patient must be motivated to use the
  reconstructed hand

Some methods available

1) Phalangisation of 1st metacarpal

Indications:
  Loss of all or most of 4 fingers
  Partial amputation of thumb
  Contracted index-thumb cleft
Requirements:
  Normal thenar muscles
  Undamaged 1st metacarpo-carpal joint

2) Phalangisation of 5th metacarpal

Indications:
  Total loss of all four fingers
  Preservation of all or part of thumb
Requirements:
  Normal hypothenar muscles
  Undamaged 5th metacarpo-carpal joint

3) Removable prosthetic gripping post
Indications:
    Loss of fingers
    Ulnar side of palm still present
    Preservation of thumb

References

Smith R J, Dworecka F 1973 Treatment of the one digit hand. Journal of Bone and Joint Surgery 55A: 113-119
Tubiana R, Roux J P 1974 Phalangisation of the first and fifth metacarpals. Journal of Bone and Joint Surgery 56A: 447-457

Wringer injuries of upper limb

General features
Uncommon up to introduction of electrical wringers
Usually young children

Clinical features
Lacerations – wide variety
Pain, swelling, deformity of fractures
Loss of function

Radiological features
Very wide variety of fractures possible
None characteristic

Pathological features
Belts or small fast rollers produce partial or total denudation
Spiked rollers shred skin and tissues
Big slow moving rollers produce lacerations and widespread flaying of soft tissues

Treatment
Wound toilet
Internal fixation of fractures
Rapid skin cover – local flap and free grafts
Diminution of edema important

References

Galasko C S B 1972 Spin dryer injuries. British Medical Journal 4: 646
Matev I 1967 Wringer injuries to the hand. Journal of Bone and Joint Surgery 49B: 722-730
Smith J R, Asturias J 1968 Card injury of the hand. Its characteristics and treatment. Journal of Bone and Joint Surgery 50A: 1161-1170

Post-traumatic osteodystrophy of hand

Synonym
Sudek's Atrophy, Algodystrophy

General features
More common when sought for
Severe cases 1 per 1,000 of all hand injuries

Clinical features
Persistent burning pain in hand
Occurs within a few days of injury
Persists long after tissues have healed
Worsened by movement or pressure
Stiffened joints
Pale, smooth, perspiring skin. Sometimes dry and warm
Atrophy of soft tissues
Hypersensitivity

Radiological features
Diffuse decalcification of skeleton of hand and forearm
"Ground-glass" appearance

Pathological features
Cause unknown
Theories:
    Exacerbation of normal post-traumatic responses
    Anti-dromic sympathetic impulses
    Vaso-motor instability
    Anxious fearful personalities

Treatment
Encouragement
Non addictive analgesics
Steroids
Vigorous prolonged physiotherapy

References

Lengenhager K 1971 Sudek's osteodystrophy. Its pathogenesis, prophylaxis and therapy. Minnesota Medicine 54:, 967-972
Plewes L W 1956 Sudek's atrophy in the hand. Journal of Bone and Joint Surgery 38B: 195-203
Sudek P 1900 Ueber die acute entzundliche knockenatrophie. Archiv Fur Klinische Chirurgie 62: 147-156

High pressure injection injuries of hand

General features
Becoming more common
Severe long term effects
Often an unskilled worker involved

Clinical features
Severe pain ⎫
Gross swelling ⎬ depending on volume injected
Loss of function
Small entry wounds visible
Neurovascular impairment in fingers
Often index and long finger worst affected

Radiological features
Scattered radio-opaque patches in soft tissues of hand

Pathological features
Grease ⎫
Diesel Oil ⎪ Track up tendon sheaths and in
Paint ⎬ soft tissue planes
Cement ⎭
Gross sepsis and later fibrosis occurs
Local gangrene frequent

Treatment
Wide incision and excision
Early decision about digital amputation
Broad spectrum antibiotics

References
Gelberman R H, Posch J L, Jurist J M 1975 High pressure injection injuries of the hand. Journal of Bone and Joint Surgery 57A: 935-937
Kaufman H D 1968 The clinico-pathological correlation of high pressure injection. Injuries of the hand. Journal of Bone and Joint Surgery 57A: 935-937
Lowry J C 1974 Industrial nail gun injuries. A Review and Case Report. Injury 5: 59-62

Electrical burns of hands

See section on burns pages 41–54

General features
Uncommon
Mostly in young children

Clinical features
Pain, charred flesh
Widespread loss of function
Vascular thrombosis in more severe burns
Flash burns look worse but are shallow
Contact burns may appear minor but are deep and widespread

Radiological features
None

Pathological features
Wide variation in size and effect of burns
Factors:
    Voltage, Amperage
    Resistance at contact and grounding
    Duration and type of current
    Pathway of current through patient
Low voltage ($< 1,000$)
    Flash burn
    Contact burn
High voltage ($> 1,000$)
    Flash burn
    Arc burn
    1. Punctate
    2. Widespread
    3. Widespread with vascular thrombosis

Treatment
Surgery:
    Early wide excision
    Early decision about amputation
    Daily inspection for swelling
    Decide daily on fasciotomy or excision of fresh necrosis

References
Peterson R A 1966 Electrical burns of the hand. Journal of Bone and Joint Surgery 48A: 407-424

Bites of the hand

General features
Human bites nearly as common as those from
   animals
Other tissues can be affected as well as hand

Clinical features
Human teeth:
   Semicircular bruising or laceration
Animal teeth:
   Irregular piercing wound
   Digit(s) ocasionally removed
Pain and swelling
Little disability at first
Untreated, serious infection can arise

Radiological features
Soft tissue swelling
Air in tissues
Rarely:
   small foreign bodies present
   Fractures or loss of phalanges

Pathological features
Bites penetrate deeper than anticipated
M-P or I-P joints may be opened if bitten in
   flexion and the opening closed when the hand
   extends

Bacteriology
Wide spectrum of organisms may be introduced
Often virulent

Treatment

Surgical
Wide excision under tourniquet and general
   anesthetic
Delayed primary suture after 5 days if clean

Antibiotics
Swab wound on admission
Give local best wide spectrum antibiotic in large
   doses
Change antibiotic at 48 hours if indicated

References
Chuinard R G, D'Ambrosia R D 1977 Human bite infections
   of the hand. Journal of Bone and Joint Surgery 59A: 416-
   418
Shields C 1975 Hand infections secondary to human bites.
   Journal of Trauma 15: 235-236

Amputations of fingers

General considerations
Function
Cosmesis
Careful planning of primary and secondary
   surgery

Each finger
Consider
   skin
   tendon
   nerve   If 3 or more tissues require
   joint   special treatment consider amputation
   bone

Multiple loss of fingers
Preserve all possible stumps. Secondary surgery
   may be required when all wounds have healed
   and future function can be fully assessed

Index finger
Minimal useful stump is $1\frac{3}{4}$ proximal phalanges
If less than this remains, the index is not used for
   pinching
Consider total amputation +/- filletting of part
   of 2nd MC
Pinching action can be strengthened by
   1) Transfer of first dorsal interosseous to long
      finger
or 2) Transfer of half of F.D.S.2 tendon into
   long finger

Long and ring fingers
Total loss of one or both leaves a gap through
   which the patient may drop small objects
   Minimal useful stump is half of basal phalanx
Cosmesis is improved in loss of one finger if the
   associated MC is filletted, at the cost of
   strength of grip
Alternative cosmetic effect in loss of long finger
   is the transfer of index ray to 3rd MC

Little finger
Minimal useful stump is the proximal $1\frac{3}{4}$
   phalanges
If less remain, consider total amputation +/-
   filletting of distal part of 5th MC

Technique
Trim phalangeal condyles if amputation through
   a joint
Palmar skin flap with dorsal scar gives good
   stump
Suture of flexor to extensor tendons over the
   stump inhibits movement of remaining finger
   thereafter

Complications
Sepsis
Dog-eared flaps
Adherent scars
Epidermoid cyst
Neuromata
Osteodystrophy

References
Eversman W W, Burkwalter W E, Dunn C 1971 Transfer of
   the long flexor tendon of the index finger to the proximal
   phalanx of the long finger during index ray amputation.
   Journal of Bone and Joint Surgery 53A: 769-773
London P S 1967 Practical guide to the care of the injured.
   P. 304. E. S. Livingstone, Edinburgh
Peacock E E 1962 Metacarpal transfer following amputation
   of a central digit. Plastic and Reconstructive Surgery 29:
   345-355

Claw hand

Synonym
Main en Griffe

Features
Hyperextension of M.P. Joints
Fixed flexion of P.I.P. and D.I.P. Joints
Lack of thumb opposition
Variable sensory loss depending on cause

Causes
Division of ulnar and median nerve at wrist
Lesion of inner cord of brachial plexus
Ischemic contracture of forearm
Syringomyelia
Peroneal muscular atrophy
Leprosy

Treatment
Many techniques available
Each hand must be considered individually

Factors:
   Muscles available for transfer
   Power of such muscle
   Joint mobility
   Degree of sensory loss
   Motivation of patient
Conservative:
Knuckle-duster splint
($+$ Opposition attachment for thumb)
Surgical
      Flexor capsulorrhaphy for M. P. Joints
   or Pulley advancement at M.P. Joints
   or F.D.S.4 → lumbrical canals
   or E.C.R.B. + E.C.U. → lumbrical canals
   or E.I. and E.D.Q. → lumbrical canals
   or E.C.R.B. extension → lumbrical canals
   or Plantaris grafts from flexor retinaculum to
      extensor expansions

References
Brand P W 1958 Paralytic claw hand, with special reference
   to paralysis in leprosy and treatment by the subclinical
   transfer of Stiles and Bunnell. Journal of Bone and Joint
   Surgery 40B: 618-632
Brand P W 1962 Tendon grafting. Journal of Bone and Joint
   Surgery 43B: 444-453
Brown P W 1970 Zancolli capsullorhaphy for ulnar claw
   hand. Journal of Bone and Joint Surgery 52A: 868-877
Bunnell S 1948 Surgery of the hand, 2nd edn. J B Lippincott
   Co., Philadelphia, p 492
Fowler S B 1953 Quoted by Riodan D C. Journal of Bone
   and Joint Surgery 35A: 313-320
Parkes A 1964 Operations for paralysis of the intrinsic
   muscles of the hand. Journal of Bone and Joint Surgery
   46B: 355-
Riordan D C 1953 Tendon transplantations in median nerve
   and ulnar nerve paralysis. Journal of Bone and Joint
   Surgery 35A: 313-320

Strangulation syndromes

Synonym
Toe/Finger tourniquet syndromes

General features
Small infants – Accidental – Caused by movement
Usually deliberate self mutilation in
Psychotic or neurotic adults
Confused elderly people

Clinical features
Pain, swelling, vascular engorgement
Constriction band
Gangrene is end result
Fingers, toes $\big\}$
$\qquad$ may be constricted
Penis, labia $\big\}$

Radiological features
Usually none unless a radio-opaque ligature has
   been used

Pathological features
Peripheral venous engorgment
Proceeds eventually to gangrene
All reported
Rubber
Cotton
Wool
Hair (patient's or relatives')
Clothing

Treatment
Immediate removal of constriction
May require anesthesia and dissection of
   edematous tissues
Ultra-conservative approach in children
Amputation as required in adults

Reference
Kerry R L, Chapman D D 1973 Strangulation of appendages
   by hair and thread. Journal of Pediatric Surgery 8: 23-27

Factitious lymphedema of hand

Synonym
Munchausen's Syndrome. (An aspect of)

General features
Adolescents or young adults affected
M : F = 1 : 2
Usually dominant hand
High incidence of pyschotics
Avoidance of work not a prime motive

Clinical features
Painless swelling of hand
May be limited by constriction ring

Occasional bruising
Function limited by swelling

Pathological features
Caused by tourniquet
   skin iritation
   blows
Histology shows non-specific inflammatory and
   extravasation of fluid and blood

Radiological features
No skeletal change
Dilated channels or lymphangiography

Treatment
Psychotherapy

Reference
Smith R J 1975 Factitious lymphedema of the hand. Journal
   of Bone and Joint Surgery 5: 7A, 89-94

16

HIP AND THIGH INJURIES

Traction lesions of lumbo-sacral plexus

General features
Uncommon
Rarer than brachial plexus lesions

Clinical features
Major injury to lower lumbar spine or pelvis
Neural deficit often overlooked initially
Variable motor and sensory losses in affected leg
Clinical lesions do not correspond always with
    myelographic lesions
Causalgia may occur

Radiological features
Fractures around sacro-iliac joint
Myelogram. Dural sacs often present from
    avulsion of nerve roots

Pathological features
Long course of lumbar and sacral nerves may
    protect them from complete avulsion, despite
    dural tears
E.M.G. and histamine axonal tests will confirm
    denervation after some weeks

Treatment
Reduction and splintage of fracture
Operative repair of nerve roots:
    rarely indicated
    unrewarding
Slow incomplete recovery to be expected

References
Finney L A, Wulfman W A 1960 Traumatic intradural
    lumbar nerve root avulsion and associated traction injury
    to the common peroneal nerve. American Journal of
    Roentgenology 84: 952-957
Harris W R et al Avulsion of lumbar roots complicating
    fracture of the pelvis. Journal of Bone and Joint Surgery
    55A: 1436-1442

Fractures of pelvis

Isolated fractures:
Acetabulum
Iliac Blade

Ring fractures:
Compression fracture with central pubic
    fragment
Hinge fractures   }(Symphysis & Sacro-
Vertical Distraction   } Iliac Joint)

Avulsions
Anterior Superior Iliac Spine
Anterior Inferior Iliac Spine
Ischial tuberosity
Iliac epiphysis

Reference
Apley A G 1973 A system of orthopaedics and fractures, 4th
    edn. ch 24, Butterworths, London, Boston

Fractures of acetabulum

General features
Young adults – victims of major violence
Old people: Minor violence
Intrapelvic visceral damage unusual

Clinical features
Pain, bruising loss of leg function
Flattening of hip soon after injury – later
    obscured by swelling

Radiological features
A-P films less helpful than oblique views
Medial displacement of femoral head often
    present
Alar projection to show anterior column of pelvis
    45° rotation to injured side
Obturator projection to show posterior column
    of pelvis 45° rotation away from injured side

Pathological features
Classification of fractures (Judet)
1) Posterior lip of acetabulum
2) Anterior column

3) Posterior column
4) Transverse with inward displacement of
   femoral head 10% have sciatic palsy
   Avascularity of femoral head uncommon –
   floor of acetabulum moves with head
Post-traumatic osteoarthrosis very common

Treatment

Youngsters:
   Open reduction and internal fixation in some
   cases
   (Major procedure, may be difficult)
Others:
   1. Traction : Longitudinal – Tibial pin
                 Lateral – Trochanteric Corkscrew
or 2. Manipulation under anesthesia with traction
   as above
       Reduction difficult to maintain
       Early active hip movements advisable
Late osteoarthrosis:
   Hip arthroplasty

References

Carnesdale P G, Stewart M J, Barnes S N 1975 Acetabular
   disruption and central fracture dislocation of the hip.
   Journal of Bone and Joint Surgery 57A: 1054-1059
Coventry M B 1974 The treatment of fracture dislocation of
   the hip by total hip arthroplasty. Journal of Bone and
   Joint Surgery 56A: 1129-1134
Judet R, Judet J, Letournel E 1964 Fractures of the
   acetabulum. Journal of Bone and Joint Surgery 46A: 1615-
   1646
Tipton W W, D'Ambrosia R D, Ryle G P 1975 Non-
   operative management of central fracture dislocation of the
   hip. Journal of Bone and Joint Surgery 57A: 888-893

Fractures disrupting pelvic ring

General features

Major violence required
High mortality particularly in oldsters
Crushing or distraction mechanism

Clinical features

Pain. Inability to move trunk or hips
Prominence of one sacro-iliac region
Hypovolemic shock
Often little initial swelling

Later massive bruising
Visceral damage common

Radiological features

Hinge fractures: (Pelvis opened at front)
Disruption of 1. symphysis or adjacent rami
            and 2. sacro-iliac joint or adjacent
                  ilium

Vertical distraction fractures
Disruption as above but cranial displacement of
   injured hind quarter

Pathological features

Pubic injuries often damage genito-urinary tract
Sacro-iliac injuries may damage the internal iliac
   vessels or lumbo-sacral nerve roots
Fractures nearly always unite

Treatment

Hinge fractures:
Reduced by side lying or compression
Pelvic sling or binder – poor control of fracture
Walking at 6-8 weeks

Vertical distraction fractures
Heavy skeletal traction to injured side
Pelvic sling or binder
No weight bearing for 8-10 weeks

For travel
Plaster spica (1½ legs)
Sacro-iliac arthrodesis rarely needed
Wait for > 3 months after injury before decision
External fixation devices still experimental

Surgery:
Internal fixation
   Persistently unstable symphysis
   Displacement of major bone fragment
Sacro-iliac arthrodesis
   Persistent instability and pain 3 months after
   injury

References

Dunn A W, Morris H D 1968 Fractures and dislocations of
   the pelvis. Journal of Bone and Joint Surgery 50B: 1639-
   1648
Harris N H, Murray R G 1974 Lesions of the symphysis
   pubis in athletes. Journal of Bone and Joint Surgery 56B:
   563-564
Morton R E, Hamilton S G I 1968 Ligature of the internal
   iliac artery for massive haemorrhage complicating fracture
   of the pelvis. Journal of Bone and Joint Surgery 50B: 376-
   379

Oppenheim W L, Tricker J, Smith R B 1978 Traumatic hemipelvectomy, The tenth survivor. A case report and a review of the literature. Injury 9: 307-312

Shanmugasandaram T K 1970 Unusual dislocation of symphysis pubis with locking. Journal of Bone and Joint Surgery 52A: 1669-1671

Sharp I K 1973 Plate fixation of disrupted symphysis pubis. Journal of Bone and Joint Surgery 55B: 618-620

Fractures of iliac blade

General features
Due to direct blow
Very painful

Clinical features
Severe pain. Local swelling later bruising, some deformity
Inability to walk or move

Radiological features
Variable fracture lines in blade of ilium
Poorly seen in A-P film of pelvis
Better seen in oblique films

Pathological features
Any movement causes pain and increased blood loss
Major loss of blood volume is frequent.
Visceral injuries rarely occur.
May be caused by metastases, especially myelomatosis

Treatment
Rest and analgesics
Manipulations +/- open reduction very rarely required for:-
1. Major displacement of very large fragment
2. Compound fracture +/- visceral injuries

References
Mackinnon W S, Lansdown E L 1972 Total dislocation of the ilium. Journal of Bone and Joint Surgery 54B: 720-722

Whiston G 1953 Internal fixation for fractures and dislocations of the pelvis. Journal of Bone and Joint Surgery 35A: 701-706

Fractures of pubic rami

General features
Usually lateral or anterior crushing injuries
Major violence required in young adults
Urethral or vesical injuries possible
Minor violence in the elderly
Very rarely compound

Clinical features:
Pain on hip movement.
Local tenderness and swelling.
Later bruising in groin and perineum.

Radiological features
Single fractures most often in old women
Double fractures on one side:
    Associated with sacro-iliac disruption
Double fractures on both sides:
    Associated with urethral damage

Pathological features:
Healing is no problem
Reduction not necessary
Little displacement because of muscular attachments

Treatment
Exclude
    sacro-iliac damage
    genito-urinary damage
Single fractures:
    Bed rest
    Early active movements
    Early walking-1-3 days
Double fractures:
    As above
    Walking 10-21 days
Quadruple fractures:
    Pelvic sling – aid to nursing
    Early active movements
    Walking at 3-4 weeks

Avulsion of pelvic apophyses

Anterior inferior iliac spine (Irving, 1964)
Attachment of M. Rectus Femoris avulsed
Due to sudden violent hip flexion and knee
extension as in kicking or high jumping
12-18 years
Local pain and tenderness
Pain on attempted hip flexion
Treatment: Rest 1-2 weeks in bed with hip
flexed

Anterior superior iliac spine e
Attachment of M. Sartorius avulsed
Rare injury
Due to sudden violent hip and knee flexion
15-25 years
Local pain, swelling and bruising
Pain on walking or attempted hip flexion
Treatment: Rest 1-2 weeks in bed with hip and
knee flexed

Ischial tuberosity (Barnes, 1972)
Attachment of hamstrings avulsed
More common than the other avulsions
Due to sudden violent hip extension and knee
flexion
Local pain and swelling
Pain when sitting or on hip flexion
Treatment:
    Rest in prone position 1-2 weeks
    Internal fixation rarely required
    Excessive callus may form

Posterior inferior iliac spine (Elton, 1972)
Attachment of M. Erector Spinae avulsed
Rare injury due to major disruption of pelvis
Persistent local pain or movement after recovery
from other injuries
Treatment: Excision of bone fragment
            or Internal Fixation

Iliac epiphysis (Godshall, 1973)
Attachment of abdominal wall muscles
Rare athletic injury
Pain and tenderness with later bruising
Treatment; Rest

References
Barnes S T, Hinds R B 1972 Pseudo tumour of ischium. A
late manifestation of avulsion of the ischial epiphysis.
Journal of Bone and Joint Surgery 54A: 645-647
Elton R C 1972 Fracture dislocation of the pelvis followed by
non-union of the posterior inferior iliac spine. Journal of
Bone and Joint Surgery 54A: 648-649
Godshall R W, Hansen C A 1973 Incomplete avulsion of a
portion of the iliac epiphysis. Journal of Bone and Joint
Surgery 55A: 1301-1302
Irving M H 1964 Exostosis formation after traumatic
avulsion of the anterior inferior iliac spine. Journal of Bone
and Joint Surgery 46B: 720-722

Visceral complications of fractures of pelvis

Rupture of diaphragm (Peltier, 1965)
Common in severe road accidents
Chest radiograph is mandatory in all trunk
injuries

Small bowel injury (Lunt, 1970, Dohian, 1966).
Arises from crushing injuries.
Mesenteric tears and tearing of walls may lead to
    Local infarcts and perforations

Bladder rupture (Reiser, 1963)
Caused by anterior crushing injuries
Full bladder: Intraperitoneal rupture
Empty bladder: Extraperitoneal rupture
Herniation of bladder is a rare complication of
    symphyseal diastasis

Urethral injury (Holdsworth, 1963)
Caused by straddle or crushing injuries
Membranous or prostatic urethra
    involved – usually ruptured

Rectal injuries (Froman, 1967)
Caused by damage to posterior part of pelvic
    ring
Tearing or perforating injuries
Potentially lethal from subsequent sepsis
Colostomy is mandatory

Vesico-vaginal fistula (Siegel, 1976)
Rare. Due to severe crushing injuries of pubic
    rami

Impotence (King, 1975)
Frequently overlooked until late reviews
15% of those with severe fractures
50% of those with urethral injuries

Herniation of bladder (Fuhs, 1978)
Rare complication of symphyseal diastasis

References
Derian P S, Purser T 1966 Herniation complicating central fracture dislocation of the hip. Journal of Bone and Joint Surgery 48A: 1614-1618
Froman C, Stein A 1967 Complicated crushing injuries of the pelvis. Journal of Bone and Joint Surgery 49B: 24-32
Fuhs S E, Herndon J H, Gould F R 1978 Herniation of the bladder, an unusual complication of traumatic diastasis of the pelvis. Journal of Bone and Joint Surgery 60A: 704-707
Holdsworth F 1963 Injuries to the genito-urinary tract associated with fractures of the pelvis. Proceedings of Royal Society of Medicine 57:, 1044-1046 et seq
King J 1975 Impotence after fractures of the pelvis. Journal of Bone and Joint Surgery 57A: 1107-1109
Lunt H R W 1970 Entrapment of the bowel within fractures of the pelvis. Injury 2: 121-126
Peltier L F 1965 Complications associated with fractures of the pelvis. Journal of Bone and Joint Surgery 47A: 1060-1069
Reiser C, Nicholas E 1963 Rupture of the bladder: unusual features. Journal of Urology 90: 53-57
Seigel R S 1971 Vesico-vaginal fistular and osteomyelitis. Journal of Bone and Joint Surgery 53A: 583-586

Posterior dislocation of hip

General features
Incidence proportional to road traffic accidents
Forces act along femoral shaft when hip is flexed and adducted
Often from a blow in the knee

Clinical features:
Extremely painful hip
Swelling posteriorly
Leg shortened, flexed, adducted and internally rotated
Sciatic palsy in 25%
Knee injuries in 50%

Radiological features
Femoral head overlies acetabulum superiorly and laterally
Shaft of femur adducted on pelvis
Acetabular marginal fracture
Osteochondral fracture of femoral head
} May be present

Lateral views difficult to take because of pain and/or deformity

Pathological features
Grades of dislocation:
  I Simple dislocation
  II Dislocation with 1 or more large fragments
    Stable on reduction
  III Fracture dislocation with severe acetabular damage and instability
  IV Dislocation with fracture of head or neck of femur
Femoral head may become ischemic 10-20%
Post traumatic osteoarthrosis in 50%
Sciatic nerve damage in 10-15%
Bone fragments may prevent reduction or cause later instability

Treatment
1. Early reduction:
  General anesthetic with relaxation
  Traction on leg for 3-4 weeks
  No weight bearing for 6 weeks
  Watch for ischemic changes to 2 years
2. Impossible reduction or Unstable reduction:
  +/- Acetabular fragment:
  +/- Femoral head fragment
} Open reduction Internal fixation of fracture
3. Sciatic paralysis
  A. No acetabular fragment and satisfactory reduction:
    Expectant attitude
    Active and passive exercises for leg
    Ankle orthosis
    Recovery may take 1-2 years
    Not always complete
  B. Large acetabular fragment and/or difficult reduction:
    Exploration of sciatic nerve
    Contusion usually found
    Division very rare:- Nerve suture

References
Chakroborti S, Miller I M 1975 Dislocation of the hip associated with fracture of the femoral head. Injury 7: 134-142
Epstein H C 1974 Posterior fracture dislocations of the hip. Long term follow up. Journal of Bone and Joint Surgery 56A: 1103-1127
Gillespie W J 1975 The incidence and pattern of knee injury associated with dislocation of hip. Journal of Bone and Joint Surgery 57B: 376-378
Kleiman S G et al 1971 Late sciatic nerve palsy following posterior fracture dislocation of the hip. Journal of Bone and Joint Surgery 53A: 781-782
Stewart M J, Milford L W 1954 Fracture dislocation of the hip – an end result study. Journal of Bone and Joint Surgery 36A: 315-342

Anterior dislocation of the hip

General features
Rare
Due to compressive forces up line of femur with hip flexed and abducted
Other injuries may be present

Clinical features
Severe pain
Swelling and later bruising in groin
Leg held abducted, externally rotated and flexed
Femoral nerve paralysis } possible
Femoral artery compression }

Radiological features
Femoral head medial and inferior to acetabulum on A-P films
Anterior in lateral films
Occasional osteochondral fracture of femoral head

Pathological features
Soft tissue stripping of femoral head and neck usually leads to avascularity and later osteoarthrosis
Recurrence and bilaterality excessively rare
Intrapelvic dislocation also reported

Treatment
Reduction immediately
Exploration of femoral neurovascular bundle if pulses do not return
Removal of osteochondral fracture if present
Bed rest on traction for 3 weeks
No weight bearing for 6 weeks
Avascular femoral head:
  Arthrodesis
  Total hip arthroplasty
Neglected anterior dislocation:
  Upper femoral osteotomy
  open reduction

References
Aggarwal N D, Singh H 1967 Unreduced anterior dislocation of the hip. Journal of Bone and Joint Surgery 49B: 288-292
Dall D, Macnab I, Gross A 1970 Recurrent anterior dislocation of the hip. Journal of Bone and Joint Surgery 52A: 574-576
Polesky R E, Poleskey F A 1972 Intrapelvic dislocation of femoral head, following anterior dislocation of the hip. Journal of Bone and Joint Surgery 54A: 1097-1098

Dislocation of hip with ipsilateral fracture of femoral shaft

General features
Uncommon
Dislocation easily overlooked, particularly in unconscious patients

Clinical features
Oligemic shock
Pain of fracture often overshadows that of dislocation
Deformity of dislocation obscured by fracture
Occasional sciatic paralysis
Other injuries may be present

Radiological features
Shaft fractures often transverse
Posterior dislocation of hip +/- acetabular marginal fracture
Persistent adduction of upper fragment of shaft may give clue to unnoticed hip dislocation

Pathological features
Major blood loss around injuries concomitant neurovascular damage possible: Femoral vessel occlusion
Later:
  Ischemia of femoral head
  Post traumatic osteo-arthrosis

Treatment
First. Reduction of dislocation
A. Manual methods difficult because of fracture (Stimson's method – patient prone hips and legs flexed over end of table)
B. Trochanteric Corkscrew or pin to act as lever
C. Open reduction:
  Additional indications
    Sciatic paralysis
    Acetabular fracture

Secondly. Reduction of fracture
Conservative: Thomas splint and skeletal traction
Surgical: Open reduction and internal fixation

References
Fina C P, Kelly P J 1970 Dislocations of the hip with fractures of the proximal femur. Journal of Trauma 10: 77-87
Helal B, Skevis X 1967 Unrecognised dislocation of the hip in fractures of the femoral shaft. Journal of Bone and Joint Surgery 49B: 293-300
Schoenecker P L, Manske P L, Sertl G O 1978 Traumatic hip dislocation with ipselateral femoral shaft fracture. Clinical Orthopaedics 130: 233-236

Neglected dislocation of hip

General features
Rare. Nearly all posterior dislocations
Due to lack of medical help
or concealment by ipselateral fracture of femoral shaft.

Clinical features
Persistent pain and swelling around hip
Leg shortened flexed, adducted and internally rotated
Inability to bear weight for 6-12 months

Radiological features
Those of any posterior dislocation
Femoral head may be ischemic (increased density) in dislocated position.

Pathological features
Acetabulum eventually fills with fibrous tissue
Capsular tear closes around femoral neck
Femoral head cartilage degenerates

Treatment:
Early:
Traction and manipulation
Late:
Heavy traction abduction in plaster
or Open reduction
or Arthrodesis
Very Late:
Upper femoral osteotomy (Schanz type)

References
Gupta R C, Shravat B P 1977 Reduction of neglected dislocation of the hip by heavy traction. Journal of Bone and Joint Surgery 59A: 249-251
Nixon J R 1976 Late open reduction of traumatic dislocation of the hip. Journal of Bone and Joint Surgery 58B: 41-43

Recurrent dislocation of hip

General features
Very rare. Nearly all posterior
Primary dislocation due to major violence
Treatment may have been delayed
Immobilisation may have been inadequate

Clinical features
Second and subsequent dislocations occur with less violence
Voluntary dislocation and reduction has been reported

Radiological features
Displaced acetabular marginal fracture may be present
Arthrography delineates:
Capsular rent
False acetabulum
Congenitally shallow acetabulum may be present

Pathological features
Ischemic necrosis of femoral head unlikely despite capsular defect and loss of ligamentum teres
Post-traumatic osteoarthrosis likely

Treatment
Surgical repair of capsular defect

References
Heinzelmann P R, Nelson C L 1976 Recurrent traumatic dislocation of hip. Journal of Bone and Joint Surgery 58A: 895-896
Liebenberg F, Domisse G F 1969 Recurrent post-traumatic dislocation of the hip. Journal of Bone and Joint Surgery 51B: 632-637

Dislocation of the hip in children

General features
Uncommon injury
Mechanisms of injury as in adults
Incidence of avascularity of femoral head is less
 (Contrast increased incidence in fractures of
 femoral neck in children)
Recurrence is excessively rare

References
Bonnemaison M F E, Henderson E D 1968 Traumatic
 anterior dislocation of the hip with acute common femoral
 occlusion in a child. Journal of Bone and Joint Surgery
 50A: 753-756
Broudy A S, Scott R D 1975 Voluntary posterior hip
 dislocation in children. Journal of Bone and Joint Surgery
 57A: 716-717
Haliburton R A, Brockenshire F A, Barber J R 1961
 Avascular necrosis of the femoral capital epiphysis after
 traumatic dislocation of the hip in children. Journal of
 Bone and Joint Surgery 43B: 43-46
Sankarankutty M 1967 Traumatic inferior dislocation of the
 hip (luxatis erecta) in a child. Journal of Bone and Joint
 Surgery 49B: 145
Schomsky J, Miller P R 1973 Traumatic hip dislocations in
 children. Journal of Bone and Joint Surgery 55A: 1057-
 1063

Soft tissue injuries of buttock and hip

General features
Rare in civilian life
Occur from gunshot wounds
 road traffic accidents
 industrial injuries

Clinical features
Flaying
Penetrating } wounds of hind quarter
Tearing
Other injuries may be present elsewhere
Major loss of blood volume
Neural and vascular damage locally
Rectal penetration or tearing very dangerous

Radiological features
Very variable range of fractures possible
Radio-opaque foreign bodies may be present

Pathological features
Infection is chief problem in recovery
Exacerbated if rectum is damaged
Tetanus and gas gangrene may occur if wound
 excision is incomplete

Treatment
Replace blood volume
Colostomy if rectum is damaged
Wound excision must be thorough
Delayed primary closure safest
Flaying injuries require skin grafting

References
Clawson D K, Seddon H J 1960 Results of repair of the
 sciatic nerve. Journal of Bone and Joint Surgery 42B: 205-
 212 et seq
London P S 1967 A practical guide to the care of the injured.
 Ch 18, E & S Livingstone, London & Edinburgh
Meester G L, Myerley W H 1975 Traumatic hemipelvectomy:
 a case report and literature review. Journal of Trauma 15:
 541-545

Traumatic separation of upper femoral epiphysis

General features
Rare
Due to major violence
Usually under 9 years
Other injuries may be present

Clinical features
Pain, swelling, tenderness
Full external rotation of leg
Minimal shortening
Ischemia of leg very rare

Radiological features
Usually Salter Type I separation
No metaphyseal fragment attached to epiphysis
Usually a severe posterior displacement

Pathological features
> 9 years more common.
Adolescent coxa vara may occur from minor
   injuries
< 9 years Premature fusion
         Non-Union   } Very frequent
         Avascular epiphysis }

Treatment

Displacement
Manipulation +/- capsulotomy of hip
Plaster spica

No Displacement (Widened epiphysis only)
Traction

References

Casey B H, Hamilton H W, Bobechko W P 1972 Reduction
   of acutely slipped upper femoral epiphysis. Journal of Bone
   and Joint Surgery 54B: 607-614
Ratliff A H C 1968 Traumatic separation of the upper
   femoral epiphysis in young children. Journal of Bone and
   Joint Surgery 50B: 757-770

Intra-capsular fractures of femoral neck

General features
Increasingly common in old age
F : M = 8 : 1
Occur from trivial violence
Rare under 50 – these are due to major violence

Clinical features
Pain around hip
Usually unable to stand
Unimpacted fractures:
   45° external rotation of leg and some
      shortening
Impacted fractures: No deformity

Radiological features
Impacted fractures sometimes difficult to
   visualise
Displaced fractures show upward shift of femoral
   neck and external rotation

Grade   I: Impaction (Incomplete fracture)
      II: Minor separation (Complete fracture)
          No displacement
     III: Moderate separation (Complete
          fracture)
          Partial displacement
      IV: Major separation (Complete fracture)
          Full displacement

Pathological features
Never occur in an arthritic hip
Very high incidence of osteoporosis
Adduction and abduction fractures are part of
   the same spiral pattern
The closer the fracture line to the articular
   surface – the greater the angulation
The longer the deformity exists the greater the
   chance of ischemia of femoral head
Security of fixation device has the greatest
   influence on union
Union may occur temporarily with an avascular
   head, but avascular bone breaks down on
   weight bearing
Late segmental collapse may occur up to 2 years
   after fracture. High incidence in young adults

Treatment
Palliative:
   Skin traction with correction of rotation
   If unfit for surgery
   To prepare for surgery
Surgical:
   Grades I and II:
      Manipulation usually not necessary
      Internal fixation by nails, pins or nail plate
         as many separate if treated conservatively
   Grade III:
      Consider internal fixation or replacement
         arthroplasty
   Grade IV:
      Replacement arthroplasty usually indicated

Problems

1. Failure of internal fixation
Due to poor technique
Osteoporotic bone
Ischemic head
Treatment: Replacement arthroplasty

2. Time of weight bearing
Early:
   If fixation is secure
   Patient is frail or confused

Delayed:
  If fixation is insecure
  If fracture is impacted
  If patient is young and can use crutches

References

Abrami G, Stevens J 1964 Early weight bearing after internal fixation of transcervical fracture of the femur. Journal of Bone and Joint Surgery 46B: 204-205

Arnold W D, Lyden J P, Minkoff J 1974 Treatment of intracapsular fractures of the femoral neck with special reference to percutaneous Knowles pinning. Journal of Bone and Joint Surgery 56A: 254-262

Barnes R et al 1976 Subcapital fractures of the femur. Journal of Bone and Joint Surgery 58B: 1-25

Bonfiglio M, Voke E M 1968 Aseptic necrosis of the femoral head and non union of the femoral neck. Journal of Bone and Joint Surgery 50A: 48-66

Chapman M W et al 1975 Treatment of intracapsular hip fractures by the Deyerle method. Journal of Bone and Joint Surgery 57A: 735-744

Colonna P C 1960 The trochanteric reconstruction operation for ununited fractures of the upper end of the femur. Journal of Bone and Joint Surgery 42B: 5-10

D'Arcy J, Devas M 1976 Treatment of fractures of the femoral neck by replacement with the Thompson prosthesis. Journal of Bone and Joint Surgery 58B: 279-286

Devas M B 1965 Stress fractures of the femoral neck. Journal of Bone and Joint Surgery 47B: 728-737

Fielding J W, Wilson S A, Ratzan S 1974 A continuing end result study of displaced intracapsular fractures of the neck of the femur treated with the Pugh nail. Journal of Bone and Joint Surgery 56A: 1464-1472

Freeman M A R, Todd R C, Pirie C J 1974 The role of fatigue in the pathogenesis of senile femoral neck fractures. Journal of Bone and Joint Surgery 56B: 698-702

Garden R S 1961 Low angle fixation in fractures of the femoral neck. Journal of Bone and Joint Surgery 43B: 647-663

Garden R S 1964 Stability and union in subcapital fractures of the femur. Journal of Bone and Joint Surgery 46B: 630-647

Hargadon E J, Pearson J R 1963 Treatment of intracapsular fracture of the femoral neck with the Chanley compression screw. Journal of Bone and Joint Surgery 45B: 305-311

Jarry L 1964 Transarticular nailing for fractures of the femoral neck. Journal of Bone and Joint Surgery 46B: 674-684

Linton P 1949 Types of displacement of fractures of the femoral neck. Journal of Bone and Joint Surgery 31B: 184-189

Protzman R R, Burkhalter W E 1976 Femoral neck fractures in young adults. Journal of Bone and Joint Surgery 58A: 689-695

Smyth E H J et al 1964 Triangle pinning for fracture of the femoral neck. Journal of Bone and Joint Surgery 46B: 664-673

Zabihi T, Kohanim M, Amir-James A K 1973 Operation in the treatment of complications of fractures of the femoral neck. Journal of Bone and Joint Surgery 55A: 129-136

Extra-capsular fractures of femoral neck

Synonym
Basal Intertrochanteric, Pertrochanteric fractures

General features:
Common in oldsters from trivial violence
Rare in youngsters from major violence.
Sometimes pathological
The only femoral neck fracture to occur in osteoarthrosis of hips

Clinical features
Pain, swelling, later bruising
90° external rotation and shortening of leg is usual but not invariable
Loss of hip movement
Inability to stand
Comminuted fractures may be internally rotated

Radiological features
Variable degrees of comminution and displacement.
Lesser trochanter may be separated.
Spiral fracture of upper femoral shaft may be present

Pathological features:
Always unite (unless pathological)
Varus angulation unless corrected
Unreducible fractures may have muscle interposed.

Treatment

Conservative
Balanced skeletal traction (Hamilton-Russell)

Surgical
A. Open reduction
   Internal fixation
      (i) Nail plate
      +/- cement as adjuvant
   or: (ii) V-Y nail for severe comminution
or: B Closed reduction
      Internal fixation with transcondylar nails

References

Conrad J J 1971 Medial displacement fixation of unstable intertrochanteric fractures of the hip. Bulletin of the Hospital for Joint Disease New York 32: 54-62

Cuthbert H, Howat T W 1977 The use of the Kuntscher Y nail in the treatment of intertrochanteric and subtrochanteric fractures of the femur. Injury 8: 135-142

Dunn E J, Skinner S R 1976 Disengagement of a sliding screw plate. Journal of Bone and Joint Surgery 58A: 1027-1028

Fordyce A 1968 False aneurysm of the profunda femoris artery following nail and plate fixation of an intertrochanteric fracture. Journal of Bone and Joint Surgery 50B: 141-143

Harrington K D 1975 The use of methylmethacylate as an adjunct in internal fixation of unstable comminuted intertrochanteric fractures in osteoporotic patients. Journal of Bone and Joint Surgery 57A: 744-750

Horn J S, Wang Y C 1964 The mechanism, traumatic anatomy, and non-operative treatment of intertrochanteric fracture of the femur. British Journal of Surgery 51: 574-580

Kaufer H, Matthews L S, Sonstegard D 1974 Stable fixation of intertrochanteric fractures. Journal of Bone and Joint Surgery 56A: 899-907

Kuderna H, Bohler N, Collon D J 1976 Treatment of intertrochanteric and subtrochanteric fractures of the hip by the ender method. Journal of Bone and Joint Surgery 58A: 604-611

Massie W K 1964 Fractures of the hip. Journal of Bone and Joint Surgery 46A: 658-690

Murray R C, Frew J F M 1949 Trochanteric fractures of the femur. A plea for conservative treatment. Journal of Bone and Joint Surgery 31B: 204-219

Pugh W L 1955 A self-adjusting nail plate for fracture about the hip joint. Journal of Bone and Joint Surgery 37A: 1085-1093

Zickel R E 1976 An intramedullary fixation device for the proximal part of the femur. Journal of Bone and Joint Surgery 58A: 866-872

Prediction of avascular necrosis of femoral head

Many methods used
Mostly unreliable and difficult to apply
Te^{99} bone scans appear promising

Methods

Injection of opaque material (Hulth, 1956)
Injection of dye (Price, 1962; Sillar, 1964)
Injection of Radioisotopes (Boyd, 1963; Holmquist, 1969)
Venous Drainage (Harrison, 1962)
Oxygen Tension (Woodhouse, 1962)
Technetium Bone Scan (Meyers, 1977)
Intra-Osseous pressure (Arnoldi, 1978)

References

Arnoldi C C, Lemperg R K 1978 Fracutre of the femoral neck. II Intra-osseous pressure measurement. Clinical Orthopaedics 129: 217-222

Boyd H B, Calundruccio R A 1963 Further observations on the use of radioactive phosphorus (P^{32}) to determine the viability of the head of the femur. Journal of Bone and Joint Surgery 45A: 445-459

Harrison M H M 1962 A preliminary report of vascular assay in prognosis of fractured femoral neck. Journal of Bone and Joint Surgery 44B: 858-868

Holmquist B, Alffram P A 1965 Prediction of avascular necrosis following cervical fracture of the femur, based on clearance of radioactive iodine from the head of the femur. Acta Orthopedica Scandinavica 36: 62-69

Hulth A 1956 Intra-osseous venographies of medial fractures of the femoral neck. Acta Chirurgica Scandinavica, Supplement 214

Meyers M H, Telfer N, Moore T M 1978 Determination of the vascularity of the femoral head with technetium 99m sulphur colloid. Journal of Bone and Joint Surgery 59A: 658-664

Price E V 1962 The viability of the femoral head after fracture of the neck of the femur. Journal of Bone and Joint Surgery 44B: 854-868

Woodhouse C F 1962 Anoxia of the femoral head. Surgery 52: 55-63

Fractures of femoral neck in children

General features

Rare. Due to major violence
Other injuries are frequently present

Clinical features

Pain, swelling
Inability to stand or move
External rotation of leg
Shortening may be present

Radiological features

Fracture may be transcervical or intertrochanteric
Usually not comminuted

Pathological features

Very high incidence of avascularity regardless of type of fracture
Probably due to hemarthrosis occluding cervical blood vessels

Treatment

Immediate:

Undisplaced:
  Capsulotomy
  Plaster Spica
Displaced:
    > 10 years Open reduction and
  capsulotomy
  Internal fixation
  < 10 years Open reduction and
  capsulotomy
  Subtrochanteric osteotomy
Non Union: Grafting procedures
Non Union and Ischemic Head:
  Subtrochanteric osteotomy and plaster spica
Union and later ischemic head:
  Arthrodesis of Hip

References

Canale S T, Bourland W L 1977 Fracture of the neck and
  intertrochanteric region of the femur in children. Journal of
  Bone and Joint Surgery 59A: 431-443
Ratliff A H C 1962 Fractures of the neck of the femur in
  children. Journal of Bone and Joint Surgery 44B: 528-542

Ipsilateral fractures of neck and shaft of femur

General features
Rare
Due to major violence
Other injuries may be present

General features
Hypovolemic shock
Pain, swelling
Loss of hip and leg function
Occasional occlusion of femoral vessels

Radiological features
Infinite variety of shaft fractures
Basal or transcervical fractures of neck
Neck fractures may be overlooked if hip is not
  fully visualised

Pathological features
Each fracture has its own group of problems

Treatment

Conservative
Manipulation

Balance skeletal traction
Difficulty in controlling upper fracture

Surgical
Internal fixation
    (a) V-Y nailing
or: (b) Posterior pins for neck
      Anterior intramedullary nail for shaft
or: (c) Nail plate for neck
      Plate for shaft

References

De Mourgues G, Fischer L P, Carret J P 1975 Fractures
  associeés homolatérales du col et de la diaphyse fémorale.
  Revue de Chirurgie Orthopedique 61: 275-284
Kimbrough E E 1961 Concomitant unilateral hip and femoral
  shaft fractures – a too frequently unrecognised syndrome.
  Journal of Bone and Joint Surgery 43A: 443-449

Subcapital fracture following pertrochanteric fracture of hip

General features
Rare

Clinical features
Symptoms of 2nd hip fracture 9-12 months after
  1st fracture
(After second minor fall)

Radiological features
Osteoporosis
Subcapital fracture
Nail plate of 1st fracture does not penetrate
  femoral head

Pathological features
Osteoporisis usually present
Local neoplasia rarely present
Stress concentration at tip of nail

Treatment
Total hip replacement with long stem femoral
    component
Excision arthroplasty if infection present

References

Baker D M 1975 Fractures of the femoral neck after healed intertrochanteric fracture. Complication of too short a nail plate. Journal of Trauma 15: 73-76

Hunter G A, Mehta A 1977 Subcapital fracture of the hip – a rare complication of intertrochanteric fracture of the femur. Canadian Journal of Surgery 20: 165-172

Fractures of greater trochanter

General features
Usually occurs in the elderly from minor trauma
Commences in diseased or osteoporotic bone

Clinical features
Pain, swelling
Limited hip movement
Pain worse on weight bearing

Radiological features
Best visualised on A-P views
Separation usually minimal

Pathological features
Wide separation of trochanteric fragment unusual – retained by fascial attachments
Usually unites by fibrous tissue
Lengthens and weakens hip abductors

Treatment
Bed rest with early active movements. Open reduction and internal rarely required for:
　Younger patients
　Good quality of bone
　Wide separation of fragment
Hip spica in full abduction sometimes feasible for young people

Avulsion of lesser trochanter

General features
Usually an athletic injury in adolescents – before fusion at 18
M > F

Clinical features
Sudden pain in groin on a powerful muscular effort
Continued pain on active hip flexion
No initial swelling or bruising
Local deep tenderness
Able to walk.

Radiological features
Avulsion of lesser trochanteric epiphysis or lesser trochanter if epiphysis has fused
Displacement proximally

Pathological features
Usually a Salter Type I epiphyseal injury
More rarely a pathological fracture from neoplasia in the elderly
Trivial violence in this instance
Fragment separated by action of ilio-psoas

Treatment
Adolescents and young adults
　Bed rest with hip and knee flexed 1-2 weeks
　Graduated exercises thereafter with temporary use of crutches
Pathological fracture:
　Consider internal fixation of femoral shaft by long nail plate or intramedullary nail

References

Dimon J H 1972 Isolated fractures of the lesser trochanter of the femur. Clinical Orthopaedics 82: 144-148

Subtrochanteric fractures of femur

General features
Youngsters:
　Normal bone Major violence
Oldsters:
　Abnormal bone
　　Porotic
　　Malacic
　　Neoplastic
　　Pagets Disease
Minor violence

Clinical feature
Pain, swelling, later bruising
Shortening and external rotation
Inability to move leg

Radiological features

May be transverse or comminuted
Oblique fractures may be displaced or
    undisplaced
Osteolysis indicates neoplasia
Paget's Disease may give a step-like fracture

Pathological features

Subtrochanteric region
    Site of high mechanical stress
    Frequent site of secondary deposits
Upper fragment
    Iliopsoas flexes and externally rotates
    Glutei abduct
Lower fragment adducted
Direction of obliquity may determine stability or
    instability of fracture

Treatment

Conservative
Children and young adults
    Manipulation
    Splintage with thigh flexed, abducted
        externally rotated and often difficult to
        maintain
    Thomas Splint with knee piece
    Plaster spica
    Traction essential for unstable oblique fracture

Surgical
Normal bone:
    Open reduction
    Internal fixation
        1. Neck nail with long plate
    or: 2. V-Y nail
    or: 3. Intra-medullary nail
Abnormal bone:
    Open reduction
    Excision Biopsy
    Internal fixation as above
    Cement filling

References

Asher M A et al 1967 Compression fixation of
    subtrochanteric fractures. Clinical Orthopaedics 117: 202-
    208
Ireland D C R, Fisher R L 1975 Subtrochanteric fractures of
    the femur in children. Clinical Orthopaedics 110: 157-166
Rybicki I E F, Simonen F A, Weis E B 1972 On the
    mathematical analysis of stress in the human femur.
    Journal of Biomechanics 5: 203-215
Seinscheimer F 1978 Subtrochanteric fractures of the femur.
    Journal of Bone and Joint Surgery 60A: 300-306

Fractures of femoral shafts in adults

General features

Major violence required
Transverse fractures: Direct blow
Oblique fractures: Twisting compressive forces
Large concealed blood loss
A fracture from trivial violence indicates bone
    pathology

Clinical features

Pain, deformity, swelling
Hypovolemic shock
Occasional neurovascular deficit
Other injuries may be present

Radiological features

Infinite variety of fracture patterns
Wide separation indicates:
    Forces acting after fracture
    Possibility of compounding
    Interposition of soft tissue
Arteriography if indicated by ischemia

Pathological features

Muscle interposition more frequent than in any
    other fracture
Compounding usually from within out
Very large bloodloss can be concealed in a
    swollen thigh

Treatment

Conservative
Manipulation
Thomas splint and skeletal traction
+/- cast brace after 3-6 weeks

Surgical
Open reduction and internal fixation
Indications:
    Reduction of hospital time
    Need to travel
    Other injuries in same leg
    Pathological fractures

Methods
Intramedullary nail:
 Transverse fractures in mid half of shaft
 Fractures in lower ¼ require cement adjuvant
Plates, Screws, Wire, etc:
 Oblique and comminuted fractures

References

Anderson R L 1967 Conservative treatment of fractures of the femur. Journal of Bone and Joint Surgery 49A: 1371-1375

Carr C R, Wingo C H 1973 Fractures of the femoral diaphysis. Journal of Bone and Joint Surgery 55A: 690-700

Grundy M 1970 Fractures of the femur in Paget's disease of bone. Their etiology and treatment. Journal of Bone and Joint Surgery 52B: 252-263

Herndon J H, Tolo T, Lamoue A C, Deffer P A 1973 Management of fractured femora in acute amputees. Journal of Bone and Joint Surgery 55A: 1600-1613

Hubbard M J S 1974 The treatment of femoral shaft fractures in the elderly. Journal of Bone and Joint Surgery 56B: 96-101

Provost R A, Morris J M 1969 Fatigue fracture of the femoral shaft. Journal of Bone and Joint Surgery 51A: 487-498

Rothwell A G, Fitzpatrick C B 1978 Closed Kuntscher nailing of femoral shaft fractures. Journal of Bone and Joint Surgery 60B: 504-509

Seimon L P 1964 Refracture of the shaft of the femur. Journal of Bone and Joint Surgery 46B: 32-39

Smith J E M 1964 The results of early and delayed internal fixation of fractures of the shaft of the femur. Journal of Bone and Joint Surgery 46B: 28-31

Stubbs B E, Matthews L S, Sonstegard D A 1975 Experimental fixation of fractures of the femur with methylmethacylate. Journal of Bone and Joint Surgery 57A: 317-321

Wardlaw D 1977 The cast brace treatment of femoral shaft fractures. Journal of Bone and Joint Surgery 59B: 411-416

Wilber M C, Evans E B 1978 Fractures of the femoral shaft treated surgically. Comparative results of early and delayed operative stabilisation. Journal of Bone and Joint Surgery 60A: 489-492

Woolson S T, Meeks L W 1974 A method of balanced skeletal traction for femoral fractures. Journal of Bone and Joint Surgery 56A: 1288-1289

Fractures of femoral shaft and head injury

General features
Common in young adults
Arise from road or machinery accidents
Other injuries may be present

Clinical features
Head Injury: Any combination of neurological or osseous lesions possible
Femoral Injury: Usually a closed fracture of shaft with deformity and swelling
Hypovolemic shock usually present

Radiological features
Any variety of cranial, facial or femoral fractures may be present

Pathological features
Femoral fractures unite rapidly with much callus, despite difficulties of fixation and splintage

Incompatibilities

Treatment:
1. Resuscitation and diagnosis
2. Observe head injury   }6-12
                                          }hours
 Apply Thomas splint and fixed traction /
Deteriorating cerebral state
 3. Craniotomy +/- internal fixation
Improving cerebral state
 4. Treat femoral fracture on its merits

References
Gibson J M C 1960 Multiple injuries, the management of the patient with a fractured femur and a head injury. Journal of Bone and Joint Surgery 42B: 425-431

	Head	Femur
Fixation	Needs mobilisation	Needs immobilisation
Treatment	Often observation	Compound fractures need operation
Fluids	Need caution	Needs copious replacement
Patient Activity	Advantageous	Deleterious
Coma	Raised intra-cranial pressure	Fat embolism.

Fractures of femoral shaft in children

General features
Common
Oblique spiral fractures occur from falling
Transverse +/- compound fractures occur from direct violence

Clinical features
Pain and swelling
Shortening and angulation
Neurovascular loss very uncommon
Not often compound
If an infant, suspect child abuse or pathological fracture

Radiological features
Oblique fractures may be long spirals with considerable shortening
Transverse fractures may be markedly displaced and/or comminuted

Pathological features
Subtrochanteric fractures:
    Upper fragment flexed and abducted by M. psoas and MM. Gluteii
Oblique fractures:
    Retain an intact periosteum despite shortening
Residual shortening:
    1-2 cm. compensated by subsequent epiphyseal growth spurt

Treatment
Infants up to 30 lb./15 Kg.: Gallows traction 3-4 weeks
Small children:
    A. Skin traction with leg on a pillow
        Liston splint on sound side from axilla to ankle
or B. Plaster spica 4-5 weeks
Larger children:
    Thomas splint with balanced skin 5-6 weeks
Internal fixation:
    Rarely required for other fractures in same leg or pathological fractures
Cast brace application at 2-3 weeks under evaluation (McCullough 1978)

References
Edvardsen P, Syversen S M 1976 Overgrowth of the femur after fracture of the shaft in childhood. Journal of Bone and Joint Surgery 58B: 339-342
Hunnberger R W, Eyring E J 1969 Proximal tibial 90-90 traction in treatment of children with femoral shaft fractures. Journal of Bone and Joint Surgery 51A: 499-503
Irani R N, Nicholson J T, Chung S M K 1976 Long term results in the treatment of femoral shaft fractures in young children by immediate spica immobilisation. Journal of Bone and Joint Surgery 58A: 945-951
McCullough N C III, Vinsant J E, Sarmiento A 1978 Functional fracture bracing of long bone fractures of the lower extremity in children. Journal of Bone and Joint Surgery 60A: 314-319

Intramedullary nailing of femur

Indications
Fractures in middle 3/5th of shaft
Transverse fractures
Short oblique fractures
Pathological fractures
Presence of other fractures
Need to travel
Need to leave hospital
Non-union
Flaying injuries

Contra-Indications
Severely contaminated fractures
Comminuted fractures
Fractures in lower $\frac{1}{5}$ of femur

Techniques
1. Open reduction
    Retrograde introduction of nail
2. Closed reduction
    Nail introduced through great trochanter under radiographic control (More exacting than open technique)

Problems
Sepsis:
    Massive antibiotics
    Rest
    Remove nail only when fracture is solid
Migration of nail: Reinsert or remove
Delayed union: Add grafts
Fracture of nail: Treat conservatively or interlock a 2nd nail.

References

Christenson N O 1973 Kutschner intramedullary reaming and nail fixation for non-union of fracture of the femur and the tibia. Journal of Bone and Joint Surgery 55B: 312-318

Debelder K R J 1968 Distal migration of the femoral intramedullary nail. Journal of Bone and Joint Surgery 50B: 324-333

Rothwell A G, Fitzpatrick C B 1978 Closed Kuntscher nailing of femoral shaft fractures. Journal of Bone and Joint Surgery 60B: 504-509

Wilson J N 1966 The management of infection after Kuntschner nailing of the femur. Journal of Bone and Joint Surgery 48B: 112-116

Ipsilateral fractures of femur and tibia

General features
Due to major violence (road or industrial accidents)
Other injuries usually present

Clinical features
Pain, swelling, deformity, loss of function
Hypovolemic shock
Neurovascular injuries often present
Major skin loss or flaying possible

Radiological features
Infinite variety of fractures of femur and tibia
Arteriography may show arterial occlusion

Pathological features
Delayed union of one fracture site is frequent
Post traumatic osteoarthrosis of knee

Treatment

Conservative
Plaster case for tibia
Balanced skeletal traction for femur
Shortening and angulation difficult to correct
Skin losses +/- ischemia may make internal fixation hazardous

Surgical
Internal fixation of one or both fractures
Allows neurovascular exploration and skin grafting if required.
Fewer complications
Faster healing
Less time in hospital

References

Fraser R D, Hunter G A, Waddell J P 1978 Ipselateral fracture of the femur and tibia. Journal of Bone and Joint Surgery 60B: 510-515

Karlstrom G, Olerud S 1977 Ipselateral fracture of the femur and tibia. Journal of Bone and Joint Surgery 59A: 240-243

Winston M E 1972 The results of conservative treatment of fractures of the femur and tibia in the same limb. Surgery Gynaecology and Obstetrics 134: 985-991

Juxta-epiphyseal fractures of lower femur

General features
Newborn:
    Obstetrical mishap in breech with extended legs
Infants:
    Child abuse
Toddlers:
    Often a pathological fracture
        Spina bifida
        Scurvy
        Polio
        Post-operative osteoporisis
Small children ⎱ Major violence
Adolescents   ⎰ Usually hyperextension of knee

Clinical features
Pain swelling deformity
Inability to bear weight or move
(Painless in spina bifida, etc.)
Popliteal vessels sometimes occluded in adolescents

Radiological features
Usually a Salter Type II injury
Other juxta epiphyseal injuries may indicate child abuse (See appropriate section)
Salter Type I injury in scurvy or infection
Wide displacement in pathological fractures

Pathological features
Diminished growth in length in 30% of patients
Later deformity related to degree of initial
    displacement

Treatment

Infants
Manipulation
Plaster spica
Treatment of cause

Spina Bifida
Splintage may cause skin ulceration
Traction may be sufficient

Others
Manipulation (Over reduction impossible)
Long leg cast
Severe hyperextension injuries held with knee
    flexed to 90° +

References

Hutchison J 1894 Lectures on injuries of the epiphyses and
    their results. British Medical Journal 1: 669
Lombardo S J, Harvey J P 1977 Fractures of the distal
    femoral epiphysis. Journal of Bone and Joint Surgery 59A:
    742-751
Stephens D C, Louis D S 1974 Traumatic separation of the
    distal femoral epiphyseal cartilage plate. Journal of Bone
    and Joint Surgery 56A: 1383-1390

Supracondylar fractures of femur

General features
Adult equivalent of a lower epiphyseal
    separation
Usually due to angulatory and compressive
    forces
Often compound

Clinical features
Pain, swelling
Inability to move knee or bear weight
Angular deformity not usually present
Femoral vessels may be occluded

Pathological features
Classification:
    I Minimal displacement
   IIA Condyles displaced medially
      Shaft lacerates extensor tendon laterally
   IIB Condyles displaced laterally
      Extensor tendon spared.
   III Extensive comminution
Transverse fractures rotated by gastronemii and
    may compress femoral vessels
Oblique fractures often contain interposed muscle
Suprapatellar bursa usually obliterated in
    healing, leading to a stiff knee

Treatment

Conservative
Balanced skeletal traction
Thomas splint and knee piece +/- later cast
    brace

Surgical
Open reduction
Internal fixation with blade plate +/- exploration
    of femoral vessels

Problems
Rotation of lower fragment
Knee stiffness
Later varus and internal rotation deformity
Delayed union

References

Mooney V et al 1970 Cast-brace treatment for fractures of
    the distal part of the femur. Journal of Bone and Joint
    Surgery 52A: 1563-1578
Neer C S, Grantham S A, Shelton M L 1967 Supracondylar
    fracture of the adult femur. Journal of Bone and Joint
    Surgery 49A: 591-613
Olerud S 1972 Operative treatment of supracondylar-condylar
    fracture of the femur. Journal of Bone and Joint Surgery
    54A: 1015-1032

Intercondylar and condylar fractures of femur

General features
Usually due to major violence in normal bone or
    trivial violence in porotic bone

Clinical features
Pain, swelling, hemarthrosis
Inability to bear weight or move knee
Occasional ischemia of lower leg

Radiological features
Single condylar fractures occur in sagittal or
    coronal plane and may be undisplaced,
    displaced or rotated.
Bicondylar fractures occur in coronal plane
Intercondylar fractures – "T" shaped
Arteriography may show popliteal occlusion

Pathological features
Avascularity never occurs
Intercondylar fractures do not separate widely
    because of ligamentous attachments
Assymmetry of joint surfaces is common, with
    later osteoarthrosis

Treatment

Undisplaced fractures
Aspiration of hemarthrosis
Padded plaster cast
Weight bearing at 6-8 weeks

Displaced fractures
Open reduction
Internal fixation
Weight bearing at 6-8 weeks

Popliteal artery occlusion
Exploration
Decompression
Reversed vein graft

Reference
Olerud S 1972 Operative treatment of supracondylar-condylar
    fractures of the femur. Journal of Bone and Joint Surgery
    54A: 1015-1032

Osteochondral fractures of lower femur

General features
Usually in adolescents
Caused by tangential blow with knee flexed
Medial > Lateral femoral condyles

Lateral fractures often associated with patellar
    dislocation

Clinical features
Pain, swelling, bruising
Hemarthrosis. Loss of movement
Weight bearing may be possible

Radiological features
Tangential or oblique views most useful
A-P and lateral views may not show fracture or
    may obscure the size of the fragment

Pathological features
In adults a tangential flake of bone and articular
    cartilage is knocked off
In adolescents a triangular segment may
    separate
Separated fragments may form loose bodies
Loose bodies may be nourished by synovial fluid
Displaced fractures may lead to later
    osteoarthrosis

Treatment:

1. Undisplaced fractures: aspirate hemarthrosis
Small fragments:
    Compression bandage
    Early active movements
Large fragments:
    Plaster cast or splintage
    Limited weight bearing

2. Displaced fractures
Open reduction
Internal fixation
Early active movements

3. Displaced fragments
Arthrotomy
Internal fixation or removal
Early active movements
Weight bearing within 2-3 weeks

References
Ahstrom J P 1965 Osteochondral fracture in the knee joint
    associated with hypermobility and dislocation of the
    patella. Journal of Bone and Joint Surgery 47A:, 1491-1502
Kennedy J C, Grainger R W, McGraw R W 1966
    Osteochondral fractures of the femoral condyles. Journal of
    Bone and Joint Surgery 48B: 436-440

Contusion of quadriceps

General features
Usually in footballers or athletes
Direct blow

Clinical features
Pain, swelling: Later bruising
Able to walk. Some loss of knee flexion
Later fibrosis or calcification

Radiological features
Soft tissue swelling
Later:
    Hazy calcification based on periosteum
Much later:
    ectopic bone formed

Pathological features
Hematoma → Resolution
    ↓
Fibrosis → Calcification
    ↓
        Bone formation

Differential diagnosis
Swelling:
    Rupture of quadriceps
    Soft tissue tumour
Calcification:
    Osteosarcoma
    Infection

Treatment
Rest: Check for hemorrhagic diathesis
Aspirate hematoma if fluctuant
Hyaluronidase by mouth or injections
Graded exercise
Biopsy: If serious doubt of diagnosis
Excision:
    Of ectopic calcification
    When mature
    Earlier if Painful
            Prominent
            Inhibiting quadriceps
Quadricepsplasty: Rarely required

Reference
Jackson D W, Feagin J A 1973 Quadriceps contusion in
    young athletes. Journal of Bone and Joint Surgery 55A:
    95-105

Comminuted fractures of patella

Synonym
Stellate fractures

General features
Caused by direct blow on patella
Often compound
In dashboard injuries, dislocation of hip may
    also be present

Clinical features
Pain, swelling, bruising
Inability to straight leg raise
No hemarthrosis if fragments separate

Radiological features
Unlimited variety of fracture patterns
Separation of fragments may occur
Tangential views not helpful

Pathological features
Impaction in flexion may cause damage to
    femoral condyles
Fragments may become loose bodies
Post-traumatic osteo-arthrosis is common

Treatment:
Compound fractures   } Patellectomy
Severely comminuted fractures } Splintage for 6
                                weeks
Closed fractures   } Circumferential wires
                           +/- pins or screws
Minor comminution   } Splintage for 6 weeks
Closed comminuted fractures in elderly and
    infirm treated by minimal splintage and early
    activity

References
Smillie I S 1970 Injuries of the knee joint. 4th edn. ch 8.
    Livingstone, Edinburgh, London
Wilkinson J 1977 Fracture of the patella treated by total
    excision. Journal of Bone and Joint Surgery 59B: 352-354

Transverse fractures of patella

General features
Common injury
Causation:
   Closed fracture: Resisted extension of knee
   Compound fracture: Sharp blow on patella

Clinical features
Pain, tenderness
Little swelling. No deformity
Fracture line may be palpable
Inability to stand
Inability to straight leg raise

Radiological features
Well visualised on AP and lateral views of knee
Fragments may be widely separated by muscular action

Pathological features:
Blood supply is least good to upper pole
Fractures untreated heal with fibrous tissue and lengthening of extensor apparatus
Irregularity of posterior surface of patella leads to later patello-femoral osteoarthrosis
Fracture may occur in lower, middle, or upper thirds
If separation occurs patellar retinacula are torn

Treatment

Undisplaced fractures
Plaster cast with knee extended for 6 weeks

Displaced fractures
Open reduction
Internal fixation (Wire, Screws, Pins)
Repair of retinacula
Splintage in extension for 2-3 weeks

References
Scapinell R 1967 Blood supply of the human patella. Journal of Bone and Joint Surgery 49B: 563-570
Smillie I S 1970 Injuries of the knee joint. 4th edn. ch 8. Livingstone, Edinburgh, London

Vertical fractures of patella

General features
Uncommon
Caused by vertical blow on edge of patella
Rarely compound

Clinical features
Pain, swelling, local tenderness
Fracture line rarely palpable
Walking and straight leg raising usually possible

Radiological features
Fracture invisible on lateral views and may be missed on AP views
Tangential views with knee flexed give clear visualisation
Fractures usually in lateral or medial third of patella
Exclude congenital bipartite patella with films of opposite knee etc.

Pathological features
Fractures will heal with fibrous union if not treated
Original injury will cause some damage to articular cartilage of femoral condyles
No damage to patellar retinacula
If untreated patello-femoral osteoarthrosis is likely

Treatment

Undisplaced fracture
Plaster cast in extension for 4-6 weeks

Displaced or compound fractures
Wound debridement
Removal of small fragment
Close internal fixation of large fragments

References
Bostrom A 1972 Fracture of the patella. Acta Orthopedica Scandinavica Supplement 143
Smillie I S 1970 Injuries of the knee joint. 4th edn. ch 8. Livingstone, Edinburgh, London

Rupture of quadriceps tendon

General features
Second half of life
Bilaterality not uncommon
Due to muscular effort
Rarely due to direct blow or laceration

Clinical features
Sudden pain
Inability to stand or to extend knee
Local swelling
Tender gap palpable above patella

Radiological features
Lateral films most useful
Fragments of upper pole of patella may be
    avulsed
Soft tissue gap may be visible
Effusion in knee joint
Upper pole of patella tilted forwards on lateral
    view

Pathological features
Some local avascularity may be present
Always heal if repaired
If neglected, extensor apparatus may be
    lengthened
Some association with rheumatoid arthritis
                          steroid therapy
                          diabetes

Treatment

Minimal lesion
Plaster cast in extension for 6 weeks

All others
Operative repair
Plaster cast in extension 6 weeks

References
Brotherton B J, Ball J 1975 Bilateral simultaneous rupture of
    the quadriceps tendon. British Journal of Surgery 62: 918-
    920
Norris M G, Leuack B 1977 Bilateral simultaneous rupture of
    quadriceps tendon: a case report. Injury 8: 315-316

Acute dislocation of patella

General features
May be first episode of recurrent dislocation
Caused by tangential blow on patella displacing it
    laterally

Clinical features
Pain, swelling, loss of knee function
Deformity from patella lying on side of lateral
    condyle (complete dislocation)
Ledged on lateral condyle (incomplete
    dislocation)
Tender gap in medial knee capsule
Local bruising here, later

Radiological features
Patella may be alongside lateral condyle
Possible fractures:
    Osteochondral fragment of lateral condyle
    Marginal fracture of patella
Rarely:
    (1) Patella rotated into intercondylar notch
    (2) Patella locked inferiorly or superiorly by
        osteophytes
Arthrography will show if a complete capsular
    tear is present

Pathological features
Dislocations occur more frequently in those with
    hypermobile joints
Lateral dislocation requires rupture of medial
    patellar retinaculum

Treatment

Conservative
Manipulation under anesthesia
Splintage in extension for 4-6 weeks

Surgical
Reduction
Medial arthrotomy:
    Removed or fixation of osteochondral
        fragments
    Repair of medial capsule
Splintage in extension 4-6 weeks

References
Ackroyd C E, Dinley R J 1976 The locked patella, an unusual complication of haemophilia. Journal of Bone and Joint Surgery 58B: 511-512
Bartlett D H, Gilula L A, Murphy W A 1976 Superior dislocation of the patella fixed by interlocked osteophytes. Journal of Bone and Joint Surgery 58A: 883-884
Frangakis E K 1974 Intra-articular dislocation of the patella. Journal of Bone and Joint Surgery 56A: 423-424
Rorabeck C H, Bobechko W P 1976 Acute dislocation of the patella with osteochondral fracture. Journal of Bone and Joint Surgery 58B: 237-240

Recurrent dislocation of patella

General features
F > M
Usually begins in childhood or adolescence
Associated with joint laxity syndromes and genu valgum

Clinical features
Usually begins with an acute episode
(If reduction is spontaneous correct diagnosis may be delayed)

Acute phase:
Sudden painful giving way of knee
Swelling and tenderness medially
Patella lies on side of lateral femoral condyle

Interphase
Apprehension sign (Patient dislikes and resists passive patellar movement)
Excessive lateral mobility of patella
Flattened femoral condyle.

Chronic phase:
Patella dislocates laterally at each knee flexion
(Dislocation in extension is rare. Tibia lies lateral to axis of femur)

Radiological features
Small high patella usually lying laterally when not dislocated
Genu recurvatum +/- genu valgum may be visible.
Tangential }Flattened lateral femoral condyle
  views: }Irregularity of medial border of patella

Pathological features

Etiology
Joint laxity
   Ehlers-Danlos Syndrome
   Marfan's syndrome
   Osteogenesis Imperfecta
   Down's syndrome
Nail-Patella syndrome
Genu Valgum
Lateral rotation of tibia
Trauma

Macroscopic changes
Lax medial capsule
Small high patella
Occasional osteochondral fracture of lateral femoral condyle

Microscopic changes
Retropatellar fibrillation of cartilage
Later, generalised osteo-arthrosis of knee

Treatment
Correct genu valgum first

Children under 12
Semitendinosus tenodesis
or Medial plication of joint capsule

Adolescents
Tibial Tuberosity transfer
Medial transfer of lateral half of patella tendon

Adults with patellofemoral degeneration
Patellectomy and plastic repair of quadriceps

References
Baker R H et al 1972 The semitendinosus tenodesis for recurrent dislocation of the patella. Journal of Bone and Joint Surgery 54B: 103-109
Dandy D J 1971 Recurrent subluxation of the patella on extension of the knee. Journal of Bone and Joint Surgery 53B: 483-487
Hampson W G J, Hill P 1975 Late results of transfer of the tibial tubercle for recurrent dislocation of the patella. Journal of Bone and Joint Surgery 57B: 209-213
Harrison M H M 1955 The results of a realignment operation for recurrent dislocation of the Patella. Journal of Bone and Joint Surgery 37B: 559-567
Hughston J C 1968 Subluxation of the patella. Journal of Bone and Joint Surgery 50A: 1003-1026
Laurin C A et al 1960 The abnormal lateral patellofemoral angle. Journal of Bone and Joint Surgery 60A: 55-60
West F E, Soto-Hall R 1958 Recurrent dislocation of the patella in the adult. Journal of Bone and Joint Surgery 40A: 386-393

Injuries of patellar ligament

General features
Usually young people < 10 years
Usually due to sudden resisted knee extension
Very rarely bilateral
Lacerations are uncommon (dashboard injuries)
Gradual detachments
  Upper: Sinding-Larsen-Johanson syndrome
  Lower: Osgood-Schlatter syndrome

Clinical features:
Pain, minor swelling
Inability to stand or to extend knee
Tender gap may be palpable

Radiological features
Upper end: Shell of patella usually avulsed
Lower end: Avulsion of part of tibial tuberosity
Soft tissue swelling
Patella lies high on femoral condyles in lateral
  view

Pathological features:
Always heal
If neglected extensor apparatus is lengthened and
  extensor lag persists
Some association with rheumatoid arthritis and
  steroid therapy

Treatment
Minor stretch (no gap detectable)
Plaster cast for 4-6 weeks with knee extended
All other injuries:
  Operative repair
  Internal fixation:
    Wiring for upper end
    Screw for lower end

References
Beddow F H, Corkery P N, Shatwell G L 1964 Avulsion of
  the ligamentous patellae from the lower pole of the patella.
  Journal of the Royal College of Surgeons of Edinburgh 9:
  66-69
Ismail A M, Balakrishnan R, Rajakumar J K 1969 Rupture
  of patellar ligament after steroid infiltration. Journal of
  Bone and Joint Surgery 51A: 503-505
Zernicke R F, Garhammer J, Jobe F W, 1977 Human
  patellar-tendon rupture. Journal of Bone and Joint Surgery
  59A: 179-183

Avulsion of tibial tuberosity

Synonym
Acute Osgood-Schlatter lesion

General features
Most acute and severe lesion of tibial tuberosity
Caused by sudden resisted extension
M > F
Commonest in adolescents
In oldsters may occur from manipulation of stiff
  knee

Clinical features
Sudden severe pain below knee during strenuous
  activity
Swelling, tenderness
Inability to extend knee or bear weight

Radiological features
Separation of tongue epiphysis of upper tibia
Superior (cranial) displacement

Pathological features
Extensor apparatus of knee gives way through
  soft epiphyseal cartilage shortly before normal
  fusion
Always unites
If neglected leads to lengthening and an extensor
  lag

Treatment
Minimal shift: Splintage in extension for 6 weeks
All other injuries:
  Open reduction
  Internal fixation
  Splintage in extension for 6 weeks

References
Hand W L, Hand C R, Dunn A W 1971 Avulsion fractures
  of the tibial tubercle. Journal of Bone and Joint Surgery
  53A: 1579-1583
Osgood R B 1903 Lesions of the tibial tubercle during
  adolescence. Boston Medical and Surgical Journal 148:
  114-117
Sclatter C 1903 Verletzungen des schnabelformigen Fortsatzes
  der Oberen. Beitrage 2, Klinische Chirurgie 38: 874-887

Investigation of internal derangement of knee

History
Precise details of previous and recent injury
Precise description of present complaints

Examination
Careful routine for deranged knee
Compare opposite knee
Examine other joints

Radiography

Conventional
A-P and lateral views
Intercondylar views
Oblique view for femoral condyles
Tangential views for patello-femoral surfaces

Cineradiography or screening
Demonstrates ligamentous laxity and patellar instability

Double contrast arthrography

Anaesthesia

Manipulation
Ligamentous laxity
Proof of locking/unlocking
Meniscal grainding tests

Arthroscopy
Meniscal injuries
Fat pad lesions
Osteochondritis Dissecans
Chondromalacia patellae

Biopsy
Synovium
Other abnormal soft tissue

Arthrotomy
Final test

References
Dandy D J, Jackson R W 1975 The impact of arthroscopy on the management of disorders of the knee. Journal of Bone and Joint Surgery 57B: 346-348
Nicholas J A, Freiberger R H, Killoran P J 1970 Double contrast arthrography of the knee. Journal of Bone and Joint Surgery 52A: 203-220

Anterior cruciate ligament injury

General features
1. Isolated injuries uncommon
   Compatible with excellent knee function
   Due to hyperextension injuries
2. Associated with other injuries
   Rupture of medial ligament
   Tears of medial meniscus
   Dislocation of knee

Clinical features
Pain, Hemarthrosis
Incomplete extension
Later:
   Rotatory instability of lateral compartment
   Anterior drawer sign positive
       (if medial ligament is also damaged)

Radiological features
Avulsion of anterior tibial spine
Normal anterior tibial movement on femur 0-5.0 mm
Rupture will allow extra movement

Pathological features
Main blood supply comes from tibia
Damage to upper ¾ will not heal
Ligament may stretch or rupture
Most repair procedures produce an avascular replacement which eventually stretches.
   Always technically difficult

Treatment
Isolated injury:
Ligament:
   No repair
   Develop quadriceps
Avulsion of spine:
   Manipulate to full extension
   Plaster cast 6 weeks
Incomplete reduction:
   Internal fixation
   Plaster cast 6 weeks

Part of associated injury:
Surgical repair less difficult
Should be attempted
Proper repair of medial ligament and posterior
   capsule most important

Old injuries:
Develop strong quadriceps
Abandon professional football

References

Kennedy J C, Weinberg H W, Wilson A S 1974 The anatomy
   and function of the anterior cruciate ligament. Journal of
   Bone and Joint Surgery 56A: 223-235
Meyers M H, McKeever F M 1970 Fracture of the
   intercondylar eminence of the tibia. Journal of Bone and
   Joint Surgery 52A: 1667-1684
Smillie I S 1970 Injuries to the knee joint. 4th edn. ch 7.
   Livingstone, Edinburgh, London
Zaricznyj B 1977 Avulsion fracture of the tibial eminence.
   Journal of Bone and Joint Surgery 59A: 1111-1114

Posterior cruciate ligament injury

General features
Uncommon as an isolated injury
Commonly overlooked
Often occurs from a direct backward blow on
   front of flexed knee

Clinical features
Pain. hemarthrosis
Limited movement especially flexion
Later:
   Posterior drawer sign positive
   Essential to compare opposite knee – interpret
      with caution

Radiological features
Avulsion of posterior upper tibial margin
   frequently seen

Pathological features
Lower attachment usually gives way
Upper attachment less often
Posterior horn of medial meniscus usually
   detached

Treatment

Avulsion
No displacement
   Plaster cast with knee extended
Displaced
   Open reduction. Internal fixation
   Plaster cast for 6 weeks
Rupture:
   Repair technically very difficult
   Durability suspect
   Plaster cast for 6 weeks

Neglected case
Develop quadriceps
Late open reduction gives poor results

References

Meyers M H 1975 Isolated avulsion of the tibial attachment
   of the posterior cruciate ligament of the knee. Journal of
   Bone and Joint Surgery 57A: 669-672
Torisu T 1977 Isolated avulsion fracture of the ribial
   attachment of the posterior cruciate ligament. Journal of
   Bone and Joint Surgery 59A: 68-72

Medial ligament injuries

General features
Common athletic and sport injury but rare in
   children
Arises from lateral stress applied to fully
   extended knee, usually when weight bearing

Clinical features
Pain, swelling, brusing
Instability on movement
Weight bearing on extended immobile knee often
   possible
Passive stretching:
   Valgus deformity
   Medial dimpling

Late effects
Pelligrini-Steida lesion
Persistent tenderness and swelling
Limited flexion

Radiological features
Widened joint space on valgus strain
1. Avulsion of bone fragments at upper or lower attachment
2. Compression fracture of lateral tibial condyle
3. Paracondylar ossification at upper insertion (Pelligrini-Steida lesion)

Pathological features
Variable range of injuries
1. Minor stretch
2. Disruption
3. Disruption
   Separation of medial meniscus) Murphy's
   Tear of anterior cruciate ligament) Triad
Pelligrini-Steida lesion due to ossification of hematoma

Treatment
M.U.A. to determine degree of damage – valgus strain
Minor Stretch:
   Plaster cast with knee extended for 6 weeks
Disruption:
   Surgical repair +/- pes anserinum transfer
Murphy's Triad:
   Meniscectomy
   Repair anterior cruciate ligament
   Repair medial ligament
Pelligrini-Stedia lesion:
   Exercise within limits of pain
   Excision when mature after 1 year
Neglected medial instability:
   Repair with fascial re-inforcements

References
Joseph K N, Pogrund H 1978 Traumatic rupture of the medial ligament of the knee in a four year old boy, case report and review of literature. Journal of Bone and Joint Surgery 60A: 402-403
Kennedy J C, Fowler P J 1971 Medial and anterior instability of the knee. Journal of Bone and Joint Surgery 53A: 1257-1270
O'Donoghue D 1969 Reconstruction for medial instability of the knee. Journal of Bone and Joint Surgery 55A: 941-955
Slocum D B, Larson R L 1968 Pes anserium trans-plantation. Journal of Bone and Joint Surgery 50A: 226-242
Smillie I S 1970 Injuries of the knee joint. 4th edn. ch 7. Livingstone, Edinburgh

Lateral ligament injuries

General features
Less common than medial ligament injuries .
Occurs from medial stress applied to fully extended knee, usually when weight bearing
Also damaged in dislocation of knee

Clinical features
Pain, swelling, bruising, on outer side of knee
Weight bearing possible on straight knee
Movement produces instability
Passive stretching:
   Varus deformity
   Lateral dimpling
Common peroneal nerve often damaged

Radiological features
Varus strain widens lateral joint space

Occasional features
1. Avulsion of head of fibula
2. Avulsion of edge of lateral tibial condyle (Indicates loss of ilio-tibial band insertion)
3. Compression fracture of medial tibial condyle

Pathological features
Lateral ligament is reinforced by ilio-tibial band and M. Biceps tendon
Variable range of injuries
1. Minor stretch
2. Disruption
Lateral meniscus rarely disturbed
Common peroneal nerve may be widely stretched

Treatment
M.U.A. to determine degree of damage – Varus strain
Minor stretch:
   Plaster cast in extension 6 weeks
Disruption:
   Surgical repair
   Plaster cast 6 weeks
Common peroneal palsy: Ankle orthosis
No recovery at 3 months: Explore nerve

References
Smillie I S 1970 Injuries of the knee joint. 4th edn. ch 7. Livingstone, Edinburgh, London
White J 1968 The results of traction injuries to the common peroneal nerve. Journal of Bone and Joint Surgery 50B: 346-350

Torn menisci

General features
Common. Medial : Lateral meniscal tears = 5 : 4
Caused by twisting movements when weight
    bearing on a flexed knee
i.e. Turning at speed : Sport injuries
      Rising from kneeling
Locking:
    Inability to achieve full extension
Giving Way:
    Sudden inability of the knee to bear weight

Clinical features

Initially
Pain, Tenderness, Effusion
Locking after injury

Later
Pain on twisting
'Giving way' of knee
Locking episodes
Grinding tests sometimes positive
Lateral compartment more 'silent' than medial

Radiological features

Initially
No changes on conventional films
Double contrast arthrography may reveal
    abnormalities

Later
Local degenerative changes

Pathological features
Menisci:
    Distribute loading forces in knee joint
      (See section on biomechanics of knee)
Youngsters:
    'Bucket handle' longitudinal tears
    'Parrot beak' free edge tears
    Peripheral detachment
Oldsters:
    As above plus – horizontal cleavage tears
Locking of longitudinal anterior tears causes
    grooving of cartilage of femoral condyles
Such tears in medial meniscus damage lower
    attachment of anterior cruciate ligament
Total removal is followed by partial regeneration

Differential diagnosis
Locking and giving way:
    Loose bodies
    Subluxation of patella

Local Tenderness:
    Ligamentous injury
    Fat pad lesion
Effusions:
    Osteochondritis Dissecans
    Rheumatoid Arthritis, etc. etc.

Treatment

Total meniscectomy
For: No hidden tears left behind
      No future tears in remaining fragment
Against: Can be difficult surgery

Partial meniscectomy
For: : Easy surgery
        May protect knee from later osteo-
        arthrosis
Against: Some meniscii have 2+ tears apart from
        the obvious one
        Future trauma may damage remaining
        part of meniscus

Post-operative problems:
Retained fragments of menisci
Prepatellar anesthesia (Medial incisions)
Instability:
    Ligamentous injury
    Unrecognised loose body
Effusion:
    Poor quadriceps
    Too early activity
    Instability
Pain:
    Hemarthrosis
    Degenerative changes
Late results:
Gradual onset of osteoarthritic changes (More
    rapidly in athletes and sportsmen)

References
Bryan R S, Dickson J N, Taylor W F 1969 Recovery of the
    knee following meniscectomy. Journal of Bone and Joint
    Surgery 51A: 973-978
Cargill A O'R, Jackson J P 1976 Bucket handle tear of the
    medial meniscus. A case for conservative surgery. Journal
    of Bone and Joint Surgery 58A: 248-257
Dandy D J, Jackson R W 1975 The diagnosis of problems
    after meniscectomy. Journal of Bone and Joint Surgery
    57B: 349-352
Dandy D J, Jackson R W 1975 Meniscectomy and
    chondromalacia of the femoral condyle. Journal of Bone
    and Joint Surgery 57A: 1116-1119
Dandy D J 1978 Early results of closed partial meniscectomy.
    British Medical Journal 1: 1099-1101
Jackson J P 1968 Degenerative changes in the knee after
    meniscectomy. British Medical Journal 2: 525-527
Smillie I S 1970 Injuries of the knee joint. 4th edn. ch 6.
    Livingstone, Edinburgh, London

Cleavage lesions of menisci

General features
Occur in middle third of life
M > F
Often associated with genu varum
Nearly all in medial menisci

Clinical features
Pain on medial side of knee
  on weight bearing after rest
  on turning while weight bearing
  on turning over in bed
  on lying on side with knees together
Onset from minimal trauma
No effusion.   Momentary instability
No locking.
Tender medial joint line
Grinding tests painful but no clicks or clunks

Radiological features
Some loss of medial tibio-femoral joint space
Double contrast arthrography rarely helpful

Pathological features
Horizontal disruption of substance of meniscus
Associated:
Collagen age changes in meniscus
  Cartilaginous degeneration in femoral and
    tibial condyles

Treatment

Conservative
(Moderate symptoms)
Heat and quadriceps exercises
Avoid, kneeling, squatting, twisting

Operative:
Severe symptoms
Failure of conservative measures

References
Noble J, Hamblen D The pathology of the degenerate
   meniscus lesion. Journal of Bone and Joint Surgery 57B:
   180-186
Smillie I S 1970 Injuries of the knee joint. 4th edn. ch 5.
   Livingstone, Edinburgh, London

Dislocation of knee

General features
Uncommon
Major violence required
Often associated with injuries elsewhere
Danger of popliteal occlusion with gangrene and
  amputation

Clinical features
Pain, deformity, swelling
Transverse medial furrow (may indicate
  irreducibility)
35% Peripheral pulses absent
35% Common peroneal palsy

Radiological features
Tibia may be rotated 90° on femur
  may lie anterior
         posterior } to femur
         medial
         lateral
Avulsion of marginal fragments of bone
Arteriograms may show popliteal artery occlusion

Pathological features
Complete disruption of ligaments
Local deformity or hematoma may occlude
  popliteal vessels
Button holing of capsule or medial hamstrings
  into intercondylar notch may prevent closed
  reduction
Nerve lesions are caused by stretching and do not
  usually recover

Treatment
1. Immediate closed or open reduction under
   anesthesia in full flexion
2. Repair of collateral ligaments with removal of
   loose menisci and other loose bodies if knee
   has been opened
3. Exploration of popliteal fossa if ischemia
   persists
4. Reversed vein graft to popliteal artery if
   required
5. Splintage of knee for 6 weeks in cylinder cast

References
Green N E, Allan B L 1977 Vascular injuries associated with dislocation of knee. Journal of Bone and Joint Surgery 59A: 236-239
Quinlan A G 1966 Irreducible posteolateral dislocation of the knee with button holing of the medial femoral condyle. Journal of Bone and Joint Surgery 48A: 1619-1621
Taylor A R, Arden G P, Rainey W A 1972 Traumatic dislocation of the knee. Journal of Bone and Joint Surgery 54B: 96-102

Penetrating injuries of knee joint

General features
Knee is most common joint to be injured
Younger age groups affected
M > F

Clinical features
Wound of varying size usually on front of knee
May be very small
24-48 hours later – swelling, pain, loss of function, pyrexia

Radiological features
Soft tissue swelling
Distension of suprapatellar bursa
Occasional gas in joint
                    Opaque foreign bodies

Pathological features
Rapidly purulent synovial effusion
Edematous inflammed synovium
Softening and fibrillation of articular cartilage

Later
Destruction of cartilage
Fibrosis of suprapatellar pouch
Fibrous ankylosis of knee in flexion

Microscopy
Dilated synovial blood vessels
Local edema
Infiltration with leucocytes

Biochemistry
Release of enzymes in synovial fluid from bacteria and leucocytes
Cathepsin   } Breakdown matrix and collagen
Hyaluronidase } in articular cartilage

Treatment
Act on suspicion of penetrating wound
Excise wound under tourniquet
Wash out knee with Saline + Penicillin
Close wound
Splint knee – no weight bearing
Systemic antibiotics
Aspirate and wash out if effusion recurs.
Change antibiotic as indicated by culture

Persistent infection:
Wide drainage
Partial synovectomy

Severely damaged joint:
Excision of infected tissues

References
Barfod B, Pers M 1970 Gastrocnemius-plasty for primary closure of compound injuries of the knee. Journal of Bone and Joint Surgery 52B: 124-127
Smillie I S 1970 Injuries of the knee joint. 4th edn. ch 11. Livingstone, Edinburgh, London

Gunshot wounds of knee

General features
Common in warfare
    urban guerilla activities
    agricultural accidents
M > F

Clinical features
Very variable damage
Wound – blood loss
Loss of function. Inability to weight bear.

Radiological features

1. Through and through injury (bullet or shrapnel)
Gas in joint
Relatively minor fractures in path of missile

2. Metallic fragments retained
Pellets or shrapnel
Gas may be present
Fragments may be in extra-articular soft tissues
No fracture may exist

3. Gross destruction.
Infinitely variable soft tissue loss and fractures

Pathological features

Bullet track may be relatively clean and
uncontaminated

Metal fragments may carry clothing etc. into
tissues with gross infection

Badly damaged knees may also conceal
neurovascular damage in popliteal fossa

Treatment

Bullet track

Excise wounds. No suture

Wash out joint with saline and antibiotic

Splintage

Repeat aspiration and wash out if required

Foreign body

Arthrotomy, Debridement,

Delayed primary suture,

Splintage. Repeat aspiration and wash out

Destruction

Aim for eventual arthrodesis

References

Ashby M E 1974 Low velocity gunshot wounds involving the
knee joint. Surgical management. Journal of Bone and
Joint Surgery 56A: 1047-1053
Barfod B, Pers M 1970 Gastrocnemius-plasty for primary
closure of compound injuries of the knee. Journal of Bone
and Joint Surgery 52B: 124-127
Buxton St J D 1944 Gunshot wounds of the knee joint.
Lancet I: 681-684
Smillie I S 1970 Injuries of the knee joint. 4th edn. ch 11.
Livingstone, Edinburgh, London

Post-traumatic stiff knee

Causes

Fracture of
  Femoral shaft
  or femoral condyles
Fracture of tibial condyles
Avulsion of collateral ligaments +/- cruciate
  ligaments
Dislocation of knee

Exacerbating factors
Infection
Ectopic ossification

Mechanisms

Adhesion of quadriceps to femoral shaft.
Adhesions of medial collateral ligament
Fibrosis of suprapatellar bursa.
Irregularities of articular surfaces
Fibrous ankylosis of knee

Prophylaxis

Accurate reduction of fractures
Avoidance of infection
Early active movements for intra-articular
  fractures

Treatment

Manipulation
Contra indications:
  Unconsolidated fractures
  Infection
  Early stages of recovery

Patello-femoral interposition arthroplasty

Plastic membrane or ⎫
Bag of iron filings   ⎬ later removed
                      ⎭

Quadriceps-plasty

References

Hesketh K J 1963 Experiences with the Thompson
quadricepsplasty. Journal of Bone and Joint Surgery 45B:
491-495
Nicoll E A 1963 Quadricepsplasty. Journal of Bone and Joint
Surgery 45B: 483-490

17

SHIN AND FOOT INJURIES

Dislocation of superior tibio-fibular joint

General features
Rare
Diagnosis often delayed
May dislocate spontaneously
May occur from trauma

Clinical features
Local pain and tenderness after injury
Passive laxity demonstrable
Spontaneous lesion:
   Girls   } self-limiting
   Adolescents }
   Lax ligament syndromes

Radiological features:
2 types of joint:
   Oblique
   Horizontal
AP films—complete separation of superior fibula
   from tibia
Compare opposite knee if necessary

Pathological features:

Subluxation
   Adolescents

Dislocations
Anterolateral:
   Commonest: From twisting injury
Posteromedial:
   Local blow
Superior:
   Associated with fracture of tibial shaft

Treatment
Acute anterolateral dislocation:
   Closed reduction
Acute posteromedial dislocation:
   Closed reduction often unstable
Persistent pain +/- instability:
   Superior tibio-fibular arthrodesis
   or Resection of proximal fibula

Reference
Ogden J A 1974 Subluxation and dislocation of proximal
   tibio-fibular joint. Journal of Bone and Joint Surgery 56A:
   145-154

Fractures of tibial condyles

General features
Caused by violent valgus or varus strain on the
   extended knee
Usually occur when weight bearing
Medial < Lateral condyle fractures
Worst injuries associated with compression

Clinical features
Pain, swelling, bruising
Inability to bear weight
Some deformity

Radiological features
Tibial condyles may be undisplaced
   depressed
   separated
Depression best shown on A. P. views taken with
   tube tilted 15° cranially.
Opposite collateral ligament is not damaged
Cruciate ligaments usually intact
Ipsilateral meniscus may be detached and
   displaced into fracture
Superior tibial articular surface may be
   fragmented and driven into fracture

Treatment

Undisplaced fractures
Aspiration of hemarthrosis
Compression bandage
Skeletal traction
Early active movements

Displaced fractures
Open reduction
Removal of meniscus
Internal fixation (Screws)
Early active movements
Weight bearing delayed for 8-12 weeks

References
Moore T M, Harvey J A 1974 Roentgenographic
   measurement of tibial plateau. Journal of Bone and Joint
   Surgery 56A: 155-160
Porter B B 1970 Crush fractures of the lateral tibial table.
   Journal of Bone and Joint Surgery 52B: 676-687
Rassmussen A S 1973 Tibial condylar fractures: improvement
   of knee joint stability as an indicator for surgical treatment.
   Journal of Bone and Joint Surgery 55A: 1331-1350

Fractures of proximal tibial metaphysis

General features
Rare
Due to direct violence – often compound
     or angulation – usually closed
Ages 2-11

Clinical features
Pain, swelling, loss of function
Little deformity
Occasional ischemia of foot

Radiological features
Little angulation
Salter Type II epiphyseal injury usually
Fibula often not injured
Interposition of fibrous tissue may occur on
   medial side

Pathological features
Premature, partial epiphyseal fusion often takes
   place
Later angulation and shortening of leg

Treatment

Minor injury
Cast for 3-4 weeks
Early weight bearing

Other injuries
Manipulation
   +/- Wound Toilet
   +/- Removal of fibrous tissue
Cast for 4-6 weeks
Delayed weight bearing

Later deformity
Tibial osteotomy

References
Jackson D W, Cozen L 1971 Genu valgum as a complication
  of proximal tibial metaphyseal fractures in children.
  Journal of Bone and Joint Surgery 53A: 1571-1578
Weber B G 1977 Fibrous interposition causing valgus
  deformity after fracture of the upper tibial metaphysis in
  children. Journal of Bone and Joint Surgery 59B: 290-292

Infra-condylar fractures of tibia

General features
Common injury of adults
Direct blow: Compound and transverse
Compressive force: Closed, comminuted

Clinical features
Pain, swelling, later bruising
Loss of function
Deformity not obvious
Occasionally:
   Ischemia of lower leg
   Neurological deficits

Radiological features
Wide variety of fracture patterns
Knee joint sometimes involved
Arteriography may show popliteal, anterior
  tibial, or posterior tibial occlusions

Pathological features
Upper fragments rotated by hamstrings
No delay in union. Much cancellous bone
  exposed
Division of popliteal vessels may be damaged
Intra-articular lesions and malunion lead to
  osteoarthrosis later

Treatment

Conservative
Closed and impacted fractures: Manipulation and
  cast 6-10 weeks often unstable

Operative
1. Compound fractures and comminuted
   fractures:
    Transverse pins above and below fracture
   Cast 6-10 weeks
2. Closed minimally comminuted fractures:
    Internal fixation. Cast 4-8 weeks

Reference
Smillie I S 1970 Injuries of the knee joint. 4th edn. ch 9.
  Livingstone, Edinburgh & London

Fractures of mid-tibial shaft

General features
Very common
Often compound
Direct and angulatory forces:
  Transverse fractures
Twisting Compressive forces:
  Oblique spiral fractures

Clinical features
Pain, swelling, deformity
Industrial and road accidents:
  Often compound and communited
  May be grossly contaminated
  May have large soft tissue and skin losses
  Other injuries may be present

Radiological features
Whole length of tibia and fibula should be
  visualised
Spiral fractures may be bottom of one bone and
  the top of the other
Infinite variety of fracture patterns
Initial films may not show full extent of
  comminution

Pathological features
Devitalised fragments may form sequestra
Upper tibial fracture may occlude popliteal
  bifurcation
Lower tibial fractures may occlude the nutrient
  tibial artery

Mechanical factors:
Indirect forces:
  low energy:
    Longitudinal fractures
    Open or closed
Direct forces:
  low energy:
    Transverse fractures
    Seldom open or comminuted
Direct forces:
  high energy:
    Often open and comminuted fractures

Treatment
1. Less severe fractures
A. *Oblique spiral fractures*
    Undisplaced
    1. Manipulation and plaster cast
    Displaced
    2. Open reduction
      Internal fixation –
        screws or
        circumferential wiring
B. *Stable transverse fractures*
    Manipulation and plaster cast
    Internal fixation may be meddlesome
C. *Compound fractures with minor skin puncture from within outwards*
    Excise wound
    Treat fracture as if it were closed.
      i.e. Manipulation and cast } as appropriate
           Internal fixation

2. Severe fractures
Treat individually:
    Factors: state of patient
    Experience of surgeon
    Materials available
A. Unstable comminuted fractures (closed)
    1. Transverse pins above and below fracture
        Manipulation and plaster cast
or: 2. Open reduction. Internal fixation
        Plates, Nails, Screws, etc.
B. Double fracture of tibial shaft
      (Other injuries elsewhere often present)
    1. Manipulation and plaster cast
or 2. Intramedullary nail
C. Unstable comminuted open fractures
    Wound toilet
    Internal fixation only if < 8 hours since injury
      and if moderate contamination
    Close skin only if no tension
    Plaster cast, well padded
D. Severe fractures with skin loss
    Debridement. No primary suture.
      Relieving incision to cover tibia if possible
    Percutaneous pins to major fragments
      A. Plaster cast with windows
    or B. External splintage on frame
    Skin grafting when wound is clean
    Bone grafting thereafter if union is delayed

Post-trauma problems
Shortening
Deformity –
  Angulation
  Scarring

Stiffness –
  Knee
  Ankle
  Foot
Clawed foot, etc. (See Compartmental
  Syndromes)

References

Alms M 1962 Medullary nailing for fracture of the shaft of
  the tibia. Journal of Bone and Joint Surgery 44B: 328-339
Christman O D, Snook G A 1968 The problem of refracture
  of the tibia. Clinical Orthopaedics 60: 217-219
Karlstrom G, Olerud S 1974 The management of tibial
  fractures in alcoholics and mentally disturbed patients.
  Journal of Bone and Joint Surgery 56B: 730-734
Karlstrom G, Olerud S 1975 Percutaneous pin fixation of
  open tibial fractures. Journal of Bone and Joint Surgery
  57A: 915-924
Laurence M, Freeman M A R, Swanson S A V 1969
  Engineering considerations in the internal fixation of
  fractures of the tibial shafts. Journal of Bone and Joint
  Surgery 51B: 754-768
Mashkow A A 1975 Distoproximal nailing of fractures of the
  tibia. Clinical Orthopaedics 109: 134-143
Moritz J R et al 1962 Spiral fractures of tibia. Long term
  results of Parham bond fixation. Journal of Trauma 2:
  147-161
Sarmiento A 1970 A functional below the knee brace for
  tibial fractures. Journal of Bone and Joint Surgery 52A:
  295-311
Vanderlinden W, Sunzel H, Larsson K 1975 Fractures of the
  tibial shaft after ski-ing and other accidents. Journal of
  Bone and Joint Surgery 57A: 321-327
Zucman J, Maurer P 1969 Two level fractures of the tibia.
  Journal of Bone and Joint Surgery 51B: 686-693.
Review; Clinical Orthopaedics, 105, 1975.

Delayed or non-union of tibial fractures

General features

Increased incidence from:
  Compound fractures
  Skin or soft tissue loss
  Local or general ischemia
Delayed Union: After 12 weeks ⎱ Arbitrary
Non-union   : After 6 months ⎰ debatable figures.

Clinical features

May not be painful or deformed, especially if
  fibula has united
  Or if fibrous union is proceeding
Some local swelling, tenderness and heat is
  always present

Radiological features

Definition of non-union: Sclerosis of medulla at
  fracture site
Sequestra may be present
United fibula may distract tibial fracture
Excessive callus indicates excessive movement
Lack of callus indicates local ischemia
Presence of intramedullary venous flow is a good
  prognostic sign

Pathological features

Local ischemia is the chief cause of non-union
Possibilities:
  1. Damage to medullary artery
  2. Local stripping of soft tissues
  3. Comminution of fracture site
Other causes:
  Persistent infection
  Loss of soft tissues
  Loss of local bone;
    At injury
    At later surgery
  Delayed or ineffective splintage

Treatment

Delayed union:
Consider patellar tendon bearing orthosis

Non-union
Divide fibula if necessary to allow tibial
  fragments to come into contact
Onlay grafting (Phemister technique) +/-
  Internal fixation

Loss of tibial shaft
Tibio-fibular synostosis
Iliac inlay grafts
Composite tissue transfers
Infection
Posterior grafting after saucerisation or
  sequestrectomy

Experimental
Pulsating Electromagnetic fields

References

Bassett C A L, Pilla A A, Pawluk R J 1977 A non-operative
  salvage of surgically resistant pseudarthroses and non-
  unions by pulsating electro-magnetic fields. Clinical
  Orthopaedics 124: 128-143
Forbes D B 1961 Subcortical iliac bone grafts in fracture of
  the tibia. Journal of Bone and Joint Surgery 43B: 672-679
Freeland A E, Mutz S B 1976 Posterior bone grafting for
  infected ununited fracture of the tibia. Journal of Bone and
  Joint Surgery 58A: 653-657

Ger R 1971 The technique of muscle transposition in the operative treatment of traumatic and ulcerative lesions of the leg. Journal of Trauma 11: 502-510, 1971

Ger R 1978 Transposition of the tendo-calcaneus for post-traumatic bone defects of the tibia. Journal of Bone and Joint Surgery 60A: 366-369

McMaster P E, Hohl M 1965 Tibiofibular cross-peg grafting. Journal of Bone and Joint Surgery 47A: 1146-1158

Puranen J, Kaski P 1974 The clinical significance of osteo-medullography in fractures of the tibial shaft. Journal of Bone and Joint Surgery 56A: 759-776

Rogers W J III, 1968 Iliac inlay-on-edge bone graft. Journal of Bone and Joint Surgery 50A: 1410-1416

Isolated fractures of fibular shaft

General features
Usually due to direct violence
May be compound
Sometimes stress or fatigue fractures

Clinical features
Pain, swelling, later bruising
No deformity. Weight bearing usually possible
High fractures may cause a common peroneal nerve palsy

Radiological features
Little displacement
Some comminution
(Ensure tibia is undamaged)

Pathological features:
Well covered by muscles
Minimal weight bearing function
Non-union very rare

Treatment

Closed fracture
Strapping
　or
Plaster cast (Patellar tendon bearing)

Compound fracture
Debridement
Plaster cast (Patellar tendon bearing)

References
Devas M B 1963 Stress fractures in children. Journal of Bone and Joint Surgery 45B: 528-541

Lambert K L 1971 The weight bearing function of the fibula. Journal of Bone and Joint Surgery 53A: 507-513

Stress fractures of tibia

Synonym
Fatigue fracture

Definition
Slowly developing fracture in normal bone caused by repetitive stress

General features
Not common
Occurs in vigorous activity
　Athletes
　Dancers
　Parachutists
But also in the elderly

Clinical features
Gradual onset of pain on weight bearing
Local tenderness and slight swelling
No deformity
Walking possible at first

Radiological feature
Firstly
　Faint cortical fissure
Later
　Fissure transverses shaft
　Periosteal thickening
Lastly
　Medullary sclerosis and healing

Pathological features
Occur in upper and lower tibia
Similar fractures occur in Paget's Disease and osteomalacia, etc.
Differential Diagnosis:
　Osteoid Osteoma
　Osteomyelitis

Treatment
Minimal pain: Rest +/- strapping
Moderate pain: Plaster cast, patellar tendon bearing

Reference

Devas M B, 1958 Stress fracture of the tibia in athletes or 'shin soreness'. Journal of Bone and Joint Surgery 40B: 227, 1958

Fractures of distal tibial epiphysis

General features
Children 6-14
Angulatory strains commonest
Compression injuries unusual

Clinical features
Pain, swelling, later bruising
Tender. Inability to walk
Minimal deformity

Radiological features
Usually:
    Salter Type II injury
Less often:
    Compression: Type V
    "Railing" fracture: type III with separation of
        medial malleolus
Rarely:
    Type I or IV
Usually:
    Postero-lateral shift of epiphysis. Little
        Displacement

Pathological features
Compression injuries often cause premature
    partial fusion of epiphysis
Later deformity and shortening of leg
Lateral epiphyseal injury at 14-16 years is rare
Rotational injuries very rare

Treatment

Angulation injuries
Manipulation
Cast for 6 weeks

"Railing" (Type III) injury
Open reduction
Intra-epiphyseal screw
Cast for 6 weeks

Compression injuries
No surgery. Cast
Delayed weight bearing
Review for 2 years after

Deformity
Lower tibial osteotomy

References

Cooperman D R, Spiegel P G, Laros G S, 1978 Tibial fractures involving the ankle in children. Journal of Bone and Joint Surgery 60A: 1040-1046
Kleiger B, Mankin J 1964 Fracture of the lateral portion of the distal tibial epiphysis. Journal of Bone and Joint Surgery 46A: 25-32
Molster A 1977 Fractures of the lateral part of the distal tibial epiphysis (Tillaux or Kleiger fracture). Injury 8: 260-263
Nevelos A B, Colton C L 1977 Rotational displacement of the lower tibial epiphysis due to trauma. Journal of Bone and Joint Trauma 59B: 331

Post-traumatic fascial compartment syndrome of leg

Synonym
Volkmann's contracture of leg
Crush syndrome

General features
Arises after fracture of tibia and/or fibula or
    crushing injuries of muscles
Becoming more generally recognised
Usually affects posterior compartments

Clinical features
Those of fracture or crushing
Pain persisting after reduction
Worse on active or passive toe or foot
    movements
Peripheral paresthesia
Peripheral ischemia

Late effects
Clawed toes
Equino-varus forefoot
Stiff toes and foot

Radiological features
Fracture(s) may or may not be present
Soft tissue swelling
Arteriography may show occlusion of anterior
    and/or posterior tibial arteries

Pathological features
Rapid rise in tissue pressure from oedema of muscle
Hematoma from injury
Ischemic necrosis of muscle with later fibrosis and shortening
Veins then arteries occluded
Peripheral gangrene may occur in severe cases

Treatment

1. Wide fascial decompression
At first treatment or when first recognised

2. Partial fibulectomy in severe cases
(Open all four fascial compartments of lower leg)

References
Garfin S, Mubarak S J, Owen C A 1977 Exertional antero-lateral compartment syndrome. Journal of Bone and Joint Surgery 59A: 404-405
Karlstrom G, Lonnerholm T, Olerud S 1975 Cavus deformity of the foot after fracture of the tibial shaft. Journal of Bone and Joint Surgery 57A: 893-900
Matsen F A, Clawson D K 1975 Compartmental syndromes. Clinical Orthopaedics 113: 2-110
Matsen F A, Clawson D K 1975 The deep posterior compartmental syndrome of the leg. Journal of Bone and Joint Surgery 57A: 34-39
Muraback S J, Owen C A 1977 Double incision fasciotomy of the leg for decompression in compartment syndromes. Journal of Bone and Joint Surgery 59A: 184-187

Anterior tibial compartment syndrome

Synonym
Shin splints. Exercise ischemia

General features
Becoming more commonly recognised
M > F
Arises from vigorous exercise, often unaccustomed
Minor symptoms repetitive on exercise

Clinical features
Pain in anterior compartment of leg
Local tenderness. Later swelling

Often:
   loss of anterior tibial pulse
   Paralysis of anterior tibial nerve
Passive flexion of foot and toes causes severe pain
If unrelieved:
   Fibrosis of muscles
   Paralysis of extension of ankle and toes

Radiological features
Soft tissue swelling anteriorly to tibia
Anteriography may show occlusion of anterior tibial artery

Pathological features
Edema of anterior fascial compartment
Progresses to ischemic necrosis of muscle
Rapid rise in tissue pressure
Occlusion of veins then arteries

Treatment
Wide fascial decompression
Skin closure

References
Horn C E 1945 Acute ischaemia of the anterior tibial muscle and the long extensor muscles of the toes. Journal of Bone and Joint Surgery 27: 615-622
Matsen F A, Clawson D K 1975 Editors, compartmental syndromes. Clinical Orthopaedics 113: 2-110
Puranen J 1974 The medial tibial syndrome. Exercise ischaemia in the medial fascial compartment of the leg. Journal of Bone and Joint Surgery 56B: 712-715
Rorabeck C H, MacNab I 1976 Anterior tibial compartment syndrome complicating fractures of the shaft of the tibia. Journal of Bone and Joint Surgery 58A: 549-550

Plastic techniques to replace skin lost from leg

Split skin graft
Easily removed
Good survival
Poor appearance
Fragile

Whole thickness skin graft
Less easily removed
Leaves a secondary deficit at donor site
Robust grafts

Fair appearance
Careful attachment required

Local flap grafts

Single pedicle
Undelayed or delayed techniques,
Small areas covered
Good to cover exposed bone
Skin fat and fascia moved in one unit
Secondary defect remains for closing

Double pedicle
Bridge Flap
Aligned longitudinally
Will cover a long strip of exposed bone
Leaves a secondary defect
Simplest form is a longitudinal relieving incision
    posteriorly to allow skin closure anteriorly

Cross leg flap grafts

Careful planning required
Both legs may be immobilised for 3-4 weeks
Contraindicated for the elderly
Secondary defects require closure or covering

Distant pedicle grafts

'Jump grafts' Abdomen – wrist – leg
Long 2 stage procedure
Requires careful planning
    Full patient co-operation
    Young patients

Microvascular techniques

Free tissue transfer of skin and fat (and bone
    occasionally)
Anastomosis of donor and recipient vessels

References

Acland R, Smith P 1976 Microvascular surgical techniques
    used to provide skin cover over an ununited tibial fracture.
    Journal of Bone and Joint Surgery 58B: 471-478
Brown R F 1965 The management of traumatic tissue loss in
    the lower limb, especially when complicated by skeletal
    injury. British Journal of Plastic Surgery 18: 26-49
Connolly J R 1956 Plastic surgery in bone problems. Plastic
    and Reconstructive Surgery 17: 129-167
Hynes W 1954 The skin dermis graft as an alternative to the
    direct or tubed flap. British Journal of Plastic Surgery 7:
    97-107
O'Brien B M 1977 Microvascular reconstructive surgery.
    Churchill Livingstone Edinburgh

Flaying injuries of legs

Synonym
Degloving injuries

General features
Due to road or machinery accident
Rolling mechanism strips soft tissues off deep
    fascia
Forceful stretching tears off skin flaps
Fractures frequently seen

Clinical features
Hypovolemic shock

Soft tissues:
Closed injury
    Massive swelling
    Later ischemia of overlying skin
        of musculofascial compartment
        of distal limb.
Open injury:
    Variable skin flaps or skin loss

Fractures
Often compound
Pain, deformity, loss of function

Radiological features
Infinite variety of fracture lines
Whole limb and other doubtful regions should be
    visualised

Pathological features
Skin flaps may be excessively contaminated
Underlying muscles may be little damaged

Treatment

Immediate
Rescusitation
Complete diagnosis

Fractures
    Internal fixation if possible
or External skeletal splintage

Soft tissue
Closed: Decompression and drainage
        Observe skin of doubtful viability

Open: Complete wound toilet
Defat smaller skin flaps and replace
Excise massive skin flaps
Later split skin grafting

References

Brown R F 1965 The management of traumatic tissue loss in the lower limb, especially when complicated by skeletal injury. British Journal of Plastic Surgery 18: 26-49
Innis C O 1958 Treatment of skin avulsions injuries of the extremities. British Journal of Plastic Surgery 10: 122-140

Classification of ankle fractures

1. Eversion (lateral rotation) fractures

A. Supination – lateral rotation
Sequence of events
1. Rupture of anterior tibio-fibular ligament
2. Oblique spinal fracture of lateral malleolus
3. Rupture of posterior tibio-fibular ligament
4. Fracture of medial malleolus

B. Pronation lateral rotation
Sequence of events
1. Fracture of medial malleolus (oblique)
2. Rupture of interosseous ligament
3. Fracture of fibula well above ankle
4. Fracture of posterior edge of tibia

2. Adduction (supination-adduction) fractures:
Sequence of events.
1. Traction fracture of lateral malleolus below ankle joint.
2. Vertical (push off) fracture of medial malleolus

3. Abduction (pronation-abduction) fractures:
Sequence of events.
1. Fracture of medial malleolus (Transverse) or rupture of medial ligament
2. Both anterior and posterior tibio-fibular ligaments rupture
3. Bending fracture of fibula just above ankle joint (Often triangular)

4. Compression (pronation-dorsiflexion) fractures
Sequence of events.
1. Fracture of medial malleolus
2. Fracture of anterior lower margin of tibia

3. Fracture of lower third of fibula
4. Fracture of tibia above previous tibial fracture

Other classifications
1. Unimalleolar fractures
Bi malleolar fractures
Tri malleolar fractures (Third malleolus is the postero-inferior tibial margin)
2. 1st Degree fracture – No talar shift
2nd Degree fracture – Minor talar shift
3rd Degree fracture – Major talar shift

References

Burwell H N, Charnley A D 1965 The treatment of displaced fractures of the ankle by rigid internal fixation and early joint movement. Journal of Bone and Joint Surgery 47B: 634-660
Lange-Hansen N 1954 Fractures of the ankle. American Journal of Roentgenology 71: 456-471

Injuries of the lateral ligament of ankle

Synonym
Sprained ankle, twisted ankle

General features
Very common
Minor adduction injury

Clinical features
Pain, swelling, later bruising
Tenderness:
localised antero-laterally to lateral malleolus
No deformity. Some loss of function

Differential diganosis
Fracture of base of 5th metatarsal

Radiological features
Soft tissue swelling
Occasional avulsion of tip of lateral malleolus
Occasional damage to supero-medial angle of talus
Stress films may show talar tilting
Arthrography may show a tear in the ankle capsule

Pathological features

Usually:

Anterior band of lateral ligament is stretched

Rarely:

Lateral ligament is ruptured

(If unrecognised may lead to persistent instability)

Treatment

1. Sprains:

Strapping and early weight bearing

Much swelling:

Local anesthetic and hyaluronidase

Much pain:

Plaster cast for 2 weeks

2. Possible rupture:

Stress inversion films under local general anesthesia +/- arthrography

3. Total rupture:

Early: Operative repair

Late: Fascial or tendinous grafting procedures

References

Brantigan J W, Pedegana L R, Lippert F G 1977 Instability of the subtalar joint. Journal of Bone and Joint Surgery 59A: 321-324

Chrisman O D, Snook G A, 1969 Reconstruction of lateral ligament tears of the ankle. Journal of Bone and Joint Surgery 51A: 904-912

Freeman M A R 1965 Treatment of ruptures of the lateral ligament of the ankle. Journal of Bone and Joint Surgery 47B: 661-668

Mehrez M, El-Geneidy S 1970 Arthrography of the ankle. Journal of Bone and Joint Surgery 52B: 308-312

Rubin G, Witten M 1960 The talar tilt angle and the fibular collateral ligaments. Journal of Bone and Joint Surgery 42A: 311-326

Staples O S 1975 Ruptures of the fibular collateral ligaments of the ankle. Journal of Bone and Joint Surgery 57A: 101-107

Supination external rotation fractures of ankle

General features

Very common

Minor violence: Fibular fracture

Major violence: Tibial and fibular fracture

Clinical features

Pain, swelling, later bruising

Tenderness over lower fibula

Little deformity

Weight bearing may be possible

Heel prominence means a tibial fracture as well as the fibular

Radiological features

Oblique fibular fracture running from level of ankle joint.

Posterior fracture of margin of lower tibia

Pathological features

Talus twisted backwards out of ankle mortice

Sequence of injuries:

1. Rupture of anterior tibio-fibular ligament

2. Oblique spiral fracture of lateral malleolus

3. Rupture of posterior tibio-fibular ligament.

4. Fracture of medial malleolus.

Deforming forces may cease to act at any point along this sequence.

Posterial entrapment of fibula-Bosworth's fracture

Treatment

Fibular fracture only

No manipulation required

4-6 weeks in cast

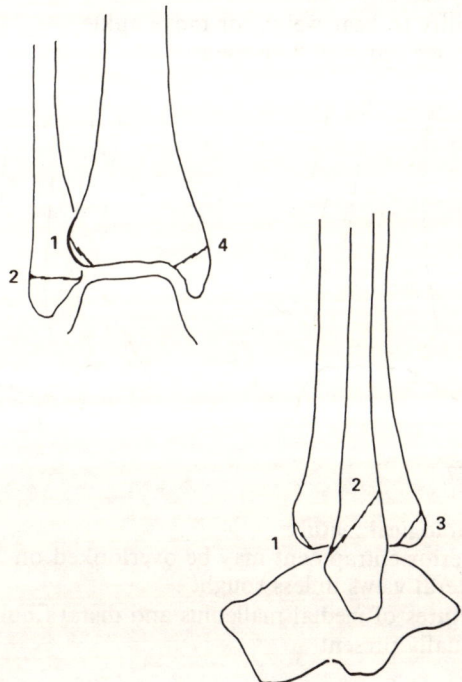

Fig. 26

Tibial fracture
Manipulation
Perfect Reduction: Full leg cast for 8-10 weeks
Imperfect Reduction: Open reduction
                               Internal Fixation of fibular
                               and tibial fractures

See Figure 26

Reference
Brodie I A O D, Denham R A 1974 The treatment of
    unstable ankle fractures. Journal of Bone and Joint
    Surgery 56B: 256-262

Bosworth fracture

Synonym
Fracture dislocation of ankle with posterior
    entrapment of fibula

General features
Rare
May be open or closed
Severe supination external rotation force applied
    to foot

Clinical features
Pain, swelling
Inability to bear weight or move ankle
Open wound may be present

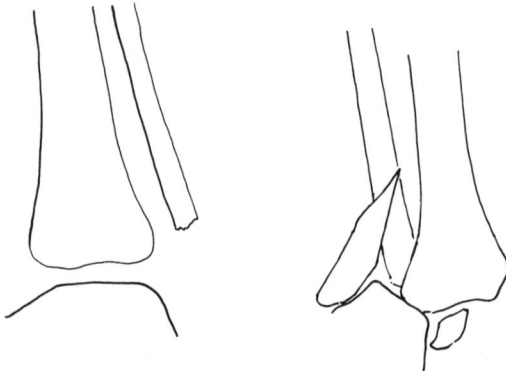

Fig. 27

Radiological features
Posterior entrapment may be overlooked on
    lateral views unless sought
Fractures of medial malleolus and distal fibula
    usually present

Pathological features
Ligaments often intact

Proximal fibular fragment caught in interosseous
    membrane or posterior malleolar fracture

Treatment
Closed injury
Closed manipulation often successful
If not – Open reduction

Open injury
Wound debridement
Open reduction
Long leg cast

See figure 27

References
Bosworth D M 1947 Fracture dislocation of the ankle with
    fixed displacement of the fibula behind the tibia. Journal of
    Bone and Joint Surgery 29: 130-135
Mayer P J, Evarts C M C 1978 Fracture dislocation of the
    ankle with posterior entrapment of the fibula behind the
    tibia. Journal of Bone and Joint Surgery 60A: 320-324

Maisonneuve s fracture dislocation of ankle

General features
Common injury
Caused by severe pronation – external rotation
    forces
    (Stage IV)

Clinical features
Pain, swelling, tenderness, later bruising
Little deformity
Inability to bear weight

Radiological features
Oblique fracture of medial malleoleus
Fracture of proximal fibula
Lateral shift of talus
Fracture of postero-inferior lip of tibia

Pathological features
Successive stages of injury
Rupture of anterior tibio-fibular ligament
    and anterior interosseous ligament

Rupture of posterior tibio-fibular ligament
Rupture of anteromedial joint capsule
Fracture of proximal fibula
Fracture of medial malleolus
Fracture of postero-inferior lip of tibia

Treatment
Open reduction
Internal fixation of medial malleolus
Cast 6-8 weeks

See Figure 28

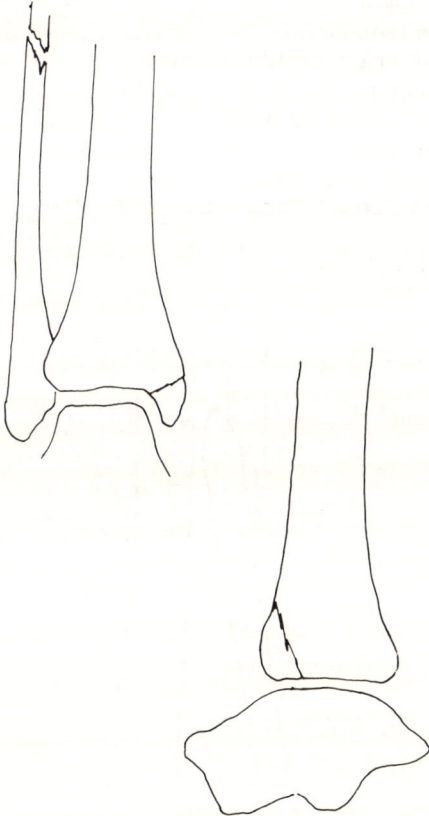

Fig. 28

References
Maisonneuve M J E 1840 Recherches sur la fracture du
  peroné. Archives de Generale Medicin 7: 165-187, 443-473
Pankovich A M 1976 Maisonneuve fracture of the fibula.
  Journal of Bone and Joint Surgery 58A: 337-342

Pronation external rotation fractures of ankle

General features
Common injuries
Due to pronation – external rotation forces

Clinical features
Pain, swelling, later bruising
Local tenderness over medial malleoleus and over
  fibular fracture above ankle joint
Variable loss of function
Deformity evident in severe injuries

Radiological features
Oblique 'pull-off' fracture of medial malleolus
Diastasis of inferior tibio-fibular joint
Fracture of fibula at a variable level well above
  ankle joint.

Pathological features
Sequence of events
  (Medial structures fail first)
1) Oblique fracture of medial malleolus
2) Rupture of interosseous ligament
3) Fracture of fibula above ankle
4) Fracture of postero-inferior edge of tibia
Deforming forces may cease at any point in this
  sequence
Upper fibular fracture:
  (Maisonneuve's fracture)   ⎞ See
  Complete tibio-fibular disruption: ⎬ Separate
  (Dupuytren's fracture)   ⎠ Sections

Treatment:
Medial malleolus:
  Open reduction
  Internal fixation
Inferior tibio-fibular diastasis
  Transverse Screw
    (Remove 6-12 weeks later because of fatigue
      fracture of screw)
Cast for 8 weeks

See Figure 29

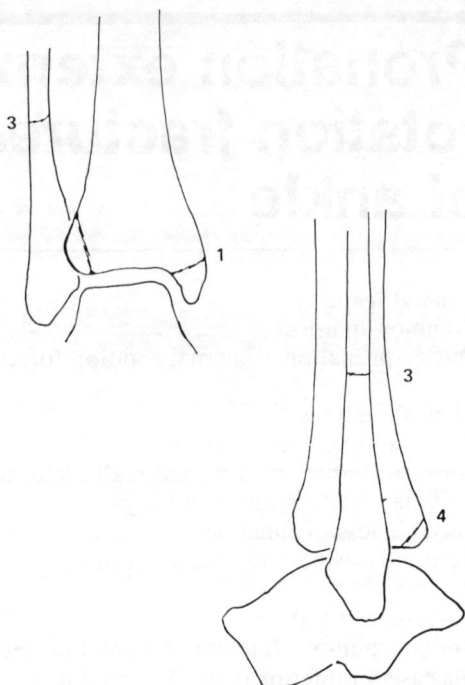

Fig. 29

Radiological features

Splaying of inferior tibio-fibular joint
Upward displacement of talus between tibia and
    fibula
Fracture of upper fibula shaft
Fracture of lower tibial articular surface and/or
    medial malleolus

Pathological features

Rarely compound
No subsequent avascularity

Treatment:

Open reduction
Transverse tibio-fibular screw
Oblique medial malleolar screw
Plaster cast 6-10 weeks
Later: Remove transverse screw by 20 weeks
    before fatigue fracture of metal
Late osteo-arthrosis: Ankle arthrodesis

See Figure 30

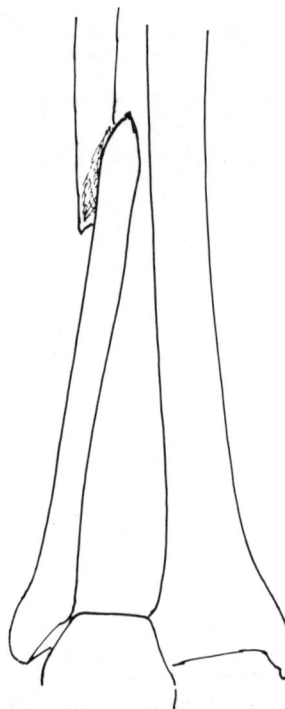

Fig. 30

References

Coonrad R W 1970 Fracture dislocations of the ankle joint
    with impaction injury of the lateral weight-bearing surface
    of the tibia. Journal of Bone and Joint Surgery 52A: 1337-
    1344
Denham R A 1964 Internal fixations for unstable ankle
    fractures. Journal of Bone and Joint Surgery 6B: 206-211

Dupuytren s fracture dislocation of ankle

General features

Uncommon
Caused by pronation – external rotation force
    (Stage IV)

Clinical features

Pain, swelling, later bruising
Deformity: Widening of ankle region
Inability to bear weight
Neurovascular damage rare

References

Colton C L 1968 Fracture diastasis of the inferior tibio-
    fibular joint. Journal of Bone and Joint Surgery 50B: 830-
    835
Colton C L, 1971 The treatment of Dupuytren's
    fracture – dislocation of the ankle. Journal of Bone and
    Joint Surgery 53B: 63-71

Dupuytren G 1819 Memoire sur la fracture de l'extremite inferieure du perone les luxations et les accidents qui en sont la suite. Annuaires Medico-Chirurgical Des Hospiteaux Et Hospices Civiles De Paris 1: 1

Goergen T G et al 1977 Roentgenographic evaluation of the tibiotalar joint. Journal of Bone and Joint Surgery 59A: 874-877

Adduction fractures of ankle

General features
Common
Inversion sprain of plantar flexed foot

Clinical features:
Pain, swelling, deformity
Loss of weight bearing ability
Medial displacement of foot on tibia

Radiological features
Tilting of talus under L.A. or G.A.
Fracture of lateral malleolus at level of ankle
  joint
Vertical fracture of medial malleolus

Pathological features
Sequence of events
1. Stretching of anterior talo-fibular ligament
2. Avulsion of lateral ligament of ankle
3. Fracture of lateral malleolus
4. Vertical "push off" fracture of medial
    malleolus and/or compression of medial
    tibial
Deforming forces may cease to act at any point
  in this sequence

Treatment:
Sprained ankle: Strapping
Ruptured lateral ligament
Fracture of lateral malleolus
} Cast 6-8 weeks in
  slight eversion
Displacement of lateral malleolus:
    Internal fixation
    Cast 6-8 weeks
Bimalleolar fractures:
    Very unstable
    Internal fixation of one or both malleoli
    Cast 10 weeks

See Figure 31

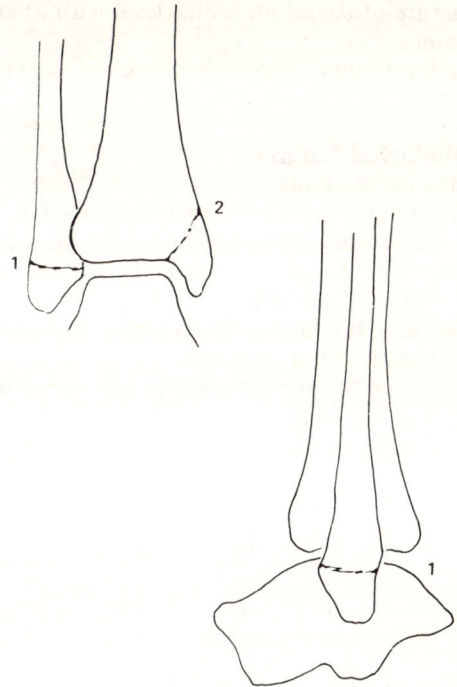

Fig. 31

References
Burwell H N, Charnley A D 1965 The treatment of displaced fractures at the ankle by rigid internal fixation and early joint movement. Journal of Bone and Joint Surgery 47B: 635-660
Ramsey P L, Hamilton W 1976 Changes in tibio talar area of contact caused by lateral talar shift. Journal of Bone and Joint Surgery 58A: 356-357

Abduction fractures of ankle

General features
Common injuries
Caused by abduction forces acting on foot

Clinical features
Pain, swelling, later bruising
Inability to bear weight
Tenderness localised over medial and lateral
    malleoli
Deformity of foot lying lateral to tibia

Radiological features
Avulsion fracture of base of medial malleolus

Fracture of lateral malleolus level with ankle joint

Comminution of outer fibular cortex at fracture site

Pathological features
Sequence of events
1. Transverse ('pull off') fracture of medial malleolus (or rupture of medial ligament)
2. Rupture of both anterior and posterior tibio-fibular ligaments.
3. Bending fracture of fibula just above ankle joint (often triangular)
Deforming forces may cease to act at any point in this sequence.

Major displacement
Internal fixation as above

See Figure 32

References
Yablon I G, Heller F G, Shouse L 1977 The key rule of the lateral malleolus in displaced fractures of the ankle. Journal of Bone and Joint Surgery 59A: 169-173

Compression fractures of ankle

General features
Uncommon
Caused by severe violence
    Usually by falling from a height
Often compound

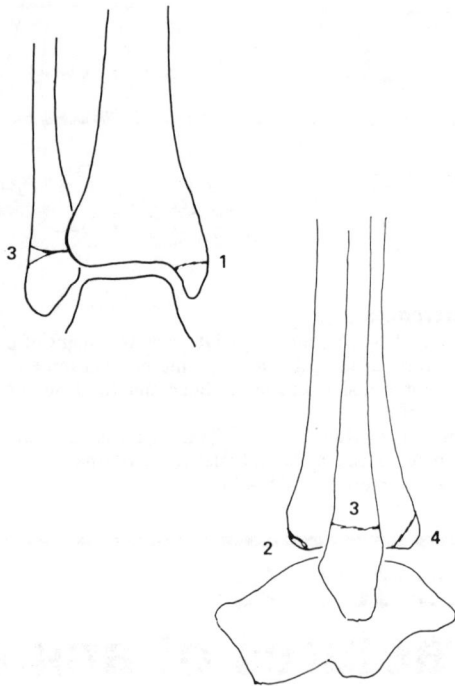

Fig. 32

Treatment

No displacement
Cast for 6-8 weeks

Minor displacement
Manipulation:
    Perfect position:
        Cast for 6-8 weeks in slight invertion
    Imperfection position:
        Internal fixation of medial malleolus
        Fibula may require a contoured plate
        Cast for 6-8 weeks

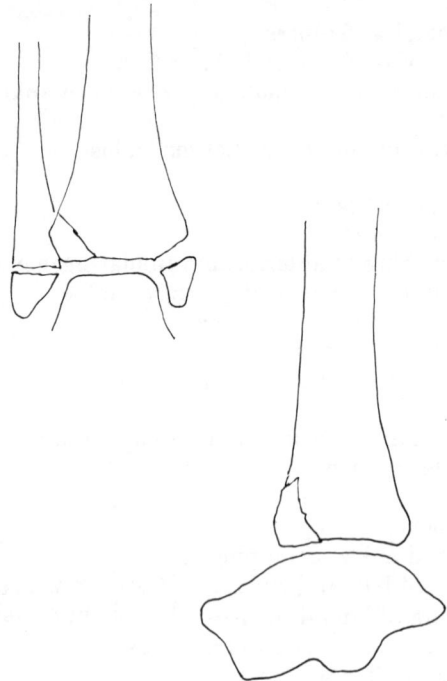

Fig. 33

Clinical features
Severe pain, tenderness and swelling
Some deformity
Complete loss of function

Radiological features

Fractures of
  lower fibula
  medial malleolus
Disruption of lower tibia

Pathological features

Considerable compression of subchondral bone
  of lower tibia
Later osteoarthrosis of ankle inevitable

Treatment

Conservative
Calcaneal traction
Compression bandage
Early active movements
Cast from 3rd to 12th or 16th week

Surgical
Open reduction
Internal fixation of malleoli
Iliac grafts to lower tibia
Early active movements
Delayed weight bearing to 12 weeks

See Figure 33

Reference:
Ruedi T P, Allgower M 1969 Fractures of the lower end of
  the tibia into the ankle joint. Injury I: 92-99

Rare injuries of ankle

1. Lateral rotatory dislocation of talus and foot
   without fracture. D'Anca (1970)
2. Subluxation of ankle without fibular
   fracture. Olerud (1971)
3. Traumatic Aneurysm of Perforating Peroneal
   Artery. Maguire (1972)

References
D'Anca A F 1970 Lateral rotatory dislocation of the ankle
  with fracture. Journal of Bone and Joint Surgery 52A:
  1643-1646
Maguire D S et al 1972 Traumatic aneurysm of perforating
  peroneal artery. Journal of Bone and Joint Surgery 54A:
  409-412
Olerud S 1971 Subluxation of the ankle without fracture of
  the fibula. Journal of Bone and Joint Surgery 53A: 594-596

Rupture of achilles tendon

General features
Incidence 1 in 20,000 per year
Age incidence 35-55 usually
M : F = 1 : 5

Etiology
Sedentary people and unusual strenuous activity
Steroid therapy – systemic or local
Push off injury
Pothole injury
Landing injury

Clinical features
Sudden pain
Palpable gap
Weakness of plantar flexion
Increased range of dorsiflexion
Squeeze test positive

Radiological features
Soft tissue lateral films ⎫
Ultransonic scan ⎭ will show gap in tendon

Pathological features
Ischemic degeneration at musculo-tendinous
  junction
Lipide deposition

Treatment

Acute rupture
Operative repair or splintage with foot in equinus
  and knee in flexion

Neglected or partial rupture
Operative repair

References
Cargill A O'R 1976 Closed rupture of the achilles tendon.
  British Journal of Hospital Medicine 16: 524-533
Jessing P, Hansen E 1975 Surgical treatment of 102 tendo-
  achilles ruptures. Suture or tenontoplasty. Acta Chirugica
  Scandinavica 141: 370-377
Nistor L 1976 Conservative treatment of fresh subcutaneous
  rupture of the achilles tendon. Acta Orthopedica
  Scandinavica 47: 459-462

Avulsion fractures of calcaneus

Synonym
Parrot-beak fracture

General features
Usually due to a blow from behind ankle
Rarely due to forceful plantar flexion of foot

Clinical features
Pain, tenderness, some swelling
Minor deformity
Standing possible, walking painful

Radiological features
Avulsion of postero-superior angle of calcaneum
Variable size and displacement of fragment

Pathological features
Separation increased by action of calf
    musculature
Fibrous union if neglected:- Resulting in
    Lengthening of Achilles tendon
    Loss of spring in gait

Treatment
Open reduction
Screw fixation
No weight bearing for 6-8 weeks

References
Lowy M 1969 Avulsion fractures of the calcaneus. Journal of
    Bone and Joint Surgery 51B: 494-497
Protheroe K 1969 Avulsion fractures of the calcaneus.
    Journal of Bone and Joint Surgery 51B: 118-122

Compression fractures of calcaneum

General features
Common injury often bilateral
(Associated with compression fractures of upper
    lumbar spine)
Rarely compound

Caused by falling from a height

Clinical features
Severe pain and swelling
Later bruising in foot and calf
Deformity of heel – swollen laterally
                                shortened
Inability to bear weight
Often overlooked in children

Radiological features

Lateral views
Loss of superior angle of calcaneum (Bohler's
    Angle)
Subtalar intra-articular fractures often present

Axial views
Broadening and comminution
Impingement of fragments on lateral or medial
    malleoli

Pathological features
Medial and lateral walls of calcaneum may
    crumble
Loss of superior angle causes secondary
    lengthening of achilles tendon
(Excessive dorsiflexion-
Weakened calf musculature-
 Loss of spring in the step)
Subtalar osteoarthrosis if joint surfaces are
    damaged

Treatment

Minimal deformity or comminution
Compression bandage
Elevation of foot
Early ankle and subtalar exercises
No weight bearing for 6-8 weeks

Comminuted fractures
    1. Manual compression
or   Compression by Bohler's clamp
      Compression bandage
      Elevation
      Early ankle and subtalar exercises
      No weight bearing 6-8 weeks
or 2. Open reduction
      Iliac or tibial bone grafts
      Plaster cast
      No weight bearing 6-8 weeks
or 3. Depression of posterior part of calcaneum
        by spike
      Plaster cast. Remove spike at 4 weeks
      No weight bearing 6-8 weeks

Post traumatic problems
Subtalar osteo-arthrosis:
    Pain on walking, especially on rough ground
Solution:
    Rigid boots
    Double irons with round ends
    Subtalar arthrodesis
Broadening of heel:
    Difficulties with shoe fitting
Solution:
    Soft wide shoe
    Custom made shoe
    Calcaneal osteotomy (very rarely required)
Valgus shift of heel:
    Flattening of long arch
    Abutment with lateral malleolus
Solution:
    Long arch support
    Removal of exostosis or part of lateral
      malleolus
Lengthening of achilles tendon:
    Lack of spring in the gait
Solution:
    Physiotherapy to strengthen calf
    Shortening of Tendo-Achilles rarely required

References

Evans J D 1966 Conservative management of os calcis fractures. Journal of Royal College of Surgeons of Edinburgh 12: 40-45

Essex-Lopresti P 1952 The mechanism reduction technique, and results in fractures of the os calcis. British Journal of Surgery 39: 395-419

Hunt D D 1970 Compression fracture of the anterior articular surface of the calcaneus. Journal of Bone and Joint Surgery 52A: 1637-1642

Isbister J F, St.C. 1974 Calcaneo-fibular abutment following crush fracture of the calcaneus. Journal of Bone and Joint Surgery 56B: 274-278

Matjeri R E, Frymoyer J W 1973 Fracture of the calcaneus in young children. Journal of Bone and Joint Surgery 55A: 1091-1094

Pridie K H 1946 A new method of treatment for severe fractures of the os calcis. Surgery, Gynaecology and Obstetrics 82: 671-675

Soeur R, Remy R 1975 Fracture of the calcaneus with displacement of the thalamic portion. Journal of Bone and Joint Surgery 57B: 413-421.

Dislocation of talus

General features:
Rare. Due to major violence.

Inversion injury: Anterolateral dislocation
Dorsiflexion injury: Postero-medial dislocation
Sometimes compound: (Anterolateral >
    Posteromedial)
Talar neck may fracture and only the body
    dislocate

Clinical features:
Pain, swelling, deformity
Inability to bear weight
Neurovascular compression in postero-medial
    dislocation occurs sometimes

Radiological features:
Talus is tilted and rotated lying posteromedial on
    calcaneus behind medial malleolus
or anterolateral in front of lateral malleolus
Fracture of talar neck may be present and only
    talar body dislocated.

Pathological features:
Talus stripped of soft tissues and usually
    avascular

Anterolateral dislocation:
Talar head directed medially and inferior surface
    backwards.

Posteromedial dislocation:
Talar head directed laterally and superior surface
    anteriorly
Talus sometimes extruded through skin wound.
Post traumatic osteoarthrosis of ankle is
    common.

Treatment:
Urgent Reduction:

1. Anterolateral manipulation:
Strong inversion and plantar flexion
+Tibio-calcaneal distraction

Posteromedial manipulation:
Full dorsiflexion with heel pulled forwards
Then evertion
Then plantar flexion with tibio-calcaneal
    distraction

2. Open reduction if unsuccessful
Plaster cast in plantigrade position
Internal fixation with wires if unstable
No weight bearing for 3 months

3. Loss of talus
Wound toilet and skin closure
Plaster cast for 3 months
Later calcaneal-tibial arthrodesis if required for
   pain.

References
Detenbeck L C, Kelly P J 1969 Total dislocation of the talus.
   Journal of Bone and Joint Surgery 51A: 283-288
Kenwright J, Taylor R E 1970 Major injuries of the talus.
   Journal of Bone and Joint Surgery 52B: 36-48

Fractures of body of talus

General features:
As isolated injuries, these are rare
Cause pain, swelling and loss of function

Lateral process of talus:

Treatment:
Removal of small fragments
Internal fixation of large fragments

Dome of talus:
Arise from inversion injuries under 30 years

Treatment:
Removal of small fragments
Internal fixation of large fragments

Posterior tubercle:
Formed by inconstant secondary centre of
   ossification
Appears 7-8 years   Fuses 18 years
Remains unfused in 8% of normals
Fracture very rarely occurs
   (Radiographic evidence of fracture
No sclerosis of contiguous margins
No separation in opposite talus)

Treatment:
Strapping
Early exercises and weight bearing

References
Mukerjee S K, Young A B 1973 Dome fracture of the talus.
   Journal of Bone and Joint Surgery 55B: 319-326
Mukerjee S K, Pringle R M, Baxter A D 1974 Fracture of
   the lateral process of the talus. Journal of Bone and Joint
   Surgery 56B: 263-273

Wood-Jones F 1949 Structure and function as seen in the
   foot. Second Edition, P. 70, Balliere, Tindall and Cox,
   London

Fractures of neck of talus

Synonym:
Aviator's Fracture

General features:
Uncommon. Rarely compound.
Caused by forced dorsiflexion
i.e. Aircraft and road crashes

Clinical features:
Pain, tenderness, swelling
Little deformity
Loss of ankle and foot movement
Inability to bear weight

Radiological features:
Classification:
1. No displacement
2. Moderate displacement
3. Displacement and dislocation of body of talus
   (Difficult to visualise well on film)
Increased density of body of talus after 8 weeks
   may indicate avascularity.

Pathological features:
Foot usually subluxes forward on body of talus.
Part or whole of body of talus may become
   avascular.
Ankle and subtalar osteo-arthrosis occurs later

Treatment:

Closed fractures:
1. Manipulation
   Cast in full equinus and eversion
   No weight bearing for 10-12 weeks
2. Failed manipulation
   Open reduction
   Internal fixation
   Cast in neutral. Weight bearing at 8-10 weeks.

Talar ischemia:
1. Bone Graft or
   Subtalar fusion
      Depending on site and extent of dead bone.
2. Talectomy or
   Pantalar arthrodesis
      If whole talus is ischaemic

References

Hawkins L G 1970 Fractures of the neck of the talus. Journal of Bone and Joint Surgery 52A: 991-1002
Kenwright J, Taylor R G 1970 Major Injuries of the talus. Journal of Bone and Joint Surgery 52B: 36-48
Mulfinger G L, Trueta J 1970 The blood supply of the talus. Journal of Bone and Joint Surgery 52B: 160-167

Subtalar dislocation

General features:
Rare
Due to major violence to foot
Forceful inversion and plantar flexion
Rarely compound
Often associated with fractures of talus

Clinical features:
Pain, swelling, later bruising.
Deformity. Inability to bear weight.
Usually no neurovascular disturbance

Radiological features:
Oblique views best show displacement
Talus lies in equinus in ankle mortise
Talus and calcaneus overlap in lateral views
Minor fractures of navicular and other tarsal
   bones often present.

Pathological features:
Foot is dilocated on talus
Talus does not become avascular
Subtalar osteoarthrosis frequently occurs later

Treatment:

1. Immediate manipulation
Plantar flexion, evertion, abduction
Unsuccessful:
   Open reduction
   Internal fixation
Cast for 6 weeks

2. Subtalar osteoarthrosis
Strong boot or
Double irons or
Subtalar arthrodesis

Reference
Kenwright J, Taylor R G 1970 Major injuries of the talus. Journal of Bone and Joint Surgery 52B: 36-48

Osteochondritis dissecans of talus

General features:
Rare
Usually affects superomedial angle of talus
May be caused by injury of moderate severity
   but may arise without recollected trauma

Clinical features:
Gradual onset of pain on ankle movement
Slight restriction of movement
No swelling, tenderness, deformity

Radiological features:
Irregularity of corner of talus on AP views
Better seen in tomographic films
Irregular small areas of increased radio density

Pathological features:
Superomedial or superolateral corner of talus
   becomes avascular
Overlying cartilage initially normal
Later bone and cartilage may separate as a small
   loose body

Treatment:

Normal cartilage
1. Insertion of Smillie pins from body of talus to
   avascular fragment

Abnormal cartilage
2. Removal of abnormal fragment

Loose bodies
3. Remove. Smooth off crater of origin
Difficulties in exposure may be overcome by
   osteotomy of medial malleolus with later screw
   fixation

References

Bernat A L, Marty M 1959 Transchondral fractures (Osteochondritis Dissecans) of the Talus. Journal of Bone and Joint Surgery 41A: 988-1020

Kappis M 1922 Weitere beitrage zur traumatisch-mechanischen entstehung der 'spontanen' knorpelablosungen (Sogen osteochondritis dissecans). Deutsche Zeitshrift fur Chirurgie 171: 13-29

Smillie I S 1960 Osteochondritis dissecans. E. & S. Livingstone, Edinburgh

Crushed foot

General features:
M > F
Usually arises from road traffic accidents
Steel toe-caps on boot reduce injuries from industrial accidents

Clinical features:
Severe pain
Inability to stand on the injured foot in most cases.
Swollen, bruised, immobile foot
Variety of soft tissue wounds can occur

Radiological features:
No fracture or dislocation may be present
But any combination of skeletal injuries can occur

Pathological features:
Massive swelling within a few hours
Subcuticular blistering is common.
Devitalised skin is not always apparent immediately.
Toes may become ischemic
Healing occurs with fibrosis on both surfaces of the foot.

Treatment:
No wound:
  Elevation
  Compression bandage
  Surgical decompression if skin or toes are in danger of necrosis
    Secondary suture later.
Soft tissue wounds:
  Debridement
  Delayed primary suture or secondary suture
Fractures:
  Reduce
  Internal fixation, (percutaneous pins)

Skin loss:
  Excise devitalised skin
  Delayed split skin grafting.
Hyaluronidase and fibrinolysins orally are of doubtful value.

Mid-tarsal fracture dislocation

General features:
Rare
Caused by angulatory forces on forefoot
Not often compound

Clinical features:
Pain, gross swelling of foot
Little deformity
Forefoot ischemia ⎫
Plantar anesthesia ⎭ may occur

Radiological features:
Wide variety of fracture lines
Oblique views essential

Pathological features:
Plantar arteries ⎫
Plantar nerves ⎭ may be compressed
Fractures may be very unstable
Post traumatic tarsal osteoarthrosis is common

Treatment:

Closed injuries:
Manipulation:
  Successful-
    Padded cast
      Unstable: Percutaneous pins
                Padded cast
Unsuccessful-
  Open reduction
  Internal fixation
  Padded cast

Compound injuries:
Wound toilet
Open reduction
+/- internal fixation
Padded cast

Later osteoarthrosis:
Midtarsal arthrodesis or
Triple arthrodesis.

References

Dewar F P, Evans D C 1968 Occult fracture subluxation of
the mid-tarsal joint 50B: 386-388
Main B J, Jowett R L, 1975 Injuries of the mid-tarsal joint.
Journal of Bone and Joint Surgery 57B: 89-97

Fractures of tarsal navicular

General features:
Uncommon
Caused by forced dorsiflexion

Clinical features:
Pain, tenderness, swelling
Minimal deformity
Inability to bear weight

Radiological features
Exclude subluxation of midtarsal joint
1. Fracture of tuberosity
    (Compare opposite foot.
    Consider os tibiale externum)
2. Fracture of dorsal lip
3. Horizontal transverse fracture.
    Dorsal fragment subluxes dorsally.

Pathological features:
Displaced fragments may become avascular
Tarsal joints all disturbed.
Malunion leads to mid tarsal osteo-arthrosis

Treatment:
Manipulation
Successful:
    Cast for 6-8 weeks
Unsuccessful:
    Open reduction
    Internal fixation
    Cast for 6-8 weeks

References

Eftekhar N M, Lyddon D W, Stevens J 1969 An unusual
fracture dislocation of the tarsal navicular. Journal of Bone
and Joint Surgery 51A: 577-581
Main B J, Jowett R L 1975 Injuries of the mid-tarsal joint.
Journal of Bone and Joint Surgery 57B: 89-97

Towne L C, Blazina M E, Cozen L N 1970 Fatigue fracture
of the tarsal navicular, Journal of Bone and Joint Surgery
52A: 376-378

Rare injuries of tarsus

Dislocation of cuneiform (Brown, 1975)
Dislocation of calcaneus (Viswanath, 1977)
Dislocation of cuboid (Drummond, 1969)
Fracture of os peroneum (Mains, 1973)

References

Brown D C, McFarland G B 1975 Dislocation of the medial
cuneiform bone in tarso-metatarsal fracture dislocation.
Journal of Bone and Joint Surgery 57A: 858-859
Drummond D S, Hastings D E 1969 Total dislocation of the
cuboid bone. Journal of Bone and Joint Surgery 51B: 716-
718
Mains D B, Sullivan R C 1973 Fracture of the os peroneum.
Journal of Bone and Joint Surgery 55A: 1529-1530
Viswanath S S, Shepherd E 1977 Dislocation of the
calcaneum. Injury 9: 50-52

Tarso-metatarsal fracture dislocations

Synonym:
Lisfranc's Fracture

General features:
Uncommon
Similar to mid-tarsal disruptions

Clinical features:
Pain, swelling, tenderness, later bruising
Deformity
Loss of ability to stand or move foot.
Plantar neurovascular damage is common.
    Ischemic toes
    Anesthetic sole

Radiological features:
Fracture of base of 2nd metatarsal allows lateral
    displacement
No Fracture: Dorsal displacement
Several other adjacent fractures may be present.

Pathological features:
Foot doubled up by
    Crushing from heel to toe when kneeling
    Crushing from toes when in full equinus
Plantar neurovascular bundle torn by local
    displacement or compressed by hematomata.
Intact bases of 1st and/or 2nd metatarsals may
    prevent reduction.

Treatment:

Ischemia:
Decompression
Open reduction
Internal fixation
Plaster cast and elevation
Weight bearing after 6 weeks

No ischemia:
Manipulation: Cast
Unsuccessful: Open Reduction
Unstable: Internal Fixation

References
Wiley J J 1971 The mechanism of tarso-metatarsal joint
    injuries. Journal of Bone and Joint Surgery 53B: 474-482
Wilson D W 1972 Injuries of the tarso-metatarsal joints.
    Etiology, classification and results of treatment. Journal of
    Bone and Joint Surgery 54ab: 677-686
Lisfranc J 1940 Fractures complique reflexions sur lepoque la
    plus opportune pour application de l'appareil. Gaz Hop 2:
    205-206

Fatigue fractures of metatarsals

Synonym:
Stress fracture, march fracture, etc.

General features:
Commonest in young people.
M > F
Occurs after unaccustomed strenuous exercise

Radiological features:
Usually 2nd metatarsal shaft affected.
3rd metatarsal shaft or other sites less often
    affected.
Early stages: No abnormality
After 1-2 days: Periosteal reaction
        5-6 days: Fracture line visible across shaft.
After 2-3 weeks: Callus formation.

Pathological features:
Minimal displacement accounts for paucity of
    radiographic changes.
Union always occurs.

Clinical features:
Gradual onset of pain and tenderness
Worsened by weight bearing
No deformity, minimal swelling.

Treatment:
Plaster cast for 6-8 weeks

Reference
Devas, M 1975 Stress fractures, ch 8. Churchill, Livingstone,
    Edinburgh
Breithaupt 1855 zur pathologue des menschlichen fusses
    Medicinische Zeitung 36: 169-177

Fractures of first metatarsal shaft

General features:
Usually due to direct violence
Often compound
Other tarsal injuries often present

Clinical features:
Pain, swelling, tenderness
Minimal deformity
Inability to stand or walk

Radiological features:
Variable fracture lines
Variable angulation and displacement

Pathological features:
Non-union very rare
Mal-union common–disturbs function of foot
Compound fractures +/- infection may cause
    adhesions of extensor and flexor tendons.

Treatment:

Closed fractures
No displacement:
    Plaster cast for 6 weeks
Displacement:
    Manipulation
    Plaster cast for 6 weeks

Unsuccessful manipulation:
Open reduction
+/- Internal fixation
Plaster cast for 6 weeks

Compound fractures:
Wound toilet
Open reduction
Plaster cast for 6-8 weeks

Fracture of metatarsal shafts 2-5

General features:
Common injury
Indirect violence – oblique fractures
Direct violence:
Often compound
Transverse or communited fractures

Clinical features:
Pain, swelling, tenderness
Little deformity
Inability to walk if more than one metatarsal is broken

Radiological features:
Variable fracture lines in neck, shafts or bases of metatarsal.
Little displacement or angulation unless other tarsal injuries are present.

Pathological features:
Fractures of neck(s) of metatarsals may disturb the balance of the forefoot for later weight bearing.
Adhesions of extensor tendons may occur at fracture sites.
Fracture of lower shaft of fifth metatarsal may be slow to unite.
Non-union of metatarsal fractures very rare.

Treatment:

Closed fractures:
One metatarsal – strapping for 6 weeks
Two or more metatarsals – Plaster cast for 6 weeks

Compound fractures:
Wound toilet. Plaster case for 6 weeks.

Reference
Watson-Jones R 1976 Fractures and joint injuries. Wilson J N (ed) 5th edn. ch 31. Churchill, Livingstone, London

Fractures of base of fifth metatarsal

Synonym:
Jones Fracture, Dancer's Fracture

General features:
Common Injury
Mechanism: Sudden inversion of foot

Clinical features:
Pain, Tenderness
No deformity, little swelling
Standing and walking possible
Distinguish from injury to lateral ligament of ankle.

Radiological features:
Best shown on oblique films
Pitfalls:
Presence of (1) Os peroneum (15%)
or (2) Os Vesalianum (0.15%)
or (3) Epiphysis at base of fifth metatarsal (8-15 years)
Films of opposite foot valuable for comparison

Pathological features:
Fibrous union is common

Treatment:
Manipulation not necessary
Moderate pain:
Strapping
Early weight bearing
Severe pain:
Plaster cast ($<$ 6 weeks)

References
Dameron J B 1975 Fractures and anatomical variations of the proximal portion of the fifth metatarsal. Journal of Bone and Joint Surgery 57A: 788-792
Jones R 1902 Fracture of the base of the fifth metatarsal bone by indirect violence. Annals of Surgery 35: 697-700
Kavanaugh J H, Brower T D, Mann R V 1978 The Jones fracture revisited. Journal of Bone and Joint Surgery 60A: 776-782

Dislocation of first metatarso- phalangeal joint

General features:
Rare
Caused by forced dorsiflexion of great toe
(Compare similar injury in thumb)

Clinical features:
Pain, tenderness, swelling
Deformity of toe
Walking painful

Radiological features:
Dorsal dislocation of proximal phalanx or first metatarsal
Sesamoids splayed on either side of head of metatarsal

Pathological features:
Usually unreducible by manipulation
Metatarsal head 'button-holes' through plantar surface of joint capsule.

Treatment:
Manipulation: Splintage for 3-4 weeks
Unsuccessful: Open reduction: +/- Internal fixation if unstable

Reference
Giannikas A C et al 1975 Dorsal dislocation of the first metatarso-phalangeal joint. Journal of Bone and Joint Surgery 57B: 384-386

Posterior tibial tendon lesions

Laceration:
Glass: Beach injuries in children.
          Window injuries in adults.
Metal: Industrial or road accidents.
Often overlooked
Give rise to unilateral pes planus.

Treatment:
Primary repair if possible
Secondary repair +/- tendon graft if septic or neglected.

Non-suppurative tenosynovitis:
Causes:
  prolonged unaccustomed exercise
  Rheumatoid arthritis
  Rarieties:
    Tuberculosis
    Pigmented villonodular synovitis.

Treatment:
1. Of cause.
2. Local Heat   Local steroid injection.
     Plaster cast 3-4 weeks.

Dislocation:
Cause:
  Injury. Usually in skiers
  May be spontaneous
  Usually becomes recurrent
  Causes instability of ankle

Treatment:
Deepening of groove behind medial malleoleus
Repair of synovial and fibrous sheath.

Spontaneous rupture:
Causes:
  Tenosynovitis: Non-suppurative or rheumatoid.
  Usually in middle age

Treatment:
Surgical repair.

Entrapment:
Cause:
  Severe fracture dislocation of ankle.

Treatment:
Open reduction
Internal fixation of fracture
Repair of synovial and fibrous sheath.

References

Coonrad R W, Bugg E I 1954 Trapping of the posterior tibial tendon and interposition of soft tissue in severe fractures about the ankle joint. Journal of Bone and Joint Surgery 36A: 744-750

Cozen L 1965 Posterior tibial tenosynovitis secondary to foot strain. Clinical Orthopaedics 42: 101-102

Griffiths J C 1965 Tendon injuries about the ankle. Journal of Bone and Joint Surgery 47B: 686-689

Kettelkamp D B, Alexander H H 1969 Spontaneous rupture of the posterior tibial tendon. Journal of Bone and Joint Surgery 51A: 759-763

Nava B E 1968 Traumatic dislocation of the tibialis posterior tendon at the ankle. Journal of Bone and Joint Surgery 50B: 150-151

Norris S H, Mankin H J 1978 Chronic tenosynovitis of the posterior tibial tendon with new bone formation. Journal of Bone and Joint Surgery 60B: 523-526

Peroneal tendon lesions

Laceration:
Rare
Usually caused by glass or metal
May not be recognised immediately until varus deformity of foot is noted
Sural nerve may also be divided

Treatment:
Acute Injury:
Immediate repair
Chronic Injury:
Repair of peroneus longus
Tendon graft of peroneus brevis

Non suppurative tenosynovitis:
Unusual. Arises after unaccustomed exercise
Pain, swelling, tenderness, crepitus

Treatment:
Local injection of steroid and local anesthetic
or
Heat and Ultrasonic Therapy
or
Plaster cast for 1 month

Rupture:
Trauma:
Resisted sudden eversion of foot
Rare
Pain, tenderness, loss of eversion

Spontaneous:
Rare
Usually due to rheumatoid arthritis
Little pain, minimal local tenderness

Treatment:
Trauma: Repair
Spontaneous: Treatment often not required

Dislocation:
Acute rupture of peroneal retinaculum
Usually in skiers

Treatment:
Early surgical repair
Plaster cast 6 weeks

References

Alm A, Lamke L O, Liljedahl S O 1975 Surgical treatment of dislocation of the peroneal tendons. Injury 7: 14-19

Burman M 1953 Stenosing tendovaginitis of the foot and ankle. Archives of Surgery 67: 686-698

Eckert W R, Davis, E A (1976) Acute rupture of the peroneal retinaculum. Journal of Bone and Joint Surgery 58A: 670-673

Evans J D 1966 Subcutaneous rupture of the tendon of peroneus longus. Journal of Bone and Joint Surgery 48B: 507-509

Griffiths J C 1965 Tendon injuries around the ankle. Journal of Bone and Joint Surgery 47B: 686-689

Laceration of toe tendons

General features:
Less common than in hand
Extensor tendons:
Objects dropped on foot
Crushing injuries
Flexor tendons:
Walking barefoot on sharp object

Clinical features:
Wound. Pain. Sensory deficit may be present.
Extensor tendon:
Drooping of toes
No extension possible
Flexor tendon:
No deformity obvious
No flexion possible

Radiological features:
None

Pathological features:
Extensor tendons retract further than in the hand
  because of no inter-connections
Flexor tendons do not retract as far as in the
  hand because of the FHL and FDL crossover
  and interconnections in the sole.
Lack of EHL and FHL gives chief disability
EDC and FDL divisions give minimal disability

Treatment:

Extensor tendons:
Wound toilet and suture
(EHL tendon requires splintage with below knee
  cast)

Flexor tendons:
Wound toilet
Lateral 4 toes
  Prolonged exploration not justified. Repair if
    found
F.H.L. tendon
  Repair if found
  Repair F.H.B. if also cut
  Below knee cast for 3 weeks.

Reference
Frenette J P, Jackson D W 1977 Lacerations of the flexor
  hallucis longus in the young athlete. Journal of Bone and
  Joint Surgery 59A: 673-676

Fracture of toes

General features:
Very common
Usually crush injuries
Often compound – often from lawn-mowers.

Clinical features:
Pain, swelling, tenderness.
Little deformity or loss of function

Radiological features:
Very variable fracture lines
Angulation not severe
Proximal phalangeal fractures angulate as in
  fingers

Pathological features:
Severe crushing may lead to ischemia.
Proximal phalangeal fractures may be angulated
  by flexor tendons

Treatment:

Prophylaxis:
Steel toe caps to industrial boots

Conservative:
2-5 toes: Wool and strapping
1st toe: Strapping or
              Below Knee plaster cast.

Surgical:
Excision of compound wounds
Amputation if viability is doubtful
Internal fixation of great toe if other leg fractures
  are present.

18

AMPUTATIONS AND PROSTHETICS

With the assistance of I. M. Troup

Functional objectives

Defined and discussed, if possible, before surgery
   with patient and relatives.
Higher aims in youth than in age

Factors:
Level of amputation
Other lesions:
   Musculo-skeletal
   Cardio-respiratory
Occupation
Intelligence
Motivation
Social setting:
   Caring relatives
   Suitable housing

Psychological aspects of amputation

A. Functional limitations
Amputee may
   Avoid performing tasks
   Compensate for loss by greater use of
      remaining limbs
   Perform task by using artificial aids

B. Functional failure:
Caused by
   design of prosthesis
   Control of prosthesis
   Lack of practice in controlling prosthesis

C. Comfort limitations:
Pain from prosthetic socket
Phantom sensations
Fatigue

D. Cosmesis of prosthesis:
Appearance
Sound of mechanical movement

E. Vocational and economic factors:
Professional jobs }
Managerial job   } rarely impaired
Intellectual jobs }
Manual jobs severely impaired

5. Social factors:
Abnormality and failure is frowned upon by
   present society
Deformity is associated with villains and crime

Younger patients:
Adapt better to loss of limb
                to use of prosthesis
Have a higher effort tolerance
Suffer more upper limb losses
Less likely to have a phantom limb

Amputee behaviour

In hospital:
Depression
Anxiety
Defiance
Cheerfulness
Resignation
Indifference

Long term:
Pyschological effects of amputation relate to
   preamputation personality of the patient
Amputees try hard to appear normal

Non-acceptance of injury
Results in
   Hostile agressive behaviour
   Timid hesitant behaviour

Acceptance of prosthesis
Results in
   Decreased sensitivity and frustrations
   Increase in social adequacy
   Greater self reliance

Psychological rehabilitation
Aims to assist patient to incorporate his
   limitations into his pattern of life with minimal
   interference of normal activities.

Aims:
Adjustment to use of prosthesis
Search for alternative goals for life satisfaction

Methods:
Early purposeful activity
Support of other more advanced amputees
Support of other staff

Reference
Amputation. 1962 S Fishman in Psychological practices with the physically disabled ed. J F Carrett E S Levine, pp1-50 Columbia Univ. Press, New York

Amputee locomotion

Pattern of an individual's walking is his solution of how to move with:
1. Minimal effort
2. Adequate stability
3. Acceptable appearance
4. Acceptable speed

Above knee gait

Stance phase:
Natural leg:
   Does not control trajectory of trunk adequately
   Makes ground contact earlier than normal sequence
   Moves forward faster than prosthetic leg
   Takes more than normal vertical load
   Bears weight longer than normal

Swing phase: amputated leg:
Initiated by hip flexors acting more strongly than normal to move the prosthesis ($\times$ 3 if knee is stiff)
Hip muscles must also control prosthetic knee to give appropriate flexion and extension
Valuting on natural leg is frequent
   Too long a prosthetic foot
   Too long a prosthesis
   Stump discomfort
   Habit
Rotational and transverse motions in a limb are absorbed by:
   Heel of a S.A.C.H. foot
   Other ankle mechanisms
   Socket/Skin interphase

Loss of major joints is compensated by exaggerated motion at other levels with increased energy expenditure

Below knee gait
Almost as usual in a young person with a comfortable prosthesis
If knee remains mobile:
   Flexion occurs from heel strike to foot flat
   Extension occurs from foot flat to mid stance
Swing phase is controlled by intact muscles
Some extra hip and knee flexion may be needed in swing-through

Energy expenditure wearing prosthesis:
Stick or Crutches
  2 point alternating gait or
  3 point partial weight bearing gait $\Big\} + 33\%$
  Swing through gait or
  3 point non weight bearing gait $\Big\} + 78\%$

References
McBeath A A, Bahrke M, Balke B 1974 Efficiency of assisted ambulation determined by oxygen consumption measurement. Journal of Bone and Joint Surgery 56A: 994-1000
Pugh L G C E 1973 The oxygen uptake and energy cast of walking before and after unilateral hip replacement with some observations of the use of crutches. Journal of Bone and Joint Surgery 55B: 742-745

Characteristics of faulty gait in amputees

Problem of each patient is individual

Common deviations:
Lateral trunk bending
Hip hiking
Internal or external hip rotation
Circumduction
Abnormal walking base
Excessive medial or lateral foot contact
Anterior trunk bending
Posterior trunk bending
Lordosis
Hyperextension of knee
Knee instability

Inadequate dorsiflexion control
Insufficient push off
Vaulting
Rhythmic disturbances
Abnormal arm motion

Immobilisation of any segment or joint of the lower extremity requires 10% increase in energy expenditure in walking.

Post-amputation problems: causing faulty gait
Infection of wound
Breakdown of ischemic scars
Ischemic pain
Stump neuromata
Formation of exostoses
Overgrowth of bone in children
Furunculosis of hair-bearing skin applied to the prosthesis.
Persistent edema of the stump
Bursa formation
Adductor roll cysts in above-knee amputees.

Phantom limb.
Incidence unknown.
Very rare in children
Commonest in adults who:
   Have viewed their mutilated limb
   Have suffered prolonged pain } before
   May benefit financially } amputation

References
Kolb L C, Frank L M, Watson E J 1952 Treatment of the acute painful phantom limb. Procedings of the Mayo Clinic 27: 110-118
Levy S W Allende M F, Barnes G H 1962 Skin problems of the leg amputee. Archives of dermatology 85: 65-81
Murdoch G 1969 Balance of the amputee. Physiotherapy 55: 405-408
Riding J 1976 Phantom limb; some theories. Anaesthesia 31: 102-106
Thompson R C, Delblanco J L, Mcallister F F 1965 Complications following lower extremity amputation. Surgery, Gynaecology and Obstetrics 120: 310-304
Waters, R L et al 1976 Energy cost of walking of amputees. The influence of the level of amputation. Journal of Bone and Joint Surgery 58A: 42-46

Faulty gait of the above-knee amputee

1. Lateral bending of trunk:
Causes:
   Short Prosthesis
   Insufficient support from lateral wall of socket
   Abducted socket
   Pain on lateral aspect of stump
   Weak abductors
   Abducted gait (vide infra)

2. Abducted gait:
Causes:
   Prosthesis too long
   Shank aligned in valgus on thigh section
   Pain in perineum
   Malignment of mechanical hip joint (if present)
   Contracted abductors
   Amputee feels insecure

3. Circumduction:
Causes:
   Insufficient knee flexion
     (i.e. Manual knee lock)
     (or Excessive friction)
     (or Tight extension aid)
   Inadequate suspension (Piston action)
   Too small a socket
   Foot set in plantar flexion
   Amputee feels insecure

4. Vaulting:
Causes:
   Excessive length of prosthesis
     (a) Inadequate suspension
     (b) Extended knee
     (c) Too small a socket
     (d) Foot set in plantar flexion
     (e) Amputee feels insecure
   Insufficient friction in prosthetic knee

5. Uneven timing:
Causes:
   Improper fitting of socket
   Too easy knee flexion with instability in extension
   Weak stump
   Poor balance
   Fear and insecurity

6. Uneven heel rise:
Cause:

A. Too much rise
Insufficient friction in prosthetic knee
(Insufficient tension or absence of extension aid)
Forceful stump flexion to ensure that prosthetic
    shank will be fully extended at heel strike

B. Too little rise
Excessive friction on prosthetic knee
(Too tight an extension aid)
Fear and insecurity
Manual knee lock

7. Terminal swing impact
Causes:
    Insufficient friction of prosthetic knee
    (Too much tension on extension aid)
    Amputee's fear of knee buckling into flexion

8. Instability of prosthetic knee
Causes:
    Knee may be in advance of line joining
        trochanter and ankle
    Insufficient initial flexion may have been built
        into socket
    Plantar flexion resistance may be too great
        causing the knee to buckle at heel strike
    Failure to limit dorsiflexion can lead to
        incomplete knee control
    Hip extensor weakness
    Severe hip flexion contracture may cause
        instability

9. Swing phase whips
Causes:
    Internal rotation of knee bolt causes 'lateral
        whip' (heel moves laterally at toe off)
    External rotation of knee bolt causes 'medial
        whip'
    Socket too tight: muscle belly contraction
        causes socket rotation
    Toe break not set at right angle to line of
        progression
    Soft flabby stump allowing socket and skin
        rotation

10. Foot slap
Cause:
    Plantar flexion bumper too soft

11. Drop off
(Downward movement of trunk as body moves
    over prosthesis)
Causes:
Inadequate limitation of dorsiflexion of foot
    Keel of S.A.C.H. foot too short
    Toe break of conventional foot too far
        posterior
    Socket placed too far anterior to foot

12. Uneven length of steps
Causes:
    Flexion contracture of hip
    Insufficient flexion of socket
    Pain or fear
    Insufficient friction in prosthetic knee

13. Lumbar lordosis
Causes:
    Flexion contracture of hip
    Insufficient initial flexion of socket
    Insufficient support from anterior socket wall
    Weak hip extensors
    Weak abdominal musculature
    Painful ischial bearing

Faulty gait of below knee amputee

Between heel strike and mid stance:

A. Excessive knee flexion:
Excessive dorsiflexion of prosthetic foot
Excessive anterior tilt of socket
Excessively stiff plantar flexion bumper or heel
    cushion
Excessive anterior displacement of socket over
    foot
Flexion contracture of knee
Posterior misplacement of suspension tabs

B. Insufficient or absent knee flexion:
Excessive plantar flexion of foot
Excessively soft plantar flexion bumper
Posterior displacement of socket over foot
Antero-distal socket discomfort
Weakness of quadriceps
Habit

Mid stance:

Excessive lateral thrust of prosthesis due to:
   Excessive medial placement of prosthetic foot
      or
   Improper medio-lateral tilt of socket

Between mid-stance and toe-off

A. Early knee flexion ('drop-off')

Excessive anterior displacement of socket over
   foot
Posterior displacement of toe break or the keel
Excessive dorsiflexion of foot
Excessive anterior tilt of socket
Soft dorsiflexion bumper

B. Delayed knee flexion:

Excessive posterior displacement of socket over
   foot
Anterior displacement of toe break or keel
Excessive plantar flexion of foot
Excessive posterior tilt of the socket
Hard dorsifexion bumper

Amputations in children

Congenital deformity:

Delay surgery until certain of its value – preserve
   length
Functional stumps of fingers and toes etc. should
   not be sacrificed for cosmesis
Overgrowth of the stump never occurs
Psychological problems are rare
Cosmesis unimportant until adolescence.

Other amputations

75% due to trauma
Growth relates to presence or absence of rapidly
   growing epiphyses,
      i.e. Distal femur, proximal tibia,
         Proximal humerus, distal radius
Epiphyseodesis rarely successful
Osteomyoplastic techniques particularly useful
Disarticulations, if feasible, give least trouble
Stump complications fewer in children
Phantom limbs are rare

References

Kay H W et al, Prosthetics and Orthrotics New York, 1967,
   New York University Postgraduate Medical School
Lakeslee B B (ed). The limb deficient child. University of
   California Press, Berkeley, 1963

Growth abnormalities in leg amputations in children

Above knee:

Hemi-atrophy of pelvis
Coxa valga
Elongation of lesser trochanter
Occasional overgrowth of femoral stump if skin
   is adherent
Spur formation on medial side of femur
An adequate stump at age 5 may be too short at
   15 because of loss of rapidly elongating distal
   femoral eiphysis

Through knee:

Ideal level for children

Below knee:

Posterior tilting of upper tibial epiphyseal plate
Anterior bowing
Varus angulation
(Valgus angulation in congenital absence of fibula)
Fibular overgrowth more common than tibial
   overgrowth.

Growth abnormalities in arm amputations in children

Above elbow:

Humeral overgrowth
Humeral varus angulation

Below elbow:

Overgrowth of radius
Pincerlike contour
Tilting of proximal radial epiphysis
Overgrowth of ulna is rare

Reference

Aitken G T, Franz C H 1953 The juvenile amputee. Journal
   of Bone and Joint Surgery 35A: 659-664

Assessment of viability of ischemic limb

Clinical examination:
Pulses
Colour
Hair presence
Warmth

Investigations:
Thermography
Oscillometry } Increasingly useful
Intra-arterial fluorescein } Invasive
Xenon 133 injection
Pulse Extinction Pressures
Doppler Ultrasound
Plethysmography
Arteriography   Minimal value

Factors in selecting level of amputation
Pathological
Anatomical
Surgical
Prosthetic
Personal: Age, Sex, Occupation

Criteria for level of amputation in occlusive vascular disease:

Above knee:
Sudden arterial occlusion in pelvic arterial tree
Absent femoral pulse
Arterial emboli in iliac or femoral vessels
Peripheral aneurysms causing gangrene at knee
    and distally

Below knee:
Each patient must be considered individually:
Slow onset of disease
Palpable femoral pulse
Functioning knee joint
Normal skin at operation site
Bleeding at operation site

References
Barnes R W, Shanik G D, Slaymaker E 1976 An index in healing in below knee amputations. Leg Blood Pressure by Doppler Ultrasound Surgery 79: 13-18
Dall J L C, McDougall A 1971 Spontaneous separation of a gangrene leg. Journal of Bone and Joint Surgery 53B: 106-107
Kelly P J, Janes J M 1970 Criteria for determining the proper level of amputation in occlusive vascular disease. Journal of Bone and Joint Surgery 52A: 1685-1688
Kostuik J P et al 1976 The Measurement of skin blood flow in peripheral vascular disease by Epicutaneous application of xenon 133. Journal of Bone and Joint Disease 58A: 833-837
Murdoch, G. 1967 Levels of amputation and limiting factors. Annals of Royal college of surgeons of England 40: 204-216
Spence V A et al Current status of thermography in peripheral vascular disease. Journal of cardiovascular Surgery 16: 572-579

Amputations around hip joint

Hindquarter amputation:

Indications:
Tumours of hemipelvis without metastases
Intractable infection
Assess patient's physical and mental state
Ensure operability by all available pre-operative
    means
General surgical assistance is desirable
Only surgical considerations are those of the
    pathology.

Disarticulation of hip

Indications:
1. Malignant Tumour of Femur
2. Intractable Sepsis of Femur
3. Trauma.
Assess pre-operative state carefully
Long posterior flap fashioned
Deep iliac glands may be removed at the same
    time.

High femoral amputation:
If within 5 cm. of lesser trochanter an above
    knee prosthesis cannot be fitted.
Indications:
    Neoplasm
    Infection
    Trauma
    Congenital deformity.

References

Elting J J, Allen J C 1972 Management of the young child with bilateral anomalous and functionless lower extremities. Journal of Bone and Joint Surgery 54A: 1523-1530

Gordon-Taylor G, Monro R 1952 The technique and management of the hindquarter amputation. British Journal of Surgery 39: 536-541

Mclean E M 1962 Avulsion of the hindquarter. Journal of Bone and Joint Surgery 44B: 384-385

Marcove R C et al 1972 Chondrosarcoma of the pelvis and upper end of the femur. Journal of Bone and Joint Surgery 54A: 561-572

Pack G T, Ehrlich H E 1946 Exarticulation of the lower extremities for malignant tumours. Annals of Surgery 123: 965-985

Pack G T, Miller T R 1964 Exarticulation of the innominate bone and corresponding lower extremity (Hemipelvectomy) for primary and metastatic cancer. Journal of Bone and Joint Surgery 46A: 91-95

Phelan J T, Nadler S H 1964 A technique of hemi-pelvectomy. Surgery, Gynaecology and Obstetrics 119: 311-318

Editorial 1974 Hindquarter amputations. British Medical Journal 4: 4-5

Above knee amputations

Second in frequency to below knee procedures

Indications:
Ischemia, Peripheral vascular disease, emboli.
Trauma
Infection
Neoplasma
Congenital abnormality

General features:
Avoid hip flexion and abduction – when severe, this deformity makes prosthesis fitting an impossibility

Myoplasty is desirable to improve post-operative circulation of stump with increased power and better function.

Knee hinge mechanisms require 10 cm. but apart from this the stump should be as long as possible.

References

Dederich R 1963 Plastic treatment of the muscles and bone in amputation surgery. Journal of Bone and Joint Surgery 45B: 60-66

Thomson R E et al 1965 Above the knee amputations and prosthetics. Journal of Bone and Joint Surgery 47A: 619-630

Hind-quarter and above-knee prostheses

Variable factors:

(A) *Suspension:*
Waist band
Shoulder suspension ⎱ separately or in
Suction socket ⎰ combination.

(B) *Socket fitting:*
Conventional
'H' type socket
Metal socket
Quadrilateral socket
Total surface bearing

(C) *Knee mechanism:*
Difficult to replace normal knee movement
Various mechanical arrangements available
(1) Minimum friction: Hinge joint.
(2) Friction resistance in swing phase
   Constant friction devices
   Variable friction devices.
   Variable friction units with cadence response.
(3) Control of swing and stance phase
   Constant friction units with weight response stabilisation.
   Variable friction units with cadence response and positive lock stabilisation.
   Variable friction units with poly-centric devices for stabilisation

(D) *Ankle – Foot Units:*
   S.A.CH. foot most commonly used.
Individual prescriptions required at each level of prosthesis

References

Gillis L 1968 A new prosthesis for disarticulation at the hip. Journal of Bone and Joint Surgery 50B: 389-391

Hensley C D 1959 The use of bilateral Canadian type disarticulation prosthesis for congenital absence of both lower extremities. Journal of Bone and Joint Surgery 41A: 417-421

Lamb D W, Simpson D C, Pirie R B 1970 The Management of lower limb phocomelia. Journal of Bone and Joint Surgery 52B: 688-691

Liao S J, Schnell A 1964 A functional above knee prosthesis for geriatric patients. Journal of Bone and Joint Surgery 46A: 1292-1294

Solomondis S E et al 1977 Biomechanics of the hip disarticulation prosthesis. Prosthetics and Orthotics International 1: 13-18

Tompson R G et al 1965 Above the knee amputations and prosthetics. Journal of Bone and Joint Surgery 47A: 619-630

Through knee amputation

Indications:
Trauma
Malignant tumours of tibia
Infection
Congenital abnormalities of lower leg
Ischemia

Advantages:
Good for children as the distal femoral epiphysis is preserved
Durable end bearing stump
Long lever arm for prosthesis
Big surface area of stump

Disadvantages:
Difficult to fit a knee hinge
Mechanism at same level as other knee
Bulky knee mechanism – but recent improvements

Modifications:
1. Patello-femoral fusion (Gritti-Stokes)
   Doubtful value now
   Difficult operation
   Longer convalescence
2. Trimming of femoral condyles to give a thinner stump

References:

Batch J W, McFaddin J G 1954 Advantages of the knee disarticulation over amputations through the thigh. Journal of Bone and Joint Surgery 36A: 921-930

Mazet R, Hennessey C A 1966 Knee disarticulations. A new technique and a new knee joint mechanism. Journal of Bone and Joint Surgery 48A: 126-139

Vitali M, Harris E E 1964 Prosthetic management of the elderly lower limb amputee. Clinical Orthopaedcis 37: 61-87

Below knee amputation

Most common of all amputations
Usually performed for ischemia in the elderly
Retention of knee joint particularly advantageous
Distal limit of stump: Musculotendinous junction of gastrocnemius
Proximal limit: Hamstring insertions

Technique
Ischemic limbs:
   Long posterior flap
   Muscles bevelled
   Anterior suture line
Vascular limbs:
   Equal flaps
   Myoplastic suture with tibio-fibular bridge improves stump
Very short stumps:
   Improved fitting of prosthesis by:
      1. Removal of whole fibula
      2. Division of hamstring insertion
In all
   Fibula sectioned proximal to talus
   Tibial sharp edges smoothed

References:

Burgess E M et al 1971 Amputations of the leg for peripheral vascular insufficiency. Journal of Bone and Joint Surgery 53A: 874-890

Ederich R 1963 Plastic treatment of the muscles and bone in amputation surgery. Journal of bone and joint surgery 45B: 60-66

McCulloch N C, Jennings J J, Sarmiento A 1972 A bilateral below the knee amputation in patients over 50 years of age. Journal of Bone and Joint Surgery 54A: 1217-1223

Mooney V et al 1976 The below the knee amputation for vascular disease. Journal of Bone and Joint Surgery 58A: 365-368

Persson B M 1974 Sagittal incision for below knee amputations in ischaemic gangrene. Journal of Bone and Joint Surgery 56B: 110-114

Immediate postsurgical prosthetic fitting

Requirements:
Meticulous surgical technique
Prosthetist available at operation

Advantages claimed
Acceleration:
  In healing of wound
  Maturation of stump
Absence of edema
Decrease of pain
Earlier ambulation
Decrease in hospitalisation
Improved psychological outlook
Earlier fitting of definitive prosthesis
Particularly applicable to B-K and T-K stumps
Also attempted with other leg stumps
May be better delayed to 7th or 10th post-
  operative day

References
Burgess E M, Romano R L, Zettle J M 1969 The managment
  of lower extremity amputations. Veterans Administration
  Report 10-6
Cohen S I et al 1974 Deleterious effect of immediate post-
  operative fitting in below knee amputations for ischaemic
  disease. Surgery 76: 992-1001
Editorial 1975 I.P.O.P.: Miracle, menace or gimmick? Lancet
  1: 620-621

Other features of post-operative care

Bandaging:
Prevents edema
Moulds stump
Requires care and expertise

Rigid dressing:
Usually a plaster cast
Prevents –
  Edema
  Stress on sutures
  Minor trauma
Requires –
  Suction drainage
  Monitoring of patient's discomfort.
  Waist or shoulder suspension

Controlled environment treatment:
Sterilised air dressing
Advantages
  Comfortable
  Allows wound inspection
           stump exercises
  Prevents edema
           infection
Disadvantage
  Expensive machinery
  Still experimental

References
Burgess E M, Tedegana L R 1977 Controlled environment
  treatment for limb surgery and trauma. A preliminary
  report. Bulletin of Prosthetic Research 10-28: 16-57
Murdoch G 1975 Research and development within surgical
  amputee care. Acta Orthopaedica Scandinavia 46, 526-547
Puddifoot, P C, Weaver L C, Marshall S A 1973 A method
  of supporting bandaging for amputation stumps. British
  Journal of Surgery 60: 729-731

Below knee prostheses

Old style:
Thigh corset.
Shoulder suspension
End-Bearing (Customised socket)
Knee hinge
Ankle hinge

New style:
Patella tendon bearing
(1) P.T.S. (La protése tibiale supra-condylienne)
(2) K.B.M. (Kondylen Bettung Munster)
(3) K.B.M. + Condylar wedge suspension.
(4) Air Cushion Socket.
Foot: Solid ankle, Cushion Heel (S.A.C.H.)

Modular assembly prosthesis (M.A.P.)—
Any prefabricated series of prosthetic parts with
customised socket.

References
Barclay W 1970 In-Prosthetic and orthotic practice.
Murdoch, G; (editor) P69. Edwin Arnold, London
Bleck E E, Canty T J, Doolittle R C 1963 Below the knee,
closed end, soft socket. Journal of Bone and Joint Surgery
45A: 967-976
Brown P W 1970 Rehabilitation of the Bilateral lower
extremity amputees. Journal of Bone and Joint Surgery
52A: 687-700
Gordon E J, Ardizzone J 1960 Clinical experiences with the
SACH foot prosthesis. Journal of Bone and Joint Surgery
42A: 226-234
Greusten S, Eriksson U 1974 Stump socket contact and
skeletal displacement in suction patellar tendon bearing
prosthesis. Journal of Bone and Joint Surgery 56A: 1692-
1696
Mazet R, Hennessey C A 1966 Knee disarticulation. Journal
of Bone and Joint Surgery 48A: 126-139
McDougall A, Emerson A 1977 The preformed socket and
modular assembly for primary amputees. Journal of Bone
and Joint Surgery 59B: 77-79

Amputation of the foot

Synonym:
Syme's amputation

Advantages:
Simple operation
Long lasting stump
No prosthesis required in certain situations

Disadvantages:
Not sufficiently proximal in peripheral vascular
disease
Difficulty in fitting a prosthesis
i.e. Thickened ankle
Condition of contra-lateral leg may be
significant.
Less suitable for women
Not every stump will bear full weight

Modifications:
Calcaneo-tibial fusion:
Whole calcaneum (Boyd, 1939)
Rotated posterior half of calcaneum (Piragoff,
(1854))
Now discarded because of difficulty in
obtaining sound Calcaneo-tibial union.

References
Boyd H B 1939 Amputation of the foot with calcaneo-tibial
arthrodesis. Journal of Bone and Joint Surgery 21: 997-
1000
Davidson W H, Bohne W H O 1975 The Syme amputation in
children. Journal of Bone and Joint Surgery 57A: 905-909
Farmer A W, Laurin C A 1960. Congenital absence of the
fibula. Journal of Bone and Joint Surgery 42A: 1-12
Harris R I 1956 Syme's amputations. The technical details
essential for success. Journal of Bone and Joint Surgery
38B: 614-632
Hormby, R, Harris W R 1975 Syme's Amputation. Journal
of Bone and Joint Surgery 57A: 346-349
Murdoch G 1976 Syme's Amputation. Journal of the Royal
College of Surgeons of Edinburgh 21: 15-30
Srinivasan H 1973 Syme's amputation in insensitive feet.
Journal of Bone and Joint Surgery 55A: 558-562

Amputations through the foot

Transmetatarsal:
Disability is proportional to length of metatarsal
removed
Thick plantar flap required to cover out stumps
of metatarsals

Tarso-metatarsal:
Lisfranc's amputation
This is the most proximal amputation to give
reasonable foot function
M. Tib. Post. and M. Peron-Long should be retained
Loss of dorsiflexors may lead to equinus

Midtarsal:
Chopart's amputation
Abandoned as it results in persistent
equinovalgus deformity

Metatarsal rays:
Only 1 or 2 may be removed as foot becomes too
thin to take weight
Unsuitable for peripheral vascular disease.

References:
Baddeley R M, Fulford J C 1965 A trial of conservative
amputations for lesions of the feet in diabetes mellitus.
British Journal of Surgery 52: 38-43
Baker W H et al 1977 Minor forefoot amputation in patients
with low ankle pressure. American Journal of Surgery 133:
331-332
Larsson U, Anderson, G B J 1978 Partial amputation of the
foot for diabetic or arteriosclerotic gangrene. Journal of
Bone and Joint Surgery 60B: 126-130
Pedersen, H E, Day A. J. (1954) The transmetatarsal
amputation in peripheral vascular disease. Journal of Bone
and Joint Surgery 36A: 1190-1199

Amputation of toes

1st toe:
Loss of leverage in rapid walking or running
Otherwise no limp

2nd toe
Removal will lead to hallux valgus
If hallux valgus is already present, amputation may remove painful pressure on displaced 2nd toe

3rd and 4th toes:
Amputation causes no diability

5th toe:
Amputation may expose 5th metatarsal head to pressure from shoes
Most frequent indication is over-riding of 5th toe or 4th toe
Beveling of metatarsal head is advantgeous

Loss of all toes:
Little disability except when
    hurrying
    squatting
    tip-toeing.
A dorsal scar is free from pressure

Loss of all but 1 or 2 toes:
Requires a well made space filler in shoes
Consider each case individually regarding removal of remaining toes

References
Flint M, Sweetnam R 1960 Amputation of all toes. Journal of Bone and Joint Surgery 42B: 90-96
Onizuka T, Noda H, Sumiya N 1976 Repair of the amoutated great toe. Journal of Trauma, 16: 836-839

Amputations around the shoulder

Forequarter amputation
Indications:
    Tumours of upper humerus or shoulder girdle
    Severe trauma to shoulder
Disadvantages:
    Always apparent
    Prosthesis has only cosmetic value

Disarticulation of shoulder
Preserves contour of shoulder for clothes
Glenoid is filled by reflecting muscle groups

High humeral amputations
Preserves shoulder and axillary contours
Stump is not effective in itself, nor with a prosthesis

References
Levinthal D H, Grossman A (1939) Interscapulothoracic amputation for malignant tumours of the shoulder region. Surgery, Gynaecology and Obstetrics, 69: 234-239
Pack G T, McNeer G, Coley B L 1942 Interscapulothoracic amputations for malignant tumours of the upper extremity. Surgery, Gynaecology and Obstetrics 74: 161-175

Above elbow amputations

Indications
Trauma
Tumours
Infection (Rarely)
Congenital abnormality (Very rarely)

Features:
Maximum length should be preserved
Any level between axillary fold and supracondylar region may be selected
Low levels function as elbow disarticulation
High levels function as shoulder disarticulation

Cineplastic techniques

Well motivated intelligent patients required.
Careful consideration of aims and methods in each individual patient
Amputation stump must be well healed and best possible function restored.
Cineplasty is a major operation requiring careful attention to detail.
Above elbow methods: M. Pectoralis Major
Below elbow methods: M. Biceps brachii
                (Most successful)

References

Brav E A et al (1957) Cineplasty: An end result study. Journal of Bone and Joint Surgery 39A: 59-76
Mazet R 1964 Double tunnel pectoral cineplasty. Journal of Bone and Joint Surgery 46A: 829-832

Below elbow amputations

Indications:
Trauma
Tumour
Infection
Congenital abnormality } Very rarely
Ischemia

Disarticulation of elbow
Broad flare of lower humerus useful for fitting prosthesis
Modern prostheses now of greater value
Lower humerus can be covered by triceps and biceps tendons to improve stump

Forearm amputations:
Preserve as much length as possible
Even stumps of 2-5 cm. are useful

Disarticulation of wrist
Better than forearm amputations
Pronation-Supination is preserved
Trans-carpal amputation will provide some flexion and extension
Difficulty in fitting appliances

Krukenberg procedure

Indications:
Bilateral loss of hands
Blind patient
Absence of prostheses. These can be fitted later if indicated and available.
Children over 2 years

Disadvantage:
Unsightly
Requires expert technique
May not be accepted by patients' family and associates
Post-surgical prosthesis (if patient changes his mind) is difficult to fit

References

Kallio K E 1948 Recent advance in Krukenberg's operation. Acta Chirurgica Scandinavica 97: 165-188
Swanson A B 1964 The Krukenberg procedure in the juvenile amputee. Journal of Bone and Joint Surgery 46A: 1540-1548

Upper limb prostheses

Features:
Low level of acceptance
Often used only for appearance
Best value for
   1. Below elbow amputees
   2. Bilateral above elbow amputees
Too little attention has been paid to sensory feed back

Types:
Dress arms-
   appearance good
   function poor
Work arms:
   Appearance poor
   function better
      Many terminal tools left at site of use

Power supply

Muscles:
Shoulder girdle for above elbow amputees
Upper arm for below elbow amputees

Electrical:
E.M.G. telemetry –
   surface electroles
   implanted electrodes
Imprecise. Many difficulties

Pneumatic:
Heavy cylinder
Requires recharging

References

Lambert T H 1967 An engineering appraisal of powered prostheses. Journal of Bone and Joint Surgery 49B: 333-341

MacDonell J A 1958 Age of fitting upper extremity prostheses in children. Journal of Bone and Joint Surgery 40A: 655-662

McKenzie D S 1965 The clinical application of externally powered artificial arms. Journal of Bone and Joint Surgery 47B: 399-410 et seq.

Mauriello G E 1968 Some electronic problems of myo electric control of powered orthotic and prosthetic appliances. Journal of Bone and Joint Surgery 50A: 524-534

Murdoch G 1970 Editor. Prosthetic and orthotic practice section 9. Edwin Arnold, London

Murray J F, Shore B, Trefler E 1972 Prostheses for children with unilateral congenital absence of the hand. Journal of Bone and Joint Surgery 54A: 1658-1664

Schmid L H 1977 The importance of information feedback in prostheses for the upper limbs. Prosthetics and orthotics international 1: 21-24

Tucker F R, Scott R N 1968 Development of a Surgically implanted myo-telemetry control system. Journal of Bone and Joint Surgery 50B: 771-779

Hemicorporectomy

Indications:
Inoperable malignancy
Intractable sepsis
   with paraplegia
   or spina bifida

Requirements:
Respiratory ⎫
Cardiac   ⎪
Renal   ⎬ normality
Hepatic   ⎪
Brachial   ⎭
Stoical co-operative patient

Problems:
Long posterior skin flap required
Diversions:
   Bowel – colostomy
   Urine – ileal bladder
Metabolic changes
Blood volume changes
Loss of body image in previously normal adults

References

Pearlman W W et al 1976 Hemicorporectomy for intractable decubitus ulcers. Archives of Surgery 11: 1139-1143

Index